Serono Symposia USA
Norwell, Massachusetts

Springer

New York
Berlin
Heidelberg
Barcelona
Hong Kong
London
Milan
Paris
Singapore
Tokyo

PROCEEDINGS IN THE SERONO SYMPOSIA USA SERIES

Continued after Index

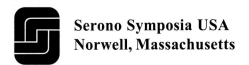

Serono Symposia USA
Norwell, Massachusetts

Daniel D. Carson

Editor

Embryo Implantation

Molecular, Cellular and
Clinical Aspects

With 70 Figures

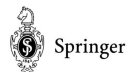

Springer

Daniel D. Carson, Ph.D.
Department of Biological Sciences
University of Delaware
Newark, DE 19716
USA

Proceedings of the International Symposium on Embryo Implantation: Molecular, Cellular and Clinical Aspects, sponsored by Serono Symposia USA, Inc., held October 3 to 6, 1997, in Newport Beach, California.

For information on previous volumes, contact Serono Symposia USA, Inc.

Library of Congress Cataloging-in-Publication Data
Embryo implantation : molecular, cellular and clinical aspects /
   edited by Daniel D. Carson.
       p.   cm.
     "Serono Symposia USA"—Series t.p.
     Includes bibliographical references and index.
     ISBN 0-387-98806-8 (alk. paper)
       1. Ovum implantation Congresses.   2. Fertilization in vitro, Human
Congresses.   I. Carson, Daniel D.   II. Symposium on Embryo
Implantation: Molecular, Cellular and Clinical Aspects (1997:
Newport Beach, Calif.)
       [DNLM: 1. Embryo Transfer Congresses.   WQ 205 E531 1999]
QP275.E43   1999
618.1'78059—dc21   99–19103

Printed on acid-free paper.

Production coordinated by Chernow Editorial Services, Inc., and managed by Francine McNeill; manufacturing supervised by Jeffrey Taub.
Typeset by KP Company, Brooklyn, NY.
Printed and bound by Maple-Vail Book Manufacturing Group, York, PA.
Printed in the United States of America.

9 8 7 6 5 4 3 2 1

ISBN 0-387-98806-8 Springer-Verlag New York Berlin Heidelberg   SPIN 10715869

SYMPOSIUM ON EMBRYO IMPLANTATION: MOLECULAR, CELLULAR AND CLINICAL ASPECTS

Scientific Committee

Daniel D. Carson, Ph.D., Chair
S.K. Dey, Ph.D.
Ari Babaknia, M.D.
Asgi Fazleabas, Ph.D.

Organizing Secretary

Leslie Nies
Serono Symposia USA, Inc.
100 Longwater Circle
Norwell, Massachusetts

Preface

Embryo implantation is a remarkable and complex process. Approaches developed from the fields of cell and developmental biology, immunology, and molecular biology have greatly enhanced our ability to study the shared as well as unique features of embryo–uterine interactions. Impressive and critical groundwork has been laid by a large and dedicated array of endocrinologists, reproductive biologists, and anatomists. These studies have set the stage to utilize sensitive and sophisticated techniques to detect and modulate protein and gene expression. Just as the symbiosis of mother and fetus is critical for the maintenance of pregnancy, so is the synergy among investigators from many disciplines, both in basic and clinical arenas, key to unraveling the mysteries of implantation and placentation. A large group of contributors in this field had the opportunity to meet and discuss the state of this art with the support of Serono Symposia USA, Inc. While it is never possible to bring together everyone who has played an important role, it was, nonetheless, both exciting and gratifying to have so many colleagues together for this event.

In the chapters that follow, the highlights of this meeting are presented as summarized by the individual presenters of seven different sessions. The topic has been considered from the broad social and ethical implications of modern in vitro fertilization and assisted reproductive technologies to detailed molecular controls over events that occur during embryonic development, uterine preparation for implantation, and placental organogenesis. These chapters demonstrate the significant and rapid progress being made in this field of biology and medicine. At the same time, they show that much more needs to be done to understand and fully appreciate this process. Lessons learned from this effort can be expected to continue to provide insights into other, related fields. Of the many contributors to our understanding of the process of implantation, none have had a larger impact than our colleague, Allen Enders. Dr. Enders has played a paramount role in developing the basic understanding of the cell biological processes underlying implantation and placentation in many species, including humans. He continues to contribute and guide thought in these areas. The participants of this symposium recognized Dr. Enders' impressive contributions by holding this event in his honor.

DANIEL D. CARSON

Contents

Contributors

CHRISTOPHER I. ACE, Department of Obstetrics and Gynecology, University of Massachusetts Medical School, Worcester, Massachusetts, USA.

SUZANNE AFONSO, Department of Cell Biology, Rutgers University, Piscataway, New Jersey, USA.

ARDESHIR BABAKNIA, Women's Health Institute of California, Costa Mesa, California, USA.

BRUCE BABIARZ, Department of Cell Biology, Rutgers University, Piscataway, New Jersey, USA.

INDRANI C. BAGCHI, Population Council, Center for Biomedical Research, New York, New York, USA.

GAIL V. BENSON, Genetics Division, Department of Medicine, Brigham and Women's Hospital, Harvard Medical School, Boston, Massachusetts, USA.

GARETH L. BLAEUER, Department of Cell Biology, Vanderbilt School of Medicine, Nashville, Tennessee, USA.

THOMAS N. BLANKENSHIP, Department of Cell Biology and Human Anatomy, University of California School of Medicine, Davis, California, USA.

D. RACHEL BREINAN, Department of Cell Biology, Vanderbilt School of Medicine, Nashville, Tennessee, USA.

ROBERT M. BRENNER, Division of Reproductive Sciences, Oregon Regional Primate Research Center, Beaverton, Oregon, USA.

DANIEL D. CARSON, Department of Biological Sciences, University of Delaware, Newark, Delaware, USA.

CHRISTOS COUTIFARIS, Department of Obstetrics and Gynecology, University of Pennsylvania Medical Center, Philadelphia, Pennsylvania, USA.

SUSAN L. CROCKIN, Newton, Massachusetts, USA.

JAMES C. CROSS, Samuel Lunenfeld Research Institute, Mount Sinai Hospital, Graduate Department of Molecular and Medical Genetics, Department of Obstetrics and Gynecology, University of Toronto, Toronto, Ontario, Canada.

CAROLINE H. DAMSKY, Departments of Stomatology and Anatomy, University of California San Francisco, San Francisco, California, USA.

SANJOY K. DAS, Department of Molecular and Integrative Physiology, Ralph L. Smith Research Center, University of Kansas Medical Center, Kansas City, Kansas, USA.

FRANCESCO J. DEMAYO, Department of Cell Biology, Baylor College of Medicine, Houston, Texas, USA.

MARY M. DESOUZA, Department of Biological Sciences, University of Delaware, Newark, Delaware, USA.

SUDHANSU K. DEY, Department of Molecular and Integrative Physiology, Ralph L. Smith Research Center, University of Kansas Medical Center, Kansas City, Kansas, USA.

KATHLEEN M. DONNELLY, Department of Obstetrics and Gynecology, University of Illinois at Chicago, Chicago, Illinois, USA.

ALLEN C. ENDERS, Department of Cell Biology and Human Anatomy, University of California School of Medicine, Davis, California, USA.

ASGERALLY T. FAZLEABAS, Department of Obstetrics and Gynecology, University of Illinois at Chicago, Chicago, Illinois, USA.

SUSAN J. FISHER, Departments of Stomatology, Obstetrics, Gynecology and Reproductive Sciences, Pharmaceutical Chemistry, and Anatomy, University of California San Francisco, San Francisco, California, USA.

MICHIKO N. FUKUDA, Glycobiology Program, The Burnham Institute, La Jolla, California, USA.

CINDEE R. FUNK, Department of Cell Biology, Baylor College of Medicine, Houston, Texas, USA.

OLGA GENBACEV, Department of Stomatology, University of California San Francisco, San Francisco, California, USA.

LOREN H. HOFFMAN, Department of Cell Biology, Vanderbilt School of Medicine, Nashville, Tennessee, USA.

JOHN HOYER, Department of Pediatrics, Children's Hospital of Philadelphia, Philadelphia, Pennsylvania, USA.

NANCY H. ING, Departments of Animal Science and Veterinary Anatomy and Public Health, Center for Animal Biotechnology of the Institute of Biosciences and Technology, Texas A&M University, College Station, Texas, USA.

SHIN-ICHI IZUMI, Department of Anatomy, Nagasaki University School of Medicine, Sakamoto, Japan.

HOWARD W. JONES, JR., Jones Institute for Reproductive Gynecology, Department of Obstetrics and Gynecology, Eastern Virginia Medical School, Norfolk, Virginia, USA.

JoANNE JULIAN, Department of Biological Sciences, University of Delaware, Newark, Delaware, USA.

LEE-CHUAN KAO, The R.W. Johnson Pharmaceutical Research Institute, Bioinformatics Program, San Diego, California, USA.

JI-YONG JULIE KIM, Department of Obstetrics and Gynecology, University of Illinois at Chicago, Chicago, Illinois, USA.

DAVID L. LACEY, Amgen, Inc., Thousand Oaks, California, USA.

DOUGLAS LEAMAN, Department of Molecular Biology, Lerner Research Institute, The Cleveland Clinic Foundation, Cleveland, Ohio, USA.

BRUCE A. LESSEY, Department of Obstetrics and Gynecology, Division of Reproductive Endocrinology and Infertility, University of North Carolina, Chapel Hill, North Carolina, USA.

HYUNJUNG LIM, Department of Molecular and Integrative Physiology, Ralph L. Smith Research Center, University of Kansas Medical Center, Kansas City, Kansas, USA.

LIMIN LIU, Department of Medicine, Duke University Medical Center, Durham, North Carolina, USA.

CHRISTOPHER LONGCOPE, Department of Obstetrics and Gynecology, University of Massachusetts Medical School, Worcester, Massachusetts, USA.

JOHN W. LUDLOW, Department of Biochemistry and Biophysics, University of Rochester Cancer Center, Rochester, New York, USA.

LIANG MA, Genetics Division, Department of Medicine, Brigham and Women's Hospital, Harvard Medical School, Boston, Massachusetts, USA.

RICHARD L. MAAS, Genetics Division, Department of Medicine, Brigham and Women's Hospital, Harvard Medical School, Boston, Massachusetts, USA.

RICHARD A. McCORMICK, Department of Theology, University of Notre Dame, Notre Dame, Indiana, USA.

MICHAEL T. McMASTER, Department of Stomatology, University of California San Francisco, San Francisco, California, USA.

DAITA NADANO, Glycobiology Program, The Burnham Institute, La Jolla, California, USA.

JUN NAKAYAMA, Central Clinical Laboratory, Shinshu University Hospital, Matsumoto, Japan.

WILLIAM C. OKULICZ, Department of Obstetrics and Gynecology, University of Massachusetts Medical School, Worcester, Massachusetts, USA.

BERT W. O'MALLEY, Department of Cell Biology, Baylor College of Medicine, Houston, Texas, USA.

AKINYINKA OMIGBODUN, Department of Obstetrics and Gynecology, University of Pennsylvania Medical Center, Philadelphia, Pennsylvania, USA.

BIBHASH C. PARIA, Department of Molecular and Integrative Physiology, Ralph L. Smith Research Center, University of Kansas Medical Center, Kansas City, Kansas, USA.

MARILYN B. RENFREE, Department of Zoology, The University of Melbourne, Parkville, Victoria, Australia.

VIRGINIA RIDER, School of Biological Sciences, University of Missouri–Kansas City, Kansas City, Missouri, USA.

R. MICHAEL ROBERTS, Department of Veterinary Pathobiology, University of Missouri, Columbia, Missouri, USA.

JANE A. ROBERTSON, Department of Animal Science, Texas A&M University, College Station, Texas, USA.

LINDA ROMAGNANO, Department of Cell Biology, Rutgers University, Piscataway, New Jersey, USA.

ZEV ROSENWAKS, The Center for Reproductive Medicine and Infertility, The New York Hospital–Cornell Medical Center, New York, New York, USA.

JEFFREY S. RUBIN, Laboratory of Cellular and Molecular Biology, National Cancer Institute, Bethesda, Maryland, USA.

IAN C. SCOTT, Samuel Lunenfeld Research Institute, Mount Sinai Hospital, Graduate Department of Molecular and Medical Genetics, University of Toronto, Toronto, Ontario, Canada.

GEOFFREY SHAW, Department of Zoology, The University of Melbourne, Parkville, Victoria, Australia.

OV D. SLAYDEN, Division of Reproductive Sciences, Oregon Regional Primate Research Center, Beaverton, Oregon, USA.

STEVEN SPANDORFER, The Center for Reproductive Medicine and Infertility, The New York Hospital–Cornell Medical Center, New York, New York, USA.

JEROME F. STRAUSS III, Center for Research on Reproduction and Women's Health, and Department of Obstetrics and Gynecology, University of Pennsylvania Medical Center, Philadelphia, Pennsylvania, USA.

GULNAR A. SURVEYOR, Department of Surgery, Wexner Institute for Pediatric Research, Children's Hospital, Columbus, Ohio, USA.

NAO SUZUKI, Glycobiology Program, The Burnham Institute, La Jolla, California, USA.

SIAMAK TABIBZADEH, Department of Pathology, Moffitt Cancer Center and the University of South Florida, Tampa, Florida, USA.

JANET TAST, Capron Park Zoo, Attleboro, Massachusetts, USA.

HAROLD G. VERHAGE, Department of Obstetrics and Gynecology, University of Illinois at Chicago, Chicago, Illinois, USA.

XINHUI ZHOU, Department of Biochemistry and Molecular Biology, University of Texas, M.D. Anderson Cancer Center, Houston, Texas, USA.

YAN ZHOU, Department of Stomatology, University of California San Francisco, San Francisco, California, USA.

PIOTR ZIOLKIEWICZ, Department of Obstetrics and Gynecology, University of Pennsylvania Medical Center, Philadelphia, Pennsylvania, USA.

Part I

Development and Future of
Human In Vitro Fertilization
and Embryo Implantation

1

Implantation in the Human as Viewed by Canon Law, Civil Law, and Natural Reason

HOWARD W. JONES, JR., RICHARD A. MCCORMICK, AND SUSAN L. CROCKIN

Implantation involves the early stages of the attachment of the conceptus to the maternal circulation. Any experimental study of this process *pari pasu* involves the conceptus, which at this stage of development may be referred to as the preembryo; the preembryo is defined as that stage of development between fertilization and the appearance of a single primitive streak. In temporal terms, this means from the 1st to the 14th day of development.

Presently, the use of Federal funds for experimental studies during this period of development is prohibited (H.R. 2880 sec 128). In addition, the Dickey–Wicker amendment (to a continuing resolution funding the NIH 1/26/96) protects the preembryo to the same degree that the fetus is protected from experimentation. According to authorities at NIH, this amendment makes it impossible to fund research involving the early preimplantation embryo.

Such an action implies that Congress and the President have decided that the early conceptus deserves protection because of its humanness or that personhood is acquired with fertilization. If the latter, it deserves protection because of its inability to give informed consent. To be sure, adults are routinely involved in experiments, but only after giving informed consent. Although it might be argued that parents should be considered responsible agents for giving informed consent for experimental studies of the conceptus, this view has not prevailed.

This discussion of the moral issues of implantation examines the nature of humanness and its acquisition, as well as the historical origin of the various views about the acquisition of personhood. From a philosophical point of view, the acquisition of the responsibilities of personhood is sometimes referred to as the acquisition of moral agency, which is defined as the cognitive ability to distinguish right from wrong without regard to self and to participate in and accept responsibility for moral decisions about persons and other moral agents (1). It is hoped that this historical approach will shed light on the moral dilemmas surrounding implantation research.

The Definition of Personhood

According to *Webster's Collegiate Dictionary* (9 ed., 1987), a person is (1) a human being: an individual; (2) the individual personality of a human being; (3) one that is recognized by law as the subject of rights and duties. In this discussion, the "rights" part of the definition is key. In practical terms, when considering the preembryo, this means protection by society from harm.

Ensoulment has certain attributes that are related to the acquisition of personhood. Although this term does not have much currency in contemporary lay society, it is a useful concept that has been much used in the past, especially in the writings of the early and medieval church fathers. In the context of this discussion, ensoulment, as used in canon law, will be considered along with the acquisition of personhood as used in civil law, or as considered by moral philosophers, biologists, and others (2).

The Acquisition of Personhood (Ensoulment)

The acquisition of ontogenetic personhood (ensoulment) has been considered by at least three disciplines in our culture:

• Canon Law

  • according to the classical tradition

  • according to the traditional tradition

• Civil Law

• Natural Reason

In addition, it is necessary to consider the phylogenetic acquisition of personhood, as this addresses the acquisition and the nature of humanness. As used here, ontogenetic refers to an individual member of the species *homo sapiens*, and phylogenetic refers to the acquisition of personhood (humanness) by the entire species *homo sapiens* during the evolutionary process.

Canon Law

The Classical Tradition

The classical tradition goes back to Aristotle—and perhaps even before. Aristotle in *de anima* stated that each individual acquires three different souls in sequence. First was a vegetable soul, then an animal soul, and finally, at birth, a rational soul. Aristotle specified a time sequence. For males, an animal soul was acquired at approximately 40 days of development, and for females, at 80 days of development.

The early church fathers adopted this concept of multiple souls, which is found in the writings of St.Thomas, St. Augustine, St. Jerome, and many others. Gratian (c. 1140 AD), who is thought to have been a monk who lived in Northern Italy, summarized the matter in his *decretum*. There, he apparently codified several revisions of canon law concerning a variety of ecclesiastical matters, but particularly abortion. His summary, therefore, is relevant to the matter at hand, as of the twelfth century. According to Gratian, abortion is not murder if the soul has not been infused. Thus, he accepted the notion that the soul was infused at some point during development. As proof of his statement, Gratian offers (1) the statement of St. Augustine about destruction of the nonanimated fetus; (2) the fact that body must be formed to accept the soul, as for example, with Adam; and, (3) the statement of St. Jerome saying murder requires a formed fetus.

Undoubtedly, the early church fathers and the fathers of the middle ages accepted the notion that ensoulment did not occur until some time during development. In modern terms, this can be interpreted as saying that the preembryo, and probably the embryo, was not considered by these early church fathers as being ensouled (i.e., they were not persons).

Although this discussion applies to the transmission of Aristotelian views to Christendom, an understanding of classical Greece views can also be found in the Islamic tradition, as well as in others, either from the study of classical Greece or of independent origin. These derivations are wonderfully summarized in *The Human Embryo: Aristotle and the Arabic and European Traditions,* by Father Gordon Dunstan as well as in the writings of others (3–6). Dunstan wrote, "The Quran left us no doubt that the fetus undergoes a series of transformations before becoming human" (p 38).

The Traditional Tradition

All living people have been born and educated in a world in which the Roman Catholic tradition of canon law states that ensoulment occurs with fertilization. This has, therefore, been referred to as the traditional concept. This concept of personhood was powerfully underlined by Pope Pius IX, whose reign, from 1846 to 1878, was longer than that of any other Roman pontiff. During his pontificate, many changes occurred. For example, when he ascended the papal throne in 1846, the Vatican exercised civil authority over a considerable area around Rome and was, in fact, one of the Italian city states that comprised Italy until unification under Garbaldi. After unification, however, the papacy's civil authority was limited to the few hundred acres that currently comprise Vatican City. Pius IX also convened the twentieth Ecumenical Council of the Roman Catholic church, commonly referred to as Vatican I, which was in session from 1869 to 1870. The Council adjourned because of the outbreak of the Franco–Prussian war. This was the first ecumenical council since the Council of Trent, which has lasted from 1542 to 1563. By approving the content of several of the pope's encyclicals and other writings, Vatican I had the effect of establishing or modifying canon law, which sets forth the basic laws of governance of the Roman Catholic church. It is inappropriate in this paper to detail the many laws (canon) promulgated by Vatican I, but it is relevant to mention the contents of (1) *Pastor aeternus*, which declared that in matters of faith or morals, the pope could speak with infallibility; and, (2) *Apostolicae Sedis* in which punishment is outlined for those who commit certain crimes. The highest punishment of excommunication is prescribed for perpetrators of several acts, including "those seeking to procure (provide/bring about) abortion if the desired effect ensues." The significant aspect of *Apostolicae Sedis* is that it no longer recognized a period during embryonic development before which excommunication did not apply. This has generally been interpreted and often cited as the concept that resulted in the modification of canon law to mean that ensoulment (i.e., personhood) was acquired with fertilization. This matter has been thoroughly reviewed in *The Crime of Abortion in Canon Law* by Father John Houser, as well as the writings of others (7–9).

It is important to distinguish between church legislation (canon law) and church practice as enunciated by clergy in good standing within the church. This is especially true at the pastoral level, but at other levels as well (10).

It is astonishing to realize that it was only in 1869, after 18 centuries of the classical tradition, that canon law concerning punishment was altered from the Aristotelian teaching, which was adopted by the early church fathers, to what we now regard as the traditional view of the Roman Catholic church and several other religious traditions.

Civil Law

Generally, U.S. civil law has not recognized the early conceptus as a person or as entitled to the full panoply of rights associated with personhood. Before medical technologies introduced the possibility of extracorporeal preembryos, U.S. jurisprudence addressed rights-related issues pertaining to a conceptus or fetus largely in the context of the procreative- or abortion-related privacy rights of the adults seeking to create or not create a child. As a long line of U.S. Supreme Court cases made clear, the "law affords constitutional protection to personal decisions relating to marriage, procreation, contraception, family relationships, child rearing, and education" (11).

The Supreme Court ruling in *Roe v. Wade* (12) clearly established the preeminent right of a woman to terminate a pregnancy up to the point of "viability," yet at the same time acknowledged the state's "important and legitimate interest in protecting the potentiality of human life" (13). On that basis, the high court has since upheld some restrictions on the rights set out in *Roe,* and courts have increasingly upheld state laws that protect viable fetuses under criminal, property, and tort laws, including criminalizing feticide of viable fetuses within homicide statutes. In *Webster v. Reproductive Health Services*, the high court declined to overturn a state law that included a preamble defining personhood as beginning at conception. Instead the court ruled that the preamble merely and legitimately stated a value judgment favoring child-birth over abortion (14). In a later decision, *Planned Parenthood of Southeastern Pennsylvania v. Casey*, the high court affirmed viability as the point of demarcation over whether a woman should be permitted to make a decision to abort or not (15). Until that point, the court ruled that a law may express "profound respect for the life of the unborn," but may not create an "undue burden" on a woman's abortion decision (16). One reason the court gave for that affirmation was that viability "is the time at which there is a realistic possibility of maintaining and nourishing a life outside the womb, so that the independent existence of the second life can in reason and all fairness be the object of state protection that now overrides the rights of the woman" (17). With medical technologies now separating the conceptus from a woman's body, the protections of *Roe* and subsequent abortion rights cases may not be wholly applicable in balancing state protections and individual rights.

The status of preembryos has been the subject of only a handful of lawsuits, all of them civil suits involving cryopreserved embryos and their disposition after a change in circumstances of the adults involved with them. The two leading cases are *Davis v. Davis* (18) and *York v. Jones* (19). In *Davis*, a divorcing couple were unable to agree whether the preembryos should be given to the wife to attempt to conceive and bear a child or children, or to the husband to destroy them and avoid unwanted parenthood. The trial court considered the preembryos as persons and awarded "custody" to the wife. The Supreme Court of Tennessee reversed and squarely rejected any characterization of preembryos as persons under either state or federal law, but concluded that they "occupy an interim category that entitles them to special respect because of their potential for human life (20). In the second case, *York v. Jones*, a 1989 case involving transportation of a preembryo from one clinic to another, the court considered the preembryos as chattel, that is, possessions in an inanimate sense, belonging to the creators of the embryo and not the clinic holding the embryo. Two other cases involving preembryos of divorcing spouses have arisen and resulted in lower court decisions. In a Massachusetts case, *A.Z. v. B.Z.* (21), the court refused to allow a wife to use cryopreserved preembryos over her husband's objection despite his previous agreement to her doing so. In that case, which is currently on appeal, the judge followed the reasoning of *Davis*, placing preembryos in a special category deserving of "special respect." In a New Jersey case, *Kass v. Kass* (22), the judge also acknowledged that preembryos are not persons but involve rights "far more precious than property rights" and ruled that the wife, not the husband, should have control over the preembryos just as if she were pregnant with the preembryos. Although these few courts have differed somewhat in their characterizations of preembryos and over who should have the right to control them, no court has recognized preembryos as persons or entities entitled to the full panoply of rights associated with personhood or even to those more limited rights associated with viable fetuses.

U.S. civil law addressing personhood has considered the responsibilities of personhood as well as the rights appertaining thereto. In this connection, it has recognized a gradation of rights and responsibilities, assigning arbitrary times when rights and responsibilities can be exercised. For example, one does not qualify for an income tax deduction until after birth. One has to be a certain age to drive a car or to vote or to be married without permission.

Natural Reason

Natural reason accepts the fact that biology is unable to identify a point in the development of an individual that signifies the acquisition of what we define as personhood or ensoulment. It furthermore rejects the external infusion of an essence, which can be defined as personhood or a soul. Personhood, therefore, develops in a Darwinian sense, that is, slowly with biological development. This point of view recognizes that for practical purposes it is necessary for society to set certain arbitrary times when a person may acquire rights and accept responsibility for various acts, as provided for in civil law. In an ideal society, these times express the will of the people, and generally do so in a democratically organized society. This point of view is elegantly set forth in *Darwin's Dangerous Idea: Evolution and the Meanings of Life* by Daniel Dennett, as well as in the writings of others (23–26).

The Phylogenetic Acquisition of Personhood

A consideration of the acquisition of personhood as we understand it and/or of humanness from a phylogenetic point of view provides an understanding of the nature of humanness and the acquisition of personhood from an ontogenetic point of view. The problem is simple to state, but difficult to solve. When, in the evolutionary tree, can one assign personhood as herein defined? For example, was Lucy, who is classified as a hominid, stood erect, and lived some 3.2 million years ago, a person in the sense that we are discussing? Do animals have souls? This discussion assumes that humanness must be acquired before or simultaneously with personhood. Most of those who have studied this believe that *homo sapiens* emerged about 100,000 years ago (27–29).

It is interesting that the distinction between man and animal is discussed very early in the Bible, "let man have dominion over ... fish ... fowl ... cattle ... and all other things upon the earth" (Genesis 2:26). Philosophers have also approached this matter. "Nature commands every animal and the creature obeys. Man feels the same impetus but . . . is free to acquiesce or resist" (Rosseau 1712–1778). Or, "Man in the system of nature . . . is exulted above any price . . . ." (Emanuel Kant 1724–1804).

Neither canon nor civil law speaks to this problem. By the Darwinian concept, personhood as defined herein has evolved over centuries, along with biological evolution. In the context of personhood, ontogeny repeats phylogeny (30,31).

The Conflict among Canon Law, Civil Law, and Natural Reason

The present conflict about embryo research is in effect a conflict between canon law on one side and civil law and natural reason on the other. For 18 centuries, the church and early church fathers adopted and supported the view of classical Greece, as expressed by Aristotle, that personhood in the sense of an entity deserving protection by society did not exist until some time well along in the developmental process of a single being of the species *homo sapiens*. In 1869, by the constitution *Apostolicae Sedis*, Pope Pius IX declared that those who caused abortion at any stage were subject to excommunication. This action has led many to accept that personhood is acquired with fertilization. It follows from *Apostolicae Sedis* that experimentation, or therapy for that matter (with special exceptions), resulting in the destruction of the conceptus at any stage during development is illicit.

Civil law, in a democratic society such as the United States, has been singularly silent on spelling out societal protection of the conceptus. To the contrary, *Roe v. Wade*, and related cases, (1973) support the view that a putative parent may have a pregnancy terminated prior to birth. The restrictive Dickey–Wicker amendment referred to above, might seem to a layman to be in conflict with *Roe v. Wade*, but there are nuances that allow them to coexist. Dickey–Wicker protects the conceptus from experimentation without informed consent. In the absence of the ability to give informed consent, the conceptus is thereby protected. However, it seems transparent that those who support Dickey–Wicker must believe that the amendment protects a human person. Thus, the segment of society that believes in the initiation of personhood with fertilization has persuaded the legislative branch of government to adopt canon law as civil law, at least in this instance.

It would perhaps take us too far afield to discuss this item in terms of the Jeffersonian struggle to separate church and state as couched in the language of religious freedom. This struggle finally resulted in the adoption by the Virginia House of Delegates of a "Bill for Establishing Religious Freedom." The Bill was written in 1777, but not adopted until 1786. The struggle also resulted in the amendment guaranteeing religious freedom in the Constitution of the United States (32).

Nevertheless, the moral status of the preembryo could be cited as a case in point. Natural reason, as noted above, accepts the inability to detect a biological moment or event that can be identified as the beginning of the human person and rejects the concept of an external infusion to establish personhood.

Rather, it recognizes the evolution of an individual essence with rights and privileges as an accompaniment of biological development. This might be called a Darwinian approach and can be applied to the ontogenetic acquisition of personhood, as well as to the phylogenetic acquisition of personhood.

One's attitude toward the ethical aspects of implantation research cannot help but be greatly influenced by the personhood issue. However, even if one rejects the concept that personhood or ensoulment begins with fertilization, it is necessary to remember that society has recognized that the origin of life is a mystery (33) and that human tissue is special. For example, human tissue removed at surgery is disposed of in a special way. Thus, a surgically removed uterus after examination by the pathologist is disposed of by cremation, but, a surgically removed uterus of a rat after being weighed as part of a bioassay for estrogen is usually disposed of by routine garbage disposal.

It follows that experimentation involving implantation of the preembryo is not to be undertaken without recognizing the special respect that society has accorded human tissue and with knowledge of the circumstance leading to the doctrine of informed consent (34). This concept leads to two straightforward principles that might be expected to govern human implantation research. These are: (1) to the extent possible the research question should be honed and refined in nonhuman species; (2) when it is necessary to turn to the human in order to improve the human condition, any experiment should be carried out in fulfilment of the doctrine of informed consent by those who "own" the preembryo. A final thought. To impose a law on implantation research on moral grounds requires us as a society to examine and debate the authority for this moral decision. It has been the intention of this discussion to contribute to that debate.

References

1. Petrinovich L. Human evolution, reproduction, and morality. New York: Plenum, 1995.
2. Goodman MF. What is a person? Clifton, NJ: Humana Press, 1988.
3. Dunstan GR. The human embryo: Aristotle and the Arabic and European traditions. Exeter: University of Exeter Press, 1990.
4. von Raffler-Engel W. The perception of the unborn across the cultures of of the world. Seattle: Hogrefe and Huber, 1994.
5. Edwards R. Life before birth: reflections on the embryo debate. London: Hutchinson, 1989.
6. Ford NM. When did I begin. Cambridge: Cambridge University Press, 1988.
7. Huser R. Crime of abortion in canon law. Washington, DC: Catholic University of America Press, 1943.
8. Hurst J. The history of abortion in the Catholic church. Washington, DC: Catholics for a Free Choice, 1989.
9. Connery J. Abortion: the Roman Catholic perspective. Chicago: Loyola University Press, 1977.
10. McCormick RA. The critical calling: reflections on moral dilemmas since Vatican II. Washington, DC: Georgetown University Press, 1989.

11. *Planned Parenthood of Southeastern Pennsylvania v. Casey*, 112 S.Ct. 2791, 2807 (1992).
12. *Roe v. Wade*, 410 U.S. 113, 93 S.Ct. 705 (1973).
13. *Roe* at 162, 93 S.Ct. at 731.
14. 492 U.S. 490, 109 S.Ct. 3040 (1989).
15. 112 S.Ct. al 2812.
16. 112 S.Ct. atl 2818, 2820.
17. 112 S.Ct. al 2818.
18. *Davis v. Davis*, 842 S.W.2d 588 (TN 1992).
19. *York v. Jones,* 717 F.Supp.421 (E.D. Va 1989).
20. *Davis*, 842 S.W.2d atl597.
21. MA. Probate Ct. 95d 1683 DV1 (Suff.Cty 1996), appeal pending.
22. No. 19658-93, 1995 WL 110368 (NY Naussau Cty.Sup.Ct. 1995).
23. Dennett DC. Darwin's dangerous idea: evolution and the meanings of life. New York: Simon and Schuster, 1995.
24. Dawkins R. River out of eden. New York: Basic Books, 1995.
25. Bronowski J. The ascent of man. Boston: Little Brown, 1973.
26. Miller RJ, Brubaker RH. Bioethics and the beginning of life. Scottsdale, PA: Herald Press.
27. Pfeiffer JE. The emergence of man. New York, Harper and Row, 1972.
28. Leakey RE, Lewin R. Origins. New York: Dutton, 1977.
29. Johanson D, Shreeve J. Lucy's child: the discovery of a human ancestor. New York: Avon, 1989.
30. Rachels J. Created from animals: the moral implications of darwinisn. Oxford: Oxford University Press, 1990.
31. Murphy MP, O'Neill LAJ. What is life? The next fifty years. Cambridge: Cambridge University Press, 1995.
32. Malone P. Jefferson and the rights of man. Boston: Little Brown, 1951.
33. John Paul II. Crossing the threshold of hope. New York: Knopf, 1994.
34. Jones HW Jr. The status of regulation of assisted reproductive technology in the United States. J Assisted Reprod Genet 1993;10:331–6.

2

The Impact of Maternal Age and Ovarian Age on Implantation Efficiency

STEVEN SPANDORFER AND ZEV ROSENWAKS

Age is perhaps the single most important variable influencing the outcome of assisted reproduction. The effect of advancing age on clinical in vitro fertilization (IVF) is manifested not only in the pattern of ovarian response to superovulation, but also in reduced implantation efficiency and an increased spontaneous abortion rate. This chapter explores the physiologic mechanisms behind this reduced implantation efficiency, its effect on IVF outcomes, and possible ways to improve embryonic implantation.

Maternal Age, Reduced Fertility, and Ovarian Reserve

A physiologic decrease in fecundity as maternal age increases has been observed. In the 1950s, a comprehensive analysis of the fertility rates of the Hutterite sect of the western United States and Canada was undertaken (1). This sect originated in Switzerland in 1528, and practically all of the living Hutterites came to South Dakota in the 1870s. Because contraception is prohibited and the communal nature of this sect removes economic burdens, there is no incentive to limit the size of families. As a result, the birth rate of the Hutterites is one of the highest on record, with an average of 11 live births per married woman. Only 5 of 209 women studied had no children, for an infertility rate of 2.4%. There was a definite decrease in fertility with advancing age; 11% of women bore no children after the age of 34, 33% of women had no children after the age of 40, and 87% of women were infertile by the age of 45. The average age of the last pregnancy was 40.9 years.

Although there is an apparent decrease in the frequency of sexual intercourse with advancing age, this does not fully account for the decline in female fertility. A French study of couples treated with donor insemination for isolated male factor infertility has revealed that the per cycle pregnancy rate declines with advancing age (2). The pregnancy rate for women under 30 was 73% after 12 insemination cycles. In women between the ages of 31 and

35, the pregnancy rate was 62% over the same time period, whereas women ages 36 to 40 had achieved only a 54% pregnancy rate. Therefore, a measurable decline in female fecundity appears to occur at least 15 years before the climacteric.

Why does this age-dependent decline in female fertility occur? Unlike their male partners, women are endowed with a finite and nonreplenishable complement of germ cells. The maximum number of germ cells actually occurs at midgestation during fetal life, at which time a total of 6 to 7 million oogonia are present. Thereafter, the germ cell content irretrievably decreases and no further de novo gametogenesis occurs. At the onset of puberty, the germ cell mass has already been reduced to approximately 300,000 oogonia. Thereafter, during the reproductive years, a number of oocytes are stimulated each month with only one or a few becoming dominant while the others undergo atresia. The absolute number of oocytes therefore continues to diminish with age.

At the age of 37 to 38, there is usually an acceleration of follicular loss. This occurs when the number of follicles reaches approximately 25,000 (3). This accelerated loss correlates with a subtle increase in serum follicle-stimulating hormone (FSH) concentration and a decrease in inhibin production. The functional capacity of the remaining follicles and germ cells has been termed the "ovarian reserve," or ovarian age. The functional ovarian age may be discordant with chronologic age, when accelerated follicular loss and/or diminished functional capacity of the remaining follicles occurs at an earlier age than expected. The subtle changes, which indicate diminished ovarian reserve, are associated with a markedly reduced fertility potential, often without apparent changes in clinically identifiable characteristics or major alterations in menstrual cyclicity.

There is evidence that oocyte quality also decreases with advancing maternal age. Studies have demonstrated a significant increase in genetically abnormal embryos after the maternal age of 35 years, suggesting an increase in aneuploidy with increasing maternal age (4). In a recent study of unfertilized oocytes after IVF, a significant rate of chromosomal degeneration was associated with advancing maternal age (5). In addition, other investigators have noted an increase in DNA fragmentation with increasing maternal age (6). These studies suggest that not only does the absolute number of oocytes diminish with advancing age, but the inherent quality deteriorates as well.

Age and IVF Outcome

Older women have a poorer prognosis for success after IVF. An analysis of our results at The Center for Reproductive Medicine and Infertility of The New York Hospital-Cornell Medical Center has revealed that the mean peak estradiol (E_2) level on the day of human chorionic gonadotropin (hCG) declines steadily with advancing age. This decline in the serum E_2 concentration is paralleled by a concomitant decrease in the mean number of oocytes retrieved per cycle. The delivery rate per embryo transfer procedure in our series dropped from 46.3% in women 30 years of age or younger to 5.2% for women 44 years of age or older. However, the mean number of embryos replaced is constant across all age groups, suggesting that it is not the embryo number per se that is the determinant of the reduced pregnancy rate seen with advancing age. Indeed, an examination of the embryo implantation rate (as assessed by the presence of a fetal heart beat per embryo transferred) reveals a decline from 33.5% in women under 34 years to 5.9% in women at age 44.

We recently analyzed 1621 consecutive cycles of IVF for implantation efficiency as a function of age (June 1995–October 1996). In this study we found an overall implantation rate of 23.3%. Table 2.1 demonstrates the implantation and delivery rates per embryo transfer throughout this study period. Implantation remained almost constant until the age of 35, and then decreased in a significant linear fashion by approximately 2.77% per year ($R^2 = 0.975$; $p < 0.0001$). Even when analyzing the subgroup of women with pure male infertility, this same response of implantation efficiency was noted.

Interestingly, we have recently discovered that while older women undergoing IVF demonstrate both a diminished response to ovarian stimulation and decreased implantation efficiency, the impaired implantation rates appear to be independent of the magnitude of the ovarian response. We re-

TABLE 2.1. Implantation and delivery rates per embryo transfer.

Age	Number	Implantation rate	Delivery/transfer
≤25	28	24.4	50.0
26	13	28.9	53.8
27	20	32.7	65.0
28	28	37.5	50.0
29	48	31.9	62.5
30	57	35.4	57.9
31	89	33.0	60.7
32	69	33.0	52.2
33	92	36.8	65.2
34	113	29.5	54.0
35	133	31.0	51.1
36	125	28.2	44.8
37	138	23.8	49.3
38	150	18.9	40.0
39	121	18.8	38.8
40	108	16.3	36.8
41	111	14.0	29.7
42	77	9.9	22.1
43	71	5.1	15.5
44	19	5.9	15.8
>44	11	2.3	0

viewed the outcome of 691 patients 40 years of age or older and compared them with 2552 women under 40 years of age. Patients from both age ranges were organized into five groups according to their serum E_2 level on the day of hCG administration. The mean number of mature oocytes retrieved and fertilized increased significantly along with the E_2 response in both groups. The mean number of embryos transferred was significantly lower only in women with the lowest E_2 response for both age categories. Delivery rates per transfer exhibited a significant linear increase with E_2 response in women less than 40, but not in women 40 years or older.

Oocyte donation serves as a useful in vivo model to further understand the impaired implantation efficiency seen in older women. Several authors have suggested that the successful implantation of oocyte donation in women older than 40 years suggests that the endometrium of older women retains normal receptivity (7,8). One investigative team failed to show a decrease in the implantation rate per transferred embryo in women older than 40 years undergoing donor oocyte transfer compared to younger recipients (9). In a subsequent report, pregnancy outcomes in younger IVF donors were compared with those in their respective older recipients who shared oocytes from the same cohort (10). There was no statistically significant difference in clinical pregnancy and delivery rates between the donors (33% and 23%, respectively) and recipients (40% and 30%, respectively). These data suggest that oocyte quality, rather than uterine factors, is the primary determinant of human implantation efficiency.

However, other investigators have suggested that uterine factors may also play a role in the age-related decline in fecundity. It has been reported that there may be a slight reduction in the embryo implantation rate in women older than 40 years undergoing oocyte donation, which can be offset by doubling the dosage of exogenous progesterone (11). We have also examined the issue of implantation efficiency in older women at our donor oocyte program. Twenty-four IVF patients who donated half of their oocytes were studied along with their respective recipients. The mean age of donors and recipients was 32.3 and 40.0 years, respectively. Although the ongoing pregnancy rate for donors (62.5%) and recipients (58.3%) was similar, there was a statistically significant decrease in the per embryo implantation rate in the recipients (25.6%) compared with the donors (42.5%). These data taken together suggest that there is a subtle decrease in implantation efficiency in older donor oocyte recipients, which may be overcome by performing multiple embryo transfers or by manipulating the hormonal milieu. Thus, although oocyte quality appears to be the major factor associated with the reduction in fecundity with advancing age, uterine factors and reduced endometrial receptivity may also play a role.

Maternal age is also a significant factor in determining the miscarriage rate in successful implantation (as defined as a positive fetal heart) after IVF. We recently reviewed 2346 consecutive IVF clinical pregnancies (1991–1995) and analyzed the pregnancy loss rate by maternal age. The overall pregnancy loss rate after demonstrating an FH during a 7-week U/S was 11.31%. A highly significant trend demonstrated an increase in fetal loss when comparing the four age groups ($\leq$ 30 yrs = 4.95% vs. 31–34 yrs = 9.46% vs. 35-39 yrs = 11.57 % vs. $\geq$ 40 yrs = 21.28%; p < 0.0001). Of the 261 losses in the study period, cytogenetic analysis was obtained on 71 (27.2%). Three specimens were nondiagnostic because of trophoblastic nonproliferation. Only 15 (22.03%) were normal (46XX or 46XY). Of the 53 (77.9%) chromosomally abnormal specimens, 45 (80.4%) were trisomies, 4 (7.14%) had 48 chromosomes, 2 were mosaics (3.57%), 2 were Turner's Syndrome (3.57%), 1 was a translocation (1.79%), and 1 was a triploidy (1.79%). The most common trisomies were 21 (7), 16 (5), 15 (5), 22 (5), and 18 (3). No differences were noted in the average age of the group with normal chromosomal losses as compared to the group with an abnormal chromosomal makeup (37.6 years old vs. 39.4 years old, p = 0.40). 91.3% of the losses in women over the age of 40 were chromosomally abnormal as compared to 71.1% of the losses in women under the age of 40 years. Thus, we have demonstrated a highly significant increase in pregnancy loss after demonstrating an FH during a 7-week U/S with increasing maternal age. The overwhelming explanation for these losses appears to be chromosomal in nature, with almost 80% having an abnormal chromosomal composition.

Ovarian Reserve and Its Relevance to In Vitro Fertilization Success

Determining basal FSH and E_2 concentrations early in the follicular phase can assess ovarian reserve. Serum FSH concentrations in the early follicular phase appear to rise several years before the menopause. It is hypothesized that elevated levels of FSH may result from the reduced secretion of inhibin from the germ-cell depleted ovaries. These subtle elevations, signaling a decline in the ovarian reserve even in women with regular menstrual cycles, have been typically associated with poor responses to gonadotropin stimulation. An elevated FSH concentration of greater than 20 mIU/mL on day 3 of the menstrual cycle has predicted a markedly diminished chance for success after IVF and related therapies (12,13). We have recently demonstrated that elevated E_2 levels in the early follicular phase also represent a poor prognostic sign for IVF outcome. There were very few successful pregnancies in women with elevated E_2 levels (>75 pg/mL) on day 3 of the menstrual cycle. It is theorized that elevated FSH concentrations in the late luteal phase of the preceding cycle may cause latter aberration.

We have further examined the relationship between basal day 3 hormonal values and IVF outcome. An analysis of 1249 gonadotropin-stimulated cycles in 782 women treated at Cornell without gonadotropin-releasing hormone agonist (GnRHa) down-regulation, where basal day 3 FSH and E_2 were determined concomitantly in the cycle of stimulation, reveals that both influence IVF outcome (14). The ongoing pregnancy rate per retrieval in this series in women with day 3 FSH levels of >20 mIU/mL was one half of that in women with day 3 FSH concentration <10 mIU/mL. The same was true for the embryo implantation rate as well. In this series, the ongoing pregnancy rate per retrieval fell by more than one half when the day 3 E_2 was >75 pg/mL, as compared to when the E_2 level was <30 pg/mL. Women with a high basal E_2 level rarely exhibit a concomitant elevation in FSH, because of feedback inhibition. In short, meaningful interpretation of basal hormonal values in the assessment of ovarian reserve requires the simultaneous determination of FSH and E_2 on day 3 of the menstrual cycle. Both have been shown to impact IVF outcome as measured by pregnancy rates and embryo implantation rates. Low early follicular phase inhibin-B concentrations may complement FSH and E_2 as markers of ovarian reserve.

Enhancing Embryonic Implantation

Several methods have surfaced as a means to diminish the embryonic loss following IVF, particularly in older women. These have included assisted hatching, preimplantation embryonic biopsy, and methods of coculture. Randomized, prospective trials of assisted hatching were undertaken at The Center for Reproductive Medicine and Infertility, in 330 couples undergoing IVF (15). The initial trials included patients with normal basal FSH levels. In these trials, assisted hatching appeared to benefit patients with thick zona (>15 μm). Further analysis of the selective assisted hatching protocol, which employed zona biometric criteria as the indication for zona drilling, indicated that women over the age of 38 appeared to derive the most benefit from this procedure. Therefore, assisted hatching techniques to facilitate embryo escape from the zona pellucida appear to facilitate embryo implantation, particularly in older patients.

In work at our center, we have demonstrated an age related increase in the rate of chromosomally abnormalities in embryos biopsied and analyzed by fluorescent in situ hybridization (FISH). This increase was noted in morphologically normal appearing embryos as well (4.0% for ages 20 to 34, 9.4% for ages 35 to 39, 23.8% for ages 40 to 47.). As the rate of chromosomal aneuploidy increases linearly with maternal age, even in embryos that otherwise appear morphologically normal, perhaps further development and refinement of embryo biopsy techniques and preimplantation genetic diagnostic procedures may allow older patients an opportunity to screen for chromosomal abnormalities and select favorable embryos for transfer. Utilizing such a strategy may then theoretically allow them to attain an improved embryo implantation rate as well as a lower early embryonic loss rate.

Utilization of coculture of human embryos with somatic cell support has been documented as beneficial. We have recently performed a study utilizing human autologous endometrial cells for coculture in patients with multiple implantation failures and have noted an increase in blastomere division and a decrease in fragmentation in embryos grown on coculture as compared to the embryos that were grown on conventional media alone. Although the exact mechanism(s) of coculture is (are) not established, growth factors are secreted by these somatic cells, and these may improve the embryonic development and, hopefully, implantation rates.

Summary

Advanced maternal age is associated with a decrease in fecundity potential. Diminutions in implantation and pregnancy rates are generally seen after the age of 35, and diminish significantly after the age of 40. Oocyte factors are felt to be primarily responsible; however, uterine factors may also play a role. Hormonal assessments of FSH and E2 levels on day 3 of the menstrual cycle are reliable measures of diminished ovarian reserve and the anticipated response to ovulation induction. A similar decrease in implantation rates and pregnancy rates are seen in older women undergoing assisted reproductive techniques, including IVF. The decrease in implantation efficiency seen in older women undergoing IVF appears to be independent of the magnitude of stimulation response. Improved implantation rates may be noted when utilizing assisted hatching, pre-implantation embryonic biopsy and methods of coculture.

References

1. Tietze C. Reproductive span and rate of reproduction among Hutterite women. Fertil Steril 1957;8:89–97.
2. Federation CECOS, Schwartz D, Mayaux JM. Female fecundity as a function of age: results of artificial insemination in 2193 nulliparous women with azoospermic husbands. N Engl J Med 1982;306:404–6.
3. Faddy MJ, Gosden RG, Gougeon A, Richardson SJ, Nelson JF. Accelerated disappearance of ovarian follicles in midlife: implications for forecasting menopause. Hum Reprod 1992;7:1342–6.
4. Munne S, Alikani M, Tomkin G, Grifo J. Embryo morphology, developmental rates and maternal age are correlated with chromosomal abnormalities. Fertil Steril 1995;64:382–91.
5. Lim AST, Tsakok MFH. Age related decline in fertility: a link to degenerative oocytes? Fertil Steril 1997;68:265–71.
6. Fujino,Y, Ozaki K, Yamamasu S et al. DNA fragmentation of oocytes in aged mice. Hum Reprod 1996;11:1480–3.
7. Sauer MV, Paulson RJ, Lobo RA. Reversing the natural decline in human fertility. An extended clinical trial of oocyte donation to women of advanced reproductive age. JAMA 1992;268:1275–9.
8. Antinori S, Versaci C, Gholami GH, Panci C, Caffa B. Oocyte donation in menopausal women. Hum Reprod 1993;8:1487–90.
9. Sauer MV, Paulson RJ, Lobo RA. Preliminary report on oocyte donation extending reproductive potential to women over 40. N Engl J Med 1990;323:1157–60.

10. Navot D, Bergh PA, Williams MA, Garrisi GJ, Guzman I, Sandler B, Grunfeld L. Poor oocyte quality rather than implantation failure as a cause of age-related decline in female fertility. Lancet 1991;337:1375–7.
11. Meldrum DR. Female reproductive aging-ovarian and uterine factors. Fertil Steril 1993;9:1–5.
12. Muasher SJ, Oehninger S, Simonetti S, Matta J, Ellis LM, Liu H-C, Jones GS, Rosenwaks Z. The value of basal and/or stimulated serum gonadotropin levels in prediction of stimulation response and in vitro fertilization outcome. Fertil Steril 1988;50:298–307.
13. Toner JP, Philput C, Jones GS, Muasher SJ. Basal follicle stimulating hormone (FSH) level is a better predictor of in vitro fertilization (IVF) performance than age. Fertil Steril 1991;55:784–91.
14. Licciardi FL, Liu H-C, Rosenwaks Z. Day 3 estradiol serum concentrations as prognosticators of stimulation response and pregnancy outcome in patients undergoing in vitro fertilization. Fertil Steril 1995;64:991–4.
15. Cohen J, Alikani M, Trowbridge J, Rosenwaks Z. Implantation efficiency by selective assissted hatching using zona drilling of human embryos with poor prognosis. Hum Reprod 1992;7:685–91.

Part II

Cellular Aspects of Implantation

3

Vascular Invasion During Implantation and Placentation

ALLEN C. ENDERS AND THOMAS N. BLANKENSHIP

In species as diverse as the golden hamster, bulldog bat, and baboon, cytotrophoblast cells originating from the embryo are thought to migrate into maternal endometrial arteries (1–5). In primates, including macaque monkeys, baboons, and humans, the cells not only migrate into the arteries but extensively modify the walls of these arteries, a process considered normal in establishing the definitive uteroplacental blood flow in these species (6–10). The functional consequences of the changes in spiral artery walls include the inability to constrict effectively in response to vasoactive stimuli. This probably helps to maintain a relatively constant maternal blood flow to the placenta regardless of changes in the physiological status of the mother. The manner in which this vascular invasion and modification occurs in macaques has been the subject of a series of recent studies in our laboratory. This chapter summarizes and interprets the results of these studies to date.

Initial Invasion of Maternal Vessels

The cellular activity that characterizes trophoblast invasion is seen almost immediately following the beginning of blastocyst implantation (gestational day 9.5). Syncytial trophoblast soon penetrates between uterine luminal epithelial cells, with which it forms cell junctions, and encounters the basal lamina (11). The syncytium and cytotrophoblast expand the implantation site within the plane of the epithelium during the subsequent trophoblastic plate stage. Syncytial trophoblast becomes organized as a thin polarized layer, the microvilli-lined apical border comprising the surface of clefts that will soon be exposed to maternal blood (12). Both the luminal epithelium and the superficial capillary plexus respond to the implanting blastocyst; the first by forming an epithelial plaque, the latter by dilation to a more venular than capillary diameter. Trophoblast first achieves contact with maternal vessels at the conclusion of the trophoblastic plate stage of embryonic development (gestational days 10.5–11), when syncytial trophoblast breaches the luminal epithelial basal lamina and the basal lamina of the dilated superficial capillaries (13). Syncytial trophoblast penetration into the superficial vessels allows maternal blood to gain access to the clefts within the trophoblastic plate. Because lacunae form at the surfaces of syncytial trophoblast, that is, where the syncytium is in contact with cytotrophoblast or endometrium, the filling of the lacunae brings cytotrophoblast in contact with maternal blood. Upon filling with maternal blood the clefts expand and become an anastomotic series of blood-filled spaces, constituting the previllous or lacunar stage of implantation (12). Syncytial trophoblast forms junctional complexes with the endothelial cells through which it intrudes, thereby forming part of the vessel wall and at the same time preserving the structural integrity of these vessels. Because there is generalized implantation site edema of the uterine stroma by this time, it is difficult to determine whether or not there is vascular leakage, but neither platelets nor erythrocytes escape the vessels at this stage. Interestingly, syncytial trophoblast does not continue to invade any maternal vessel beyond the areas of initial perforation.

Within one day of the initial penetration of the maternal capillaries, cytotrophoblast cells are found in the lumina of some arterioles close to the implantation site, having migrated from the superficial capillaries (13,14). The small size of the arterioles and the large size of the intraluminal cytotrophoblast cells results in at least transitory occlusion of these vessels by the formation of cytotrophoblast plugs. However, maternal blood retains access to the lacunae because of the widespread anastomosis of the superficial capillary plexus, although the ingress of blood to the implantation site is probably from the periphery of the plexus rather from the underlying arterioles at this stage.

Three to four days after the onset of implantation, cytotrophoblast proliferates rapidly in the septae between lacunae and extends into the endometrium, around clusters of epithelial plaque cells, and into adjacent endometrial vascular spaces (gestational days 13–14). These cells occupy the spaces between the basal surfaces of syncytial trophoblast septae and extend to the endometrial stroma, thus forming anchoring villi. The accumulation of cytotrophoblast cells from the anchoring villi cell columns spreads across the surface of the uterine stroma to form the trophoblastic shell (15). Trophoblast cells of the shell synthesize and secrete large amounts of extracellular matrix (ECM), together forming the "floor" of the placenta (16,17), opposite the "ceiling" formed by the chorionic plate (18). Cytotrophoblast located at the interface with the endometrial stroma continues to penetrate into the endometrium, often using vascular channels. Nevertheless, as the shell develops, apertures remain, providing the continuity of maternal blood flow into the lacunae, which become the intervillous space of the placenta.

Cytotrophoblast Invasion of the Artery Wall

The cytotrophoblast cells are initially contained entirely within the lumen of the invaded arterioles and spiral arteries (Fig. 3.1a, b). These cells migrate rapidly along the luminal surfaces of endothelial cells, and by day 14 can be found within arteries deep in the endometrium well beyond the level of the trophoblastic shell (14). As these cells move along the endothelium, they are subjected to shear forces generated by the flow of arterial blood. The means by which intraluminal cytotrophoblast cells maintain adhesion between themselves, as well as adhesion to maternal endothelium, may be partially explained by their expression of neural cell adhesion molecule (NCAM), which is expressed only on cytotrophoblast cells, and platelet-endothelial cell adhesion molecule (PECAM), which is expressed on the surfaces of both cytotrophoblast cells and endothelium (19,20). Each of these adhesion molecules possess homophilic binding properties. Intraluminal cytotrophoblast cells are frequently closely packed, devoid of intercellular junctions, possess abundant polyribosomes, moderate amounts of rough endoplasmic reticulum, and euchromatic nuclei. Only a few at a time show ectoplasmic pseudopodia of the type usually associated with locomotion.

Shortly after filling the lumen in areas near the trophoblastic shell, the plug of cytotrophoblast cells within a spiral artery begins to disassociate as some of these cells penetrate between endothelial cells, through the basal lamina, and migrate into the artery wall, becoming intramural cytotrophoblast cells (Fig. 3.1c). Other trophoblast cells that formed the plug continue to migrate distally (toward the myometrium), against the flow of arterial blood. No morphologically defined junctions are formed between these cytotrophoblast cells and the endothelium. This movement of cytotrophoblast from the lumen outward (extravasation) is not to be confused with the initial invasion of the capillaries by syncytial trophoblast (intravasation). With the migration of cytotrophoblast cells into the artery wall the lumen is reestablished, and arterial blood is confluent with the intervillous space. Further description of the invasion of the arterial wall and the formation of intramural cells is given below.

As the arterial flow supplying maternal blood into the intervillous space is established, the tapped veins provide the outflow from the placenta. Cytotrophoblast cells extend only a short distance into the lumina of veins (Fig. 3.1d), with modification of the venous wall restricted to the immediate vicinity of the trophoblastic shell (14,21). The extensive migration seen in the arterial limb of the placental blood supply does not occur in the veins. The mechanism by which cytotrophoblast cells discriminate between arteries and veins and determine the correct direction for migration is currently unknown, but in vitro studies using human cytotrophoblast suggest that local differences in oxygen tension may play a role (22). The only trophoblast reported to pass through the veins for any distance beyond the shell is that which

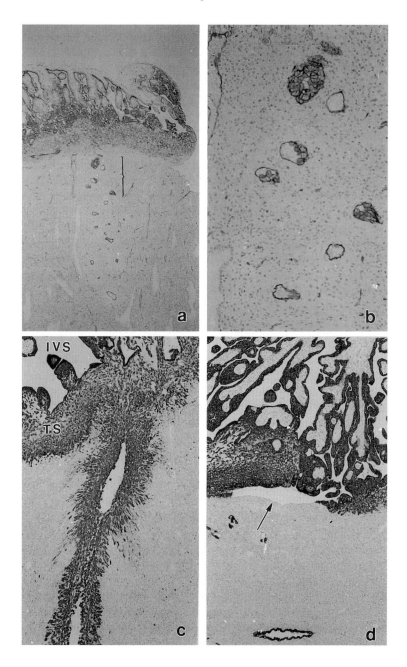

FIGURE 3.1. (a), (b) An early placentation site, day 16 of gestation stained with antibody to PECAM. (a) Spiral arteries are approximately perpendicular to the surface of the endometrium, and the upper coils (bracket) of one artery have been invaded by cytotrophoblast cells. (b) At a higher magnification it can be seen that four coils of the artery have been invaded by PECAM-positive cytotrophoblast cells. Note that the coil proximal to the placenta is largely filled cytotrophoblast cells. (c), (d) Developing placenta at

breaks away from its normal position in the placenta (deported trophoblast) and is swept into veins solely by blood flow pressure gradients (23).

At 15 to 17 days of gestation, several spiral arteries are located within the endometrium subjacent to the placenta (Fig. 3.1a), which measures approximately 0.5 cm in diameter at this stage (at term the placenta will measure approximately 8 cm in diameter). However, only a subset of these will be modified by trophoblast cells. The arteries pass as a series of asymmetrical coils from the uterine radial arteries toward the surface of the endometrium, with the terminal coils near the surface being smaller in diameter than those in the basal region. These arteries, with their adjacent endometrial stroma, comprise "Streeter's columns" (6,24), which are separated from one another by intervening uterine glands. The arteries invaded by intramural cytotrophoblast show substantial increases in the diameter of the vessel and the thickness of its wall. In portions of the artery closer to the trophoblastic shell, intramural cells form a complete collar, completely displacing the endothelium and largely displacing the smooth muscle cells. Because there is no evidence of cytotrophoblast replication within the invaded vessels intraluminal cytotrophoblast cells must migrate from the regions of proliferation in the anchoring villi cell columns, through the trophoblastic shell, and into the deeper regions of the arteries. The trophoblast cells within an artery take the form of a large, continuous, cohesive mass. The stages of cytotrophoblast-mediated modifications are depicted in Figures 3.2 and 3.3.

This pattern of proximal to distal progressive invasion, followed by cytotrophoblast-mediated modification of artery walls, is repeated in each of the arteries invaded regardless of the time of onset of invasion. As the continuous group of trophoblast cells extends deeper into the artery, distal to the trophoblastic shell, only a portion of the artery is filled, and intramural cells are formed where the trophoblast contacts and penetrates between endothelial cells. This pattern may be explained by a continuous column of cytotrophoblast cells extending into the spiral arteries, with individual cells penetrating through the endothelium and into the tunica media in a "first-come, first-in" sequence. These intramural cells accumulate in the wall, consequently expanding the diameter of the vessel. The advancing tip of the trophoblast cell column tapers to a thin layer only one cell deep, where intraluminal cells are found adherent to the endothelium but no intramural cells are formed. Intraluminal cells show little tendency to migrate into the branches of spiral arteries, but continue to move against the flow of blood. Although endothelial cells are displaced from their basal lamina, they do not appear to by lysed at the time of release. Cytotrophoblast cells are not nota-

---

27 days of gestation stained with antibody to cytokeratin. (c) An invaded spiral artery entering the trophoblastic shell (TS). Note that the entire wall of the vessel is composed of cytokeratin-positive cytotrophoblast cells. Intervillous space (IVS). (d) A vein from the same placenta as (c). Although the vein is patent to the intervillous space, cytotrophoblast has not replaced the wall of the vessel where it remains in contact with the endometrium (arrow). a: X 26;b: X 100;c, d: X 42.

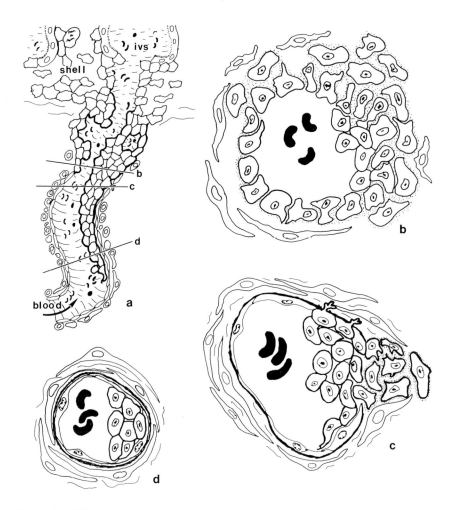

FIGURE 3.2. The sequence of cytotrophoblast cell activities involved in intraarterial invasion. (a) Cells from the anchoring villus cell column (located just above the top of the figure) are recruited to the trophoblastic shell, and then proceed as an irregular column of cells (heavy outline) into the artery, moving against the flow of blood, the latter flowing toward the intervillous space (IVS). (b) Proximal to the trophoblastic shell the cytotrophoblast cells have completely displaced the endothelium of the artery and form a lining to the vessel. Cytotrophoblast cells have also entered the vessel wall where they form a pad of cells and extracellular matrix (right). (c) Farther along the vessel, more distal to the shell, cytotrophoblast cells breach the endothelium (upper right) and enter the artery wall where they form a pad of cells and extracellular matrix (right). Much of the endothelium and artery wall remains intact. (d) Near the end of the intraarterial cytotrophoblast column the cells lie wholly within the arterial lumen.

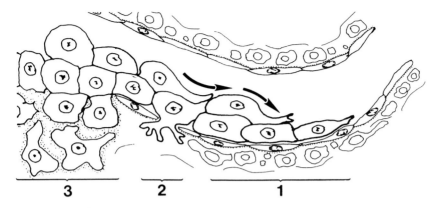

FIGURE 3.3. Diagram of a column of cytotrophoblast cells progressing into a spiral artery (*arrows* indicate the direction of migration). (1) Area of intraluminal cytotrophoblast cell adhesion to, and migration upon, the luminal surface of endothelium. (2) Region of cytotrophoblast cell penetration into the artery wall. (3) Area of intramural cell hypertrophy and extracellular matrix synthesis.

bly phagocytic at any stage of artery modification, nor is macrophage or granulocyte activity increased in the areas of vessel wall penetration.

Modification and Replacement of the Tunica Media

The first region penetrated by extravasating cytotrophoblast cells is that region first occupied by intraluminal cells (i.e., the portion of the vessel adjacent to the trophoblastic shell). Their passage through the endothelial basal lamina (Figs. 3.4 and 3.5) and ECM of the tunica media is probably facilitated by the matrix metalloproteinases identified in these cells (25,26). The region of invaded tunica media is extended from the shell commensurate with progression of the column of intraluminal trophoblast cells. In areas proximal to the shell, where the cellular plug earlier filled the entire lumen, the tunica media conversion involves the entire cross-section. More distally, where the column of intraluminal cytotrophoblast cells occupies only a portion of the lumen, the intramural cells occupy a more restricted region.

The first trophoblast cells to enter the wall at a specific level of an artery initially interdigitate with the cells and the normal ECM of the tunica media (Fig. 3.5). As more cells penetrate into the wall, the normal components of the tunica media are displaced or replaced. Smooth muscle cells lose their normal extended, circumferential orientation and appear dispersed, contracted, and disorganized (Figs. 3.6 and 3.7). However, there is little sign of smooth muscle cell death. Coincident with tunica intima penetration, intramural cytotrophoblast cells begin to secrete ECM (Fig. 3.8) containing, at least, laminin

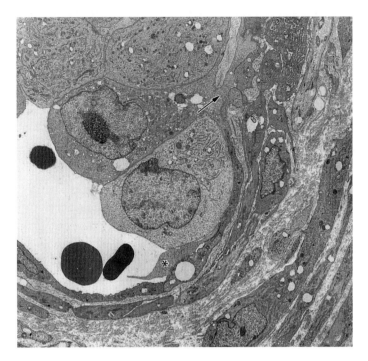

FIGURE 3.4. Large intraluminal cytotrophoblast cells show ectoplasmic processes extending into the wall of an arteriole (*arrow*) and along the endothelium (*) in a 15-day implantation site. × 2600.

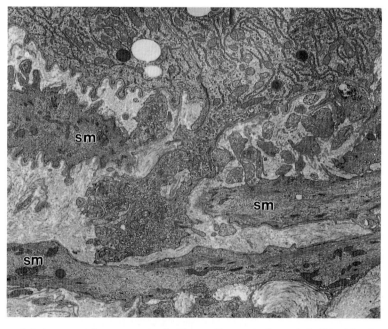

FIGURE 3.5. A process from a cytotrophoblast cell extends through the basal lamina and between adjacent smooth muscle cells (sm). The endothelium has already been displaced from this area of the artery. × 7400.

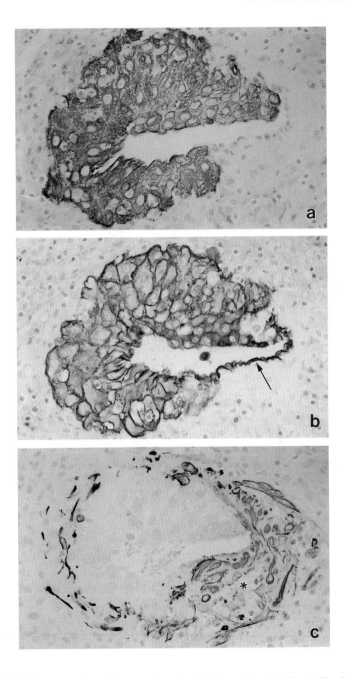

FIGURE 3.6. Adjacent sections from an artery invaded by cytotrophoblast cells, day 40 of pregnancy. (a) Cytotrophoblast cells immunoreactive for cytokeratin are located both along the lumen and adjacent to the endometrial stroma. (b) PECAM stains both endothelial cells (*arrow*) and the surfaces of cytotrophoblast cells. (c) Actin staining of the smooth muscle cells of the artery. Note the abundance of smooth muscle cells where the endothelium is intact (*) and the interruption of the muscle layer around the rest of the artery. × 240.

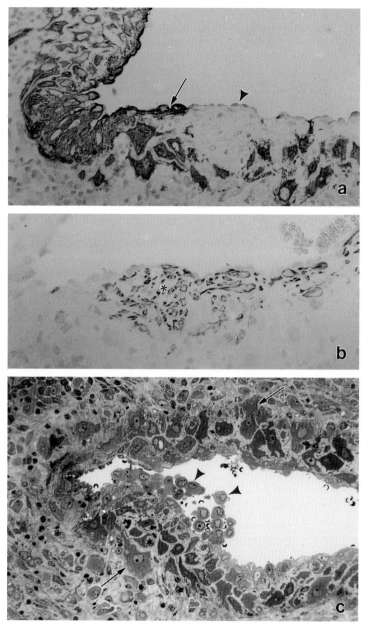

FIGURE 3.7. Invaded arteries from 57 days of pregnancy. The distribution of both cytotrophoblast cells (a) and smooth muscle cells (b) is irregular around the circumference of the artery. (a) Cytokeratin-stained cytotrophoblast cells are present in the wall of the vessel and along the lumen (*arrow*). On the right (*arrowhead*) the endothelium is present and cytotrophoblast does not form this part of the surface of the vessel. (b) Section adjacent to (a) stained for smooth muscle actin showing a group of smooth muscle cells (*) where cytotrophoblast does not form part of the surface of the vessel. (c) A plastic section prepared from the same specimen seen in (a) and (b). Cytotrophoblast cells are located within the lumen (*arrowheads*) and as larger cells in the wall of the vessel (*arrows*). Intact endothelial cells are still present at the right side of this vessel. × 240.

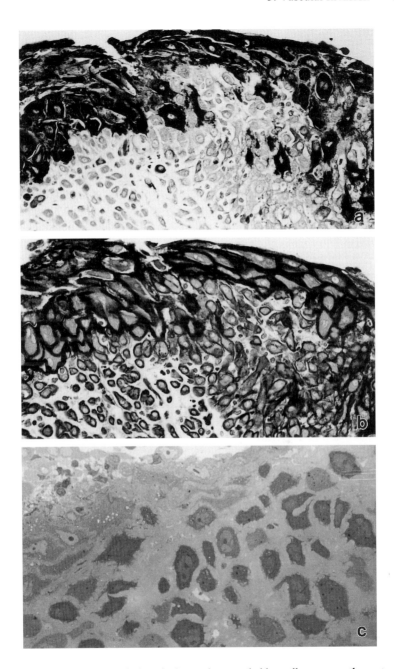

FIGURE 3.8. Extracellular matrix is deposited around cytotrophoblast cells as soon as they enter the wall of the artery, thus forming a cell and matrix pad that is particulary well developed later in pregnancy. (a) Cytokeratin staining of cytotrophoblast cells in an invaded artery on day 50 of gestation. (b) In this section located adjacent to that seen in (a), antibody to type IV collagen reveals thick layers of collagen-rich matrix around individual cytotrophoblast cells (above) and thinner layers around decidualized stromal cells (below). (c) In this plastic section prepared from tissue collected on day 129 of pregnancy, the space separating intramural cytotrophoblast cells increased with the deposition of extracellular matrix between them. (a,b) × 240: c: × 600.

and type IV collagen, although relatively deficient in fibronectin (10). The ECM is first seen as small accumulations interspersed between the membranes of intramural cells located near the lumen (Enders and Blankenship, unpublished observations). As intramural cells come to lie more deeply within the artery wall the amount of ECM separating the cells increases substantially, forming thick layers that segregate each cell. In addition, the amount of ECM increases as pregnancy proceeds (Fig. 3.8c), even between intramural cells located next to the lumen. Cytoplasmic processes of intramural cells traverse the ECM walls, sometimes forming gap junctions. In areas near the trophoblastic shell the intramural cells of the modified artery merge with those of the shell, with the ECM of each compartment continuous with the other (Fig. 3.1c). The number of intramural cell layers making up the wall may number up to about eight, with cells added to the luminal surface as new intraluminal cells arrive from areas more proximal to the trophoblastic shell. No evidence of mitotic activity is seen among these cells and they remain mononuclear throughout gestation.

Intramural cells replace all or part of the tunica intima and tunica media (Figs. 3.6–3.8). As they become sequestered within ECM, these cells undergo substantial hypertrophy which, combined with the deposition of ECM, serves to increase both the thickness of the arterial wall and the circumference of the vessel. These cells retain an extensive Golgi system and dilated rough endoplasmic reticulum throughout pregnancy. They also maintain their intense immunoreactivity for cytokeratins and positive, although reduced, reactions for NCAM and PECAM. As the ECM "capsules" are synthesized the metalloproteinases become heterogeneous in distribution, with some of the individual intramural cells heavily reactive, and others unreactive (26).

The groups of intramural cells intercalated within the artery wall at the site of extravasation typically span the entire wall, with some cells maintaining direct contact with the lumen and other cells in contact with the uterine stroma (Figs. 3.6 and 3.7). This "pad" of intramural cells constitutes a greater or lesser fraction of the artery wall. Smooth muscle cells and their native matrix (containing fibers characteristic of type I collagen) are not seen within these wedges of intramural cells (Figs. 3.6 and 3.7). Thus, the portion of wall containing intramural cytotrophoblast probably comprises new tissue. In addition, the smooth muscle cells found in the uninvaded, but adjacent, portion of the tunica media lose their normal organization and cease to form a discrete circumferential layer. In some cases the pad of cytotrophoblast cells extends circumferentially within the wall (Fig. 3.7a). These intramural cells may lie just beneath the endothelium, in which case adjacent smooth muscle cells tend to be rounded. When these cells encroach beneath the smooth muscle, between the tunica media and uterine stroma, the smooth muscle cells appear unusually thin but remain fusiform. In either case the attenuation of the smooth muscle cells and the wide spacing between the cells renders an image more typical of veins than a muscular artery.

Discussion and Conclusions

Trophoblast cells encounter maternal blood very soon after blastocyst attachment to the endometrium. Immediately after penetrating the uterine epithelial basal lamina, syncytial trophoblast penetrates the superficial endometrial capillaries. Because these vessels are approached through the stroma, this represents an example of intravasation. Upon gaining access to the maternal vasculature, intraluminal cytotrophoblast cells discriminate between arteries and veins, migrating extensively only within the former. Within the spiral arteries, cytotrophoblast cells invade the tunica intima and tunica media, escaping the lumen via extravasation. The often used term "endovascular trophoblast" could indicate mononuclear cells, multinuclear cells, cells residing in capillaries, sinusoids, veins, arteries, or the walls of arteries. Because the trophoblast cells involved with each of these vascular components probably represent different states of differentiation and interact with their immediate environments in distinct ways, it may be useful to precisely identify these cells with respect to their location.

Evidence indicates that intraarterial cells do not replicate (27). The most likely origin, therefore, for the many cytotrophoblast cells found in the arteries throughout gestation is the proliferative regions of the cell columns (15,27). Within the columns, proliferation of cells is limited to the first few layers next to the mesenchymal core of the contiguous anchoring villus. From this site of origin, cytotrophoblast cells destined to contribute to arterial modification must migrate through the ECM-rich distal cell column (15,17,28,29), into the trophoblastic shell, and locate the lumen of an artery. These trophoblast cells then enter the very different environment of a maternal blood vessel, resist dispersion due to the forces of arterial blood flow, and migrate significant distances along fetal and maternal substrata. During migration, invasive cytotrophoblast must interpret signals that determine whether the cell will continue to migrate or convert to the intramural phenotype and engage in the process of extravasation. Soon after the cell enters the artery wall it ceases to migrate and begins to synthesize and secrete ECM, and remains in this position for the duration of pregnancy. In this respect the intramural cytotrophoblast pads are repeating processes involved with the formation of a trophoblastic shell. Similar cytotrophoblast deposition of ECM is seen in the chorionic plate during late gestation (18).

There is surprisingly little evidence in the macaque of adverse reaction by endometrial tissues during vascular invasion by trophoblast. In the second half of gestation occasional regions of the arterial lumina where cytotrophoblast is present show small amounts of fibrin deposition or platelet adhesion. Throughout the modification of vessel walls there is very little evidence of necrosis or apoptosis, although the latter could occur rapidly and thus not be easily detected. Nevertheless, there is no recruitment of leukocytes to the area of trophoblast invasion and the slightly increased accumulations of macrophages appears confined to the outer margins of Streeter's columns, rather than in contact with the artery walls. It is difficult to determine whether or not the greater amount of cytotrophoblast-associated artery wall damage reported for the human is the result of the greater length of gestation, actual species differences in the mechanisms of artery adaptation, or differences in interpretation. It does appear, however, that some of the earlier investigators did not recognize that the cytotrophoblast cells are probably synthesizing large amounts of ECM. Instead, they may have interpreted the accumulation of such material as a response of the artery wall to damage induced by the invading cytotrophoblast.

There is little evidence in macaques that cytotrophoblast cells that migrate extensively through the endometrial stroma (interstitial trophoblast; 30) contribute to the modification of spiral artery walls. Many more cytokeratin positive interstitial cells are present in the human than in the macaque (31). Although cytokeratin positive interstitial cells are found around the spiral arteries during the first month of pregnancy in macaques, they do not appear to interact directly with these vessels. Therefore we consider that the majority, or perhaps all, of the arterial changes described result from those cells migrating through the lumen.

Some intramural cytotrophoblast cells maintain direct contact with the lumen and share the arterial lining with endothelial cells. Both cell types coexist in close proximity throughout pregnancy. Because endothelial cells were rarely observed as a monolayer overlying intramural trophoblast cells, reendothelialization in invaded arteries is doubtful prior to parturition. The situation with invaded veins is less clear. Monolayers of endothelium, identified with antibody to factor VIII-related antigen, are seen on surfaces of trophoblast cells that are apposed to the venous channels through the trophoblastic shell. By contrast, at the endometrial front of the shell cytotrophoblast often replaces the endothelium over part of the circumference of the veins.

The expression of select adhesion molecules (PECAM, VE-cadherin, integrins $\alpha 1\beta 1$ and $\alpha V\beta 3$) by human invasive cytotrophoblast and the positions of these cells within the lining of arteries has prompted some investigators to consider intraarterial cytotrophoblast as demonstrating the acquisition of an endothelialized phenotype (32). However, because the cytotrophoblast displaces the endothelium and colonizes the tunica media, it is not simply an endothelial lining. Other investigators have described invasive cytotrophoblast as exhibiting epithelial-mesenchymal transition (33). While it is certainly true that invasive cytotrophoblast cells display behavior atypical of epithelium, the general validity of these characterizations is limited, however, by their retention of cytokeratins and the tendency for intramural cells to form microvilli lined vacuoles.

Although macaque monkeys and baboons are the most closely related species to the human that are readily available for study, it is necessary to pay equal attention both to the similarities and the differences. The perforation of vessels by syncytial trophoblast, formation of a placental disc, subsequent intraluminal invasion of spiral arteries by cytotrophoblast, and modification of the spiral artery walls are features common to the macaque and human. However, the human placenta is larger, gestation is longer, and the start of invasion of the arteries by intraluminal cytotrophoblast is apparently slightly later than in the macaque. Furthermore, there are many more interstitial trophoblast cells in the human, and these cells may also be involved in artery remodeling, especially in the later stages. Unfortunately, little information is available concerning the first six to seven weeks after implantation in the human. It appears likely, however, that much of the early modification of arterial walls in the human uterus occurs in a similar fashion to that reported here for the more orderly and rapidly developing placenta of macaques.

References

1. Pijnenborg R, Robertson WB, Brosens I. The arterial migration of trophoblast in the uterus of the golden hamster, *Mesocricetus auratus*. J Reprod Fert 1974;40:269–80.
2. Pijnenborg R, Robertson WB, Brosens I, Dixon G. Review article: invasion and the establishment of haemochorial placentation in man and laboratory animals. Placenta 1981;2:71–92.
3. Rasweiler JJ IV. Pregnancy in chiroptera. J Exp Zool 1993;266:495–513.
4. Carpenter SJ. Trophoblast invasion and alteration of mesometrial arteries in the pregnant hamster: light and electron microscopic observations. Placenta 1982;3:219–42.
5. Tarara R, Enders AC, Hendrickx AG, Gulamhusein N, Hodges JK, Hearn JP et al. Early implantation and embryonic development of the baboon: stages 5, 6, and 7. Anat Embryol 1987;176:267–75.
6. Harris JWS, Ramsey EM. The morphology of human uteroplacental vasculature. Contrib Embryol Carnegie Inst 1966;38:43–58.
7. Ramsey EM, Harris JWS. Comparison of uteroplacental vasculature and circulation in the rhesus monkey and man. Contrib Embryol Carnegie Inst 1966;38:58–70.
8. Brosens IA, Robertson WB, Dixon HG. The physiological response of the vessels of the placental bed to normal pregnancy. J Pathol Bact 1967;93:569–79.
9. Ramsey EM, Houston ML, Harris JWS. Interactions of the trophoblast and maternal tissues in three closely related primate species. Am J Obstet Gynecol 1976;124: 647–52.
10. Blankenship TN, Enders AC, King BF. Trophoblastic invasion and the development of uteroplacental arteries in the macaque: Immunohistochemical localization of cytokeratins, desmin, type IV collagen, laminin, and fibronectin. Cell Tissue Res 1993;272:227–36.
11. Enders AC, Hendrickx AG, Schlafke S. Implantation in the rhesus monkey: initial penetration of endometrium. Am J Anat 1983;167:275–98.
12. Enders AC. Trophoblast differentiation during the transition from trophoblastic plate to lacunar stage of implantation in the rhesus monkey and human. Am J Anat 1989;186: 85–98.
13. Enders AC, King BF. Early stages of trophoblastic invasion of the maternal vascular system during implantation in the macaque and baboon. Am J Anat 1991;192:329–46.
14. Enders AC, Lantz KC, Schlafke S. Preference of invasive cytotrophoblast for maternal vessels in early implantation in the macaque. Acta Anat 1996;155:145–62.

15. Enders AC. Cytodifferentiation of trophoblast in the anchoring villi and trophoblastic shell in the first half of gestation in the macaque. Micros Res Tech 1997;38:3–20.
16. Enders AC. The transition from lacunar to villous stage of implantation in the macaque, including establishment of the trophoblastic shell. Acta Anat 1995;152:151–69.
17. Blankenship TN, Enders AC, King BF. Distribution of laminin, type IV collagen, and fibronectin in the cell columns and cytotrophoblastic shell of early macaque placentas. Cell Tissue Res 1992;270:241–8.
18. King BF, Blankenship TN. Differentiation of the chorionic plate of the placenta: cellular and extracellular matrix changes during development in the macaque. Anat Rec 1994;240:267–76.
19. Blankenship TN, King BF. Macaque intra-arterial trophoblast and extravillous trophoblast of the cell columns and cytotrophoblastic shell express neural cell adhesion molecule (NCAM). Anat Rec 1996;245:525–31.
20. Blankenship TN, Enders AC. Expression of platelet-endothelial cell adhesion molecule-1 (PECAM) by macaque trophoblast cells during invasion of the spiral arteries. Anat Rec 1997;247:413–9.
21. Blankenship TN, Enders AC, King BF. Trophoblastic invasion and modification of uterine veins during placental development in macaques. Cell Tissue Res 1993;274:135–44.
22. Genbacev O, Zhou Y, Ludlow JW, Fisher SJ. Regulation of human placental development by oxygen tension. Science 1997;277:1660–72.
23. Hawes CS, Suskin HA, Petropoulas A, Latham SE, Mueller UW. A morphologic study of trophoblast isolated from peripheral blood of pregnant women. Am J Obstet Gynecol 1994;170:1297–300.
24. Boyd JD, Hamilton WJ. The human placenta. Cambridge: Heffer, 1970.
25. Blankenship TN, King BF. Identification of 72-kilodalton type IV collagenase at sites of trophoblastic invasion of macaque spiral arteries. Placenta 1994;15:177–87.
26. Blankenship TN, Enders AC. Trophoblast cell-mediated modifications to uterine spiral arteries during early gestation in the macaque. Acta Anat 1997;158:227–36.
27. Blankenship TN, King BF. Developmental expression of Ki-67 antigen and proliferating cell nuclear antigen (PCNA) in macaque placentas. Devel Dynamics 1994;201:324–33.
28. Blankenship TN, King BF. Developmental changes in the cell columns and trophoblastic shell of the macaque placenta: an immunohistochemical study localizing type IV collagen, laminin, fibronectin and cytokeratins. Cell Tissue Res 1993;274:457–66.
29. King BF, Blankenship TN. Ultrastructure and development of a thick basement membrane-like layer in the anchoring villi of macaque placentas. Anat Rec 1994;238:498–506.
30. Kurman RJ, Main CS, Chen HC. Intermediate trophoblast: a distinctive form of trophoblast with specific morphological, biochemical and structural features. Placenta 1984;5:349–70.
31. Enders AC. Cytotrophoblast invasion of the endometrium in the human and macaque stage of implantation. Troph Res 1997;10:83–95.
32. Zhou Y, Fisher SJ, Janatpour M, Genbacev O, Dejana E, Wheelock M et al. Human cytotrophoblasts adopt a vascular phenotype as they differentiate: a strategy for successful endovascular invasion? J Clin Invest 1997;99:2139–51.
33. Vicovac L, Aplin JD. Epithelial-mesenchymal transition during trophoblast differentiation. Acta Anat 1996;156:202–16.

4

Oxygen Regulates Human Cytotrophoblast Proliferation, Differentiation, and Invasion: Implications for Endovascular Invasion in Normal Pregnancy and Preeclampsia

Olga Genbacev, Yan Zhou, Michael T. McMaster, John W. Ludlow, Caroline H. Damsky, and Susan J. Fisher

Morphological Aspects of Normal Human Placentation/Cytotrophoblast Invasion In Vivo, with Special Emphasis on Endovascular Invasion

The human placenta's unique anatomy (Fig. 4.1) is the result, in large part, to differentiation of its epithelial stem cells, termed cytotrophoblasts (reviewed in (1)). How these cells differentiate determines whether chorionic villi, the placenta's functional units, float in maternal blood or anchor the conceptus to the uterine wall. In floating villi, cytotrophoblasts differentiate by fusing to form multi-nucleate syncytiotrophoblasts whose primary function—transport—is ideally suited to their location at the villus surface. In anchoring villi, cytotrophoblasts also fuse, but many remain as single cells that detach from their basement membrane and aggregate to form cell columns (Fig. 4.1A). Cytotrophoblasts at the distal ends of these columns attach to, then deeply invade, the uterus (interstitial invasion; Fig. 4.1A, C) and its arterioles (endovascular invasion; not shown). As a result of endovascular invasion, the cells replace the endothelial and muscular linings of uterine arterioles, a process that initiates maternal blood flow to the placenta and greatly enlarges the vessel diameter. Paradoxically, the cells invade only the superficial portions of uterine venules. How this unusual behavior is regulated is unknown.

Cells that participate in endovascular invasion have two types of interactions with maternal arterioles. In the first type, large aggregates of these fetal cells are found primarily inside the vessel lumen. These aggregates can either lie adjacent

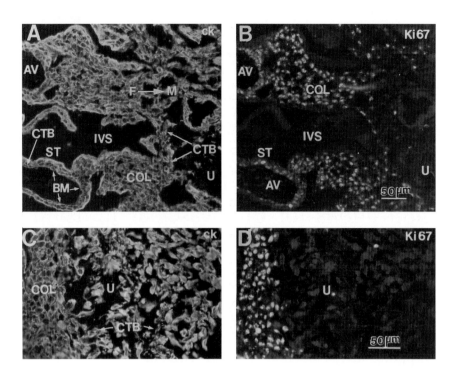

FIGURE 4.1. Tissue sections of the maternal-fetal interface at 10 weeks of gestation. (A) Cytokeratin (ck) staining shows the placental trophoblast populations. In anchoring villi (AV) cytotrophoblast (CTB) stem cells are attached to the trophoblast basement membrane (BM). These cells fuse to form multinucleate syncytiotrophoblasts (ST) which cover most of the villus surface of the placenta, where they are in direct contact with maternal blood in the intervillous space (IVS). In certain areas a subpopulation of cytotrophoblast stem cells aggregates to form cell columns (COL). These fetal cells invade maternal tissue (F→M), thereby attaching the anchoring villi to the uterus (U). (B) Cytotrophoblast stem cells and those in cell columns react with an antibody against Ki67, an antigen indicative of DNA synthesis. Cells in the column also begin to switch their expression of stage-specific antigens to those indicative of invasion (not shown). (C) Cytokeratin staining shows that once the cell columns contact the uterus, the cytotrophoblasts disaggregate and invade the uterus, where they intermingle with maternal cells. (D) Once they disaggregate, Ki67 staining abruptly stops. Reprinted from Genbacev et al. (14) by permission of AAAS.

to the apical surface of the resident endothelium or replace it such that they appear directly attached to the vessel wall. In the second type, cytotrophoblasts are found within the vessel wall rather than in the lumen. In this position, they colonize the smooth-muscle layer of the vessel and lie subjacent to the endothelium. These different types of interactions may be progressive stages in a single process, or indicative of different strategies by which cytotrophoblasts accomplish endovascular invasion. In either case, the stage in which fetal cytotrophoblasts cohabit with maternal endothelium in the spiral arterioles is transient. By late second trimester these vessels are lined exclusively by cytotrophoblasts, and endothelial cells are no longer visible in either the endometrial or the superficial portions of their myometrial segments.

Morphological Aspects of Abnormal Human Placentation/Cytotrophoblast Invasion in Preeclampsia

Preeclampsia is a disease that adversely affects 7% to 10% of first pregnancies in the United States (reviewed in [2]). The mother shows signs and symptoms that suggest widespread alterations in endothelial function (e.g., high blood pressure, proteinuria and edema [3]). In some cases the fetus stops growing, which leads to intrauterine growth retardation. The severity of the disease varies greatly. In its mildest form, the signs/symptoms appear near term and resolve after birth, with no lasting effects on either the mother or the child. In its most severe form, the signs/symptoms occur in the second trimester. If they cannot be controlled, the only option is delivery, with consequent iatrogenic fetal prematurity. Because of the latter form of the disease, preeclampsia and hypertensive diseases of pregnancy are leading causes of maternal death and contribute significantly to premature deliveries in the United States (4).

Although the cause of preeclampsia is unknown, the accumulated evidence strongly implicates the placenta (5). Anatomic examination shows that the specific area of the placenta most affected by this syndrome is the fetal–maternal interface. Cytotrophoblast invasion of the uterus is shallow, and endovascular invasion does not proceed beyond the terminal portions of the spiral arterioles. The effect of preeclampsia on endovascular invasion is particularly evident when interactions between fetal cytotrophoblasts and maternal endothelial cells are studied in detail (6,7). Serial sections through placental bed biopsies of all the patients we have studied shows that few of the spiral arterioles contain cytotrophoblasts. Instead, most cytotrophoblasts remain at some distance from these vessels. Where endovascular cytotrophoblasts are detected, their invasion is limited to the portion of the vessel that spans the superficial decidua. Thus, there is little difference between cytotrophoblast interactions with veins and arterioles in the uterus. Even if the cytotrophoblasts gain access to the lumen, they usually fail to form tight aggregates among themselves, or to spread out on the vessel wall, as is observed for cytotrophoblasts in control samples matched for gestational age. Instead they tend to remain as individual rounded cells, suggesting that they are poorly anchored to the vessel wall. Thus, cytotrophoblasts in preeclampsia not only have a limited capacity for endovascular invasion, but also display an altered morphology in their interactions with maternal arterioles.

Because of these alterations in endovascular invasion, the maternal vessels of preeclamptic patients do not undergo the complete spectrum of physiologic changes that normally occur (e.g., loss of endothelial lining and musculoelastic tissue); the mean external diameter of the myometrial vessels is less than half that of similar vessels from uncomplicated pregnancies (8–10). In addition, not as many vessels show evidence of cytotrophoblast invasion (11). Thus, the architecture of these vessels precludes an adequate response to gestation-related fetal demands for increased blood flow.

Oxygen Tension Regulates Human Cytotrophoblast Proliferation and Differentiation In Vitro

We used information about the morphological aspects of cytotrophoblast invasion in normal pregnancy and in preeclampsia to formulate hypotheses about the regulatory factors involved. Specifically, in normal pregnancy cytotrophoblasts invade large-bore arterioles, where they are in contact with well-oxygenated maternal blood. But in preeclampsia, invasive cytotrophoblasts are relatively hypoxic. We also took into account that blood flow to the placenta changes dramatically in early pregnancy. During much of the first trimester there is little endovascular invasion, so maternal blood flow to the placenta is at a minimum. The oxygen pressures of the intervillus space (that is, at the uterine surface) and within the endometrium are estimated to be (mean $\pm$ SD) 17.9 ± 6.9 mm Hg and 39.6 ± 12.3 mm Hg, respectively, at 8 to 10 weeks of gestation (12). Afterward, endovascular invasion proceeds rapidly; cytotrophoblasts are in direct contact with blood from maternal spiral arterioles, which could have a mean oxygen pressure as high as 90 to 100 mm Hg. Thus, as cytotrophoblasts invade the uterus during the first half of pregnancy, they encounter a steep, positive oxygen tension gradient. These observations, together with the results of initial experiments we conducted on isolated cytotrophoblasts (13), suggested that oxygen tension might regulate cytotrophoblast proliferation and differentiation along the invasive pathway (14).

First, we used immunolocalization techniques to study the relationship between cytotrophoblast proliferation and differentiation in situ. Cytotrophoblasts in columns (i.e., cells in the initial stages of differentiation) reacted with an antibody against the Ki67 antigen (Fig. 4.1B, (14)), which is indicative of DNA synthesis (15). Distal to this region, anti-Ki67 staining abruptly stopped (Fig. 4.1D), and the cytotrophoblasts intricately modulated their expression of stage-specific antigens (data not shown), including integrin cell adhesion molecules (16), matrix metalloproteinase-9 (17), HLA-G (a cytotrophoblast class Ib major histocompatibility complex molecule (18)), and human placental lactogen (19). These results suggested that during differentiation along the invasive pathway, cytotrophoblasts first undergo mitosis, then exit the cell cycle and modulate their expression of stage-specific antigens.

As an in vitro model system for testing this hypothesis, we used organ cultures of anchoring villi explanted from early gestation (6 to 8 week) placentas onto an ECM substrate. Some of the anchoring villi were cultured for 72 h in a standard tissue culture incubator (20% O_2 or 98 mm Hg). Figure 4.2A shows a section of one such control villus that was stained with an antibody that recognizes cytokeratin to demonstrate syncytiotrophoblasts and cytotrophoblasts. The attached cell columns were clearly visible. To assess the cells' ability to synthesize DNA, the villi were incubated with BrdU. Incorporation was detected in the cytoplasm, but not the nuclei, of syncytiotrophoblasts. Few or none of the cells in columns incorporated BrdU (Fig. 4.2B). Other anchoring villi were maintained in an hypoxic atmosphere

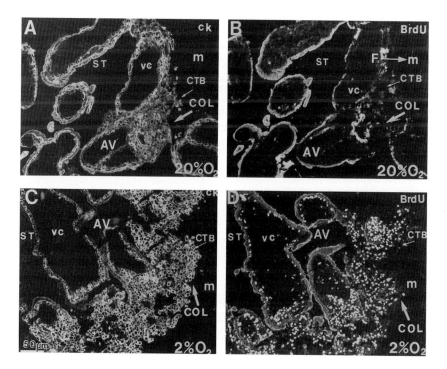

FIGURE 4.2. Low oxygen (2% O_2) stimulates cytotrophoblast BrdU incorporation in vitro. Anchoring villi (AV) from 6–8 week placentas were cultured on Matrigel (m) for 72 h in either 20% O_2 (A, B) or 2% O_2 (C, D). By the end of the culture period, fetal cytotrophoblasts migrated into the Matrigel (F→m). To assess cell proliferation, BrdU was added to the medium. Tissue sections of the villi were stained with anti-cytokeratin (ck; A, C), which recognizes syncytiotrophoblasts (ST) and cytotrophoblasts (CTB) but not cells in the villus core (vc); and with anti-BrdU (B, D), which detects cells in S phase. Villus explants maintained in 2% O_2 (C) formed much more prominent columns (COL) with a larger proportion of CTB nuclei that incorporated BrdU (D) than explants cultured in 20% O_2 (A, B). Reprinted from Genbacev et al. (14) by permission of AAAS.

(2% O_2 or 14 mm Hg). After 72 h, cytokeratin staining showed prominent cell columns (Fig. 4.2C), and the nuclei of many of the cytotrophoblasts in these columns incorporated BrdU (Fig. 4.2D). Because cytotrophoblasts were the only cells that entered S phase, we also compared the ability of anchoring villus explants cultured under standard and hypoxic conditions to incorporate [^{3}H]thymidine. Villus explants ($n = 21$ per group; dissected from 7 placentas) cultured under hypoxic conditions (2% O_2) incorporated 3.3 ± 1.2 times more [^{3}H]thymidine than villi cultured under standard conditions (20% O_2). In contrast, [^{3}H]thymidine incorporation by explants ($n = 8$ per group; dissected from 4 placentas) cultured in a 6% O_2 atmosphere (40 mm Hg) was no different than in control villi. Taken together, these results suggest that a hypoxic atmosphere, comparable to that encountered by early gestation cytotrophoblasts in the intervillous space, stimulates the cells to enter S phase.

Cytokeratin staining also showed that the cell columns associated with anchoring villi cultured under hypoxic conditions were larger than cell columns of control villi cultured under standard conditions (compare Figs. 4.2A and 4.2C). We made serial sections of columns attached to two villus explants maintained for 72 h in 20% O_2 and two that were maintained in 2% O_2, and then counted the number of cells in each column ($n = 8$ per group; dissected from 2 placentas). Under standard tissue culture conditions, the columns contained a mean of 516 ± 72 cells. In hypoxic conditions, they contained a mean of 1476 ± 156 cells. These results indicate that hypoxia stimulates cytotrophoblasts in cell columns to proliferate.

We reasoned that the hypoxia-induced changes in the cells' proliferative capacity would be reflected by changes in their expression of proteins that regulate passage through the cell cycle. With regard to the G2-M transition, we were particularly interested in their cyclin B expression, because threshold levels of this protein are required for cells to enter mitosis (20). Immunoblotting of cell extracts showed that after 3 days in culture, anchoring villi maintained in 2% O_2 contained 3.1 times more cyclin B than did villi maintained in 20% O_2 (Fig. 4.3a). Immunolocalization experiments confirmed that cyclin B was primarily expressed by cytotrophoblasts (not shown). Because p21[WF1/CIP1] abundance has been correlated with cell cycle arrest (21), we also examined the effects of oxygen tension on cytotrophoblast expression of this protein. Very little p21[WF1/CIP1] expression was detected in cell extracts of anchoring villi maintained for 72 h in 2% O_2 (Fig. 4.3b), but expression increased 3.8-fold in anchoring villi maintained for the same time period in 20% O_2. Immunolocalization experiments confirmed that p21[WF1/CIP1] was primarily expressed by cytotrophoblasts (not shown). These results, replicated in 5 separate experiments, confirm that culturing anchoring villi in 20% O_2 induces cytotrophoblasts in the attached cell columns to undergo cell cycle arrest, whereas culturing them in 2% O_2 induces them to enter mitosis.

Changes in proliferative capacity are often accompanied by concomitant changes in differentiation. Accordingly, we investigated the effects of hy-

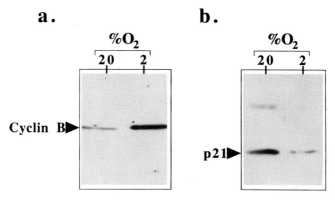

FIGURE 4.3. Hypoxia induces changes in cytotrophoblast expression of proteins that regulate progression through the cell cycle. (a) Villus explants cultured for 72 h in 2% O_2 contained 3.1 times more cyclin B than did villi maintained under standard culture conditions (20% O_2) for the same length of time. (b) Expression of p21 increased 3.8-fold in anchoring villi cultured for 72 h in 20% O_2 as compared to 2% O_2. Reprinted from Genbacev et al. (14) by permission of AAAS.

poxia on the ability of cytotrophoblasts to differentiate along the invasive pathway (Fig. 4.4). Under standard tissue culture conditions, cytotrophoblasts migrated from the cell columns and modulated their expression of stage-specific antigens, as they do during uterine invasion in vivo (16). For example, they began to express integrin $\alpha 1$, a laminin-collagen receptor that is required for invasiveness in vitro (22). Both differentiated cytotrophoblasts and villus stromal cells expressed this antigen (Fig. 4.4B). When cultured under hypoxic conditions, cytotrophoblasts failed to stain for integrin $\alpha 1$, but stromal cells continued to express this molecule, suggesting the observed effects were cell-type specific (Fig. 4.4E). Hypoxia also reduced cytotrophoblast staining for human placental lactogen, another antigen that is expressed once the cells differentiate (not shown). However, lowering the O_2 tension did not change cytotrophoblast expression of other stage-specific antigens, such as HLA-G (Figs. 4.4C and 4.4F), and integrins $\alpha 5/\beta 1$ and $\alpha V/\beta 3$ (not shown). These results suggest that hypoxia produces selective deficits in the ability of cytotrophoblasts to differentiate along the invasive pathway.

The effects of oxygen tension on the proliferative capacity of cyto-trophoblasts could help explain some of the interesting features of normal placental development. Before cytotrophoblast invasion of maternal vessels establishes the uteroplacental circulation (≤ 10 weeks), the conceptus is in a relatively hypoxic atmosphere. During this period, placental mass increases much more rapidly than that of the embryo proper. Histological sections of early-stage pregnant human uteri show bilaminar embryos surrounded by thousands of trophoblast cells (23). The fact that hypoxia stimulates

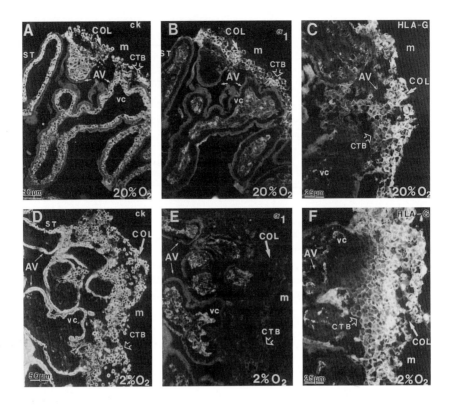

FIGURE 4.4. Some aspects of cytotrophoblast differentiation/invasion are arrested in hypoxia. Anchoring villi (AV) from 6–8 week placentas were cultured on Matrigel (m) for 72 h in either 20% O_2 (A–C) or 2% O_2 (D–F). Tissue sections of the villi were stained with anti-cytokeratin (ck; A, D), anti-integrin $\alpha 1$ (B, E) or anti-HLA-G (C, F). Cytotrophoblasts (CTB) that composed the cell columns (COL) of villus explants that were cultured in 20% O_2 upregulated both integrin $\alpha 1$ (B) and HLA-G expression (C). In contrast, cytotrophoblasts in anchoring villus columns maintained in 2% O_2 failed to express integrin $\alpha 1$, although constituents of the villus core continued to express this adhesion molecule (E). But not all aspects of differentiation were impaired; the cells upregulated HLA-G expression normally (F). ST, syncytiotrophoblast; vc, villus core. Reprinted from Genbacev et al. (14) by permission of AAAS.

cytotrophoblasts, but not most other cells (24), to undergo mitosis could help account for the discrepancy in size between the embryo and the placenta, which continues well into the second trimester of pregnancy (25). Although we do not as yet understand this phenomenon at a mechanistic level, we have recently shown (see below) that cytotrophoblasts within the uterine wall mimic a vascular adhesion molecule phenotype (7). In other tissues hypoxia induces vascular endothelial growth factor production which stimulates endothelial cell proliferation (26), raising the possibility that similar regulatory pathways operate during placental development.

We suspect that the effects of oxygen tension on cytotrophoblast differentiation/invasion could also have important implications. Relatively high oxygen tension promotes cytotrophoblast differentiation and could help explain why these cells extensively invade the arterial rather than the venous side of the uterine circulation. Conversely, if cytotrophoblasts do not gain access to an adequate supply of maternal arterial blood, their ability to differentiate into fully invasive cells may be impaired. We suggest that the latter scenario could be a contributing factor to pregnancy-associated diseases, such as preeclampsia, that are associated with abnormally shallow cytotrophoblast invasion and faulty differentiation, as evidenced by their inability to upregulate integrin $\alpha 1$ expression (6). These results also prompted us to consider the possibility that the profound effects of oxygen on invasive cytotrophoblasts might be indicative of their ability to assume a vascular-like phenotype.

During Normal Pregnancy, Invasive Cytotrophoblasts Modulate Their Adhesion Molecule Repertoire to Mimic That of Vascular Cells

Recently, we tested the hypotheses that invasive cytotrophoblasts mimic broadly the adhesion phenotype of the endothelial cells they replace and that these changes in adhesion phenotype have the net effect of enhancing cytotrophoblast motility and invasiveness (7). To test these hypotheses, we first stained tissue sections of the fetal-maternal interface for specific integrins, cadherins, and immunoglobulin family adhesion receptors that are characteristic of endothelial cells and leukocytes. We then tested the functional consequences for cytotrophoblast adhesion and invasion of expressing the particular adhesion receptors that were upregulated during cytotrophoblast differentiation.

First, we examined the distribution patterns of αV integrin family members. We were particularly interested in these molecules because of their regulated expression on endothelial cells during angiogenesis and their upregulation on some types of metastatic tumor cells. αV family members displayed unique and highly specific spatial staining patterns on cytotrophoblasts in anchoring villi and the placental bed. An $\alpha V \beta 5$-complex-specific antibody stained the cytotrophoblast monolayer in chorionic villi. Staining was uniform over the entire cell surface. The syncytiotrophoblast layer, and cytotrophoblasts in cell columns and the placental bed, did not stain for $\alpha V \beta 5$. In contrast, anti-$\alpha V \beta 6$ stained only those chorionic villus cytotrophoblasts that were at sites of column formation. The cytotrophoblast layer still in contact with basement membrane stained brightly, while the first layer of the cell column showed reduced staining. The rest of the cytotrophoblasts in chorionic villi, cytotrophoblasts in more distal regions of cell columns, and cytotrophoblasts within placental bed and vasculature did not stain for αVβ6, documenting a specific association of this integrin with initiation of column formation. In yet a different pattern, staining for anti-αVβ3 was weak or not detected on villus cytotrophoblasts or on cytotrophoblasts in the initial layers of cell columns. However, strong staining was detected on cytotrophoblasts within the uterine wall and vasculature. Thus, individual members of the αV family, like those of the β1 family (16), are spatially regulated during cytotrophoblast differentiation. Of particular relevance is the observation that αVβ3 integrin, whose expression on endothelial cells is stimulated by angiogenic factors, is prominent on cytotrophoblasts that have invaded the uterine wall and maternal vasculature.

Because blocking αVβ3 function suppresses endothelial migration during angiogenesis, we determined whether perturbing its interactions also affects cytotrophoblast invasion in vitro. Freshly isolated first trimester cytotrophoblasts were plated for 48 h on Matrigel-coated Transwell filters in the presence of control mouse IgG or the complex-specific anti-αVβ3 IgG, LM609. Cytotrophoblast invasion was evaluated by counting cells and cellular processes that had invaded the Matrigel barrier and extended through the holes in the Transwell filters. LM609 reduced cytotrophoblast invasion by more than 75% in this assay, indicating that this receptor, like the α1β1 integrin (22), contributes significantly to the invasive phenotype of cytotrophoblasts.

Next, we examined cadherin switching during cytotrophoblast differentiation in vivo. The cytotrophoblast epithelial monolayer stained strongly for the ubiquitous epithelial cadherin, E-cadherin, in a polarized pattern. Staining was strong on the surfaces of cytotrophoblasts in contact with one another and with the overlying syncytiotrophoblast layer and was absent at the basal surface of cytotrophoblasts in contact with basement membrane. In cell columns, E-cadherin staining intensity was reduced on cytotrophoblasts near the uterine wall and on cytotrophoblasts within the decidua. This reduction in staining was particularly pronounced in second trimester tissue. At this stage, E-cadherin staining was also very weak or undetectable on cytotrophoblasts that had colonized maternal blood vessels and on cytotrophoblasts in the surrounding myometrium. All locations of reduced E-cadherin staining were areas in which invasion is active during the first half of gestation. Interestingly, the staining intensity of E-cadherin was strong on cytotrophoblasts in all locations in term placentas, at which time cytotrophoblast invasive activity is poor. Taken together, these data are consistent with the idea that cytotrophoblasts transiently reduce E-cadherin function at times and places of their greatest invasive activity.

Cadherin switching occurs frequently during embryonic development when significant morphogenetic events take place. We therefore stained sections of first and second trimester placental tissue with antibodies to other classical cadherins. These tissues did not stain with antibodies against P-cadherin. However, they did stain with three different monoclonal antibodies that recognize the endothelial cadherin, VE–cadherin. In chorionic villi, antibody to

VE cadherin did not stain villus cytotrophoblasts, although it stained the endothelium of fetal blood vessels within the villus stroma. In contrast, anti-VE-cadherin stained cytotrophoblasts in cell columns and in the decidua, the very areas in which E-cadherin staining was reduced. VE-cadherin staining was stronger in these areas in second trimester tissues. In maternal vessels that had not yet been modified by cytotrophoblasts, anti-VE-cadherin stained the endothelial layer strongly. Following endovascular invasion, cytotrophoblasts lining maternal blood vessels also stained strongly for VE-cadherin. Thus, cytotrophoblasts that invade the uterine wall and vasculature express a cadherin characteristic of endothelial cells.

Next, we used function-perturbing anti-cadherin antibodies, in conjunction with the Matrigel invasion assay, to assess the functional consequences of cadherin modulation for cytotrophoblast invasiveness. We plated isolated second trimester cytotrophoblasts for 48 h on Matrigel-coated filters in the presence of control IgG or function-perturbing antibodies against VE-cadherin or E-cadherin. By 48 h, significant invasion was evident in control cytotrophoblasts. In cultures treated with anti–E-cadherin, cytotrophoblast invasiveness increased more than three fold, suggesting that E-cadherin normally has a restraining effect on invasiveness. In contrast, antibody against VE-cadherin reduced the invasion of cytotrophoblasts to about 60% of control. This suggests that the presence of VE cadherin normally facilitates cytotrophoblast invasion. Taken together, these functional data suggest that as they differentiate, the cells modulate their cadherin repertoire to one that contributes to their increased invasiveness.

Our data presented thus far indicate that, as they differentiate, cytotrophoblasts downregulate adhesion receptors highly characteristic of epithelial cells (integrin $\alpha6\beta4$ (16) and E-cadherin) and upregulate analogous receptors that are expressed on endothelial cells (integrins $\alpha1\beta1$ (16) and $\alpha V\beta3$, and VE-cadherin). These observations support our hypothesis that normal cytotrophoblasts undergo a comprehensive switch in phenotype so as to resemble the endothelial cells they replace during endovascular invasion.

We hypothesize that this unusual phenomenon plays an important role in the process which these cells form vascular connections with the uterine vessels. Ultimately these connections are so extensive that the spiral arterioles become hybrid structures in which fetal cytotrophoblasts replace the maternal endothelium and much of the highly muscular tunica media. As a result, the diameter of the spiral arterioles increases dramatically, allowing blood flow to the placenta to keep pace with fetal growth. Circumstantial evidence suggests that several of the adhesion molecules whose expression we studied could play an important role in forming these novel vascular connections. In the mouse, for example, targeted disruption of either vascular cell adhesion molecule (VCAM)-1 or $\alpha4$ expression results in failure of chorioallantoic fusion. It is interesting to find that cytotrophoblasts are the only cells, other than the endothelium, that express VE-cadherin. In addition, VE-cadherin and platelet-endothelial cell adhesion molecule (PECAM)-1 are the first adhesion receptors expressed by differentiating endothelial cells during early development. $\alpha V\beta 3$ expression is upregulated on endothelial cells during angiogenesis by soluble factors that regulate this process. Thus, adhesion receptors that are upregulated as normal cytotrophoblasts differentiate/invade play vital roles in differentiation and expansion of the vasculature.

Invasive Cytotrophoblasts Fail to Switch Their Adhesion Molecule Repertoire to Mimic That of Vascular Cells in Preeclampsia

Next we tested the hypothesis that preeclampsia negatively affects the ability of cytotrophoblasts to express adhesion molecules that are normally modulated during the unique epithelial-to-vascular transformation that occurs in normal pregnancy (27). First, we compared cytotrophoblast expression of three members of the αV family ($\alpha V\beta 5$, $\alpha V\beta 6$, and $\alpha V\beta 3$) in placental bed biopsies obtained from control and preeclamptic patients that were matched for gestational age. We found that preeclampsia changed cytotrophoblast expression of all three αV-family members. When samples were matched for gestational age, fewer preeclamptic cytotrophoblast stem cells stained with an antibody that recognized integrin $\beta 5$. In contrast, staining for $\beta 6$ was much brighter in preeclamptic tissue and extended beyond the column to include cytotrophoblasts within the superficial decidua. Of greatest interest, staining for $\beta 3$ was weak on cytotrophoblasts in all locations; cytotrophoblasts in the uterine wall of preeclamptic patients failed to show strong staining for $\beta 3$, as did cytotrophoblasts that penetrated the spiral arterioles. Thus, in preeclampsia, differentiating/invading cytotrophoblasts retain expression of $\alpha V\beta 6$, which is transiently expressed in remodeling epithelium, and fail to upregulate $\alpha V\beta 3$, which is characteristic of angiogenic endothelium. Therefore, as was the case for integrin $\alpha 1$ (6), our analyses of the expression of αV-family members suggest that in preeclampsia, cytotrophoblasts start to differentiate along the invasive pathway but cannot complete this process.

Preeclampsia also had a striking effect on cytotrophoblast cadherin expression. In contrast to control samples, cytotrophoblasts in both the villi and decidua showed strong reactivity with anti-E-cadherin, and staining remained strong even on cytotrophoblasts that had penetrated the superficial portions of uterine arterioles. Interestingly, in preeclampsia we consistently found that cytotrophoblasts within the uterine wall tended to exist as large aggregates, rather than as smaller clusters and single cells, as is the case in normal pregnancy. This observation is in accord with the likelihood that E-cadherin mediates strong intercellular adhesion between cytotrophoblasts, as it does in all other normal epithelia examined.

Strikingly, no VE-cadherin staining was detected on cytotrophoblasts in any location in placental bed specimens obtained from preeclamptic patients;

neither cytotrophoblasts in the cell columns nor the few cells that were found in association with vessels in the superficial decidua expressed VE-cadherin. However, staining for this adhesion molecule was detected on maternal endothelium in the unmodified uterine vessels in preeclamptic placental bed biopsy specimens. Thus, cadherin modulation by cytotrophoblasts in preeclampsia was defective, as shown by the persistence of strong E-cadherin staining and the absence of VE-cadherin staining on cytotrophoblasts in columns and in the superficial decidua.

Our results raise the interesting possibility that the failure of preeclamptic cytotrophoblasts to express vascular-type adhesion molecules, as normal cytotrophoblasts do, impairs their ability to form connections with the uterine vessels. This failure ultimately limits the supply of maternal blood to the placenta and fetus, an effect thought to be closely linked to the pathophysiology of the disease. We also hypothesize that the failure of preeclamptic cytotrophoblasts to make a transition to a vascular cell adhesion phenotype might be part of a broader-spectrum defect in which the cells fail to function properly as endothelium. Such a failure would no doubt have important effects on the maintenance of vascular integrity at the maternal-fetal interface. Clearly, in preeclampsia undifferentiated cytotrophoblasts that fail to mimic the adhesion phenotype of endothelial cells are present in the termini of maternal spiral arterioles. Whether their presence affects the phenotype of maternal endothelium in deeper segments of the same vessels and/or is linked to the maternal endothelial pathology that is a hallmark of this disease is an interesting question that remains to be investigated.

Acknowledgments. This work was supported by HD 30367, HD 22210, and 3RT-0324 from The University of California Tobacco-related Disease Program to S.J.F., a Rockefeller Foundation Postdoctoral Fellowship to Y.Z., and CA 56940 to J.W.L. We thank R. Joslin for excellent technical assistance and E. Leash for excellent editorial assistance.

References

1. Cross JC, Werb Z, Fisher SJ. Implantation and the placenta: key pieces of the development puzzle. Science 1994;266:1508–18.
2. Roberts JM, Taylor RN, Friedman SA, Goldfien A. New developments in pre-eclampsia. In: Dunlop W, ed. Fetal medical review. London: Edward Arnold, 1993.
3. Roberts JM, Taylor RN, Musci TJ, Rodgers GM, Hubel CA, McLaughlin MK. Preecampsia: an endothelial cell disorder. Am J Obstet Gynecol 1989;161:1200–4.
4. Berg CJ, Atrash HK, Koonin LM, Tucker M. Pregnancy-related mortality in the United States, 1987–1990. Obstet Gynecol 1996;88:161–7.
5. Redman CW. Current topic: pre-eclampsia and the placenta. Placenta 1991;12:301–8.
6. Zhou Y, Damsky CH, Chiu K, Roberts JM, Fisher SJ. Preeclampsia is associated with abnormal expression of adhesion molecules by invasive cytotrophoblasts. J Clin Invest 1993;91:950–60.

7. Zhou Y, Fisher SJ, Janatpour M, Genbacev O, Dejana E, Wheelock M et al. Human cytotrophoblasts adopt a vascular phenotype as they differentiate: a strategy for successful endovascular invasion? J Clin Invest 1997;99:2139–51.

8. Brosens IA, Robertson WB, Dixon HG. The role of the spiral arteries in the pathogenesis of preeclampsia. Obstet Gynecol Annu 1972;1:177–91.

9. Gerretsen G, Huisjes HJ, Elema JD. Morphological changes of the spiral arteries in the placental bed in relation to pre-eclampsia and fetal growth retardation. Br J Obstet Gynaecol 1981;88:876–81.

10. Moodley J, Ramsaroop R. Placental bed morphology in black women with eclampsia. S Afr Med J 1989;75:376–8.

11. Khong TY, De WF, Robertson WB, Brosens I. Inadequate maternal vascular response to placentation in pregnancies complicated by pre-eclampsia and by small-for-gestational age infants. Br J Obstet Gynaecol 1986;93:1049–59.

12. Rodesch F, Simon P, Donner C, Jauniaux E. Oxygen measurements in endometrial and trophoblastic tissues during early pregnancy. Obstet Gynecol 1992;80:283–5.

13. Genbacev O, Joslin R, Damsky CH, Polliotti BM, Fisher SJ. Hypoxia alters early gestation human cytotrophoblast differentiation/invasion in vitro and models the placental defects that occur in preeclampsia. J Clin Invest 1996;97:540–50.

14. Genbacev O, Zhou Y, Ludlow JW, Fisher SJ. Regulation of human placental development by oxygen tension. Science 1997;277:1669–72.

15. Schwarting R. Little missed markers and Ki-67 (Editorial). Lab Invest 1993;68: 597–9.

16. Damsky CH, Fitzgerald ML, Fisher SJ. Distribution patterns of extracellular matrix components and adhesion receptors are intricately modulated during first trimester cytotrophoblast differentiation along the invasive pathway, in vivo. J Clin Invest 1992;89:210–22.

17. Librach CL, Werb Z, Fitzgerald ML, Chiu K, Corwin NM, Esteves RA et al. 92-kD type IV collagenase mediates invasion of human cytotrophoblasts. J Cell Biol 1991;113:437–49.

18. McMaster MT, Librach CL, Zhou Y, Lim KH, Janatpour MJ, Demars R et al. Human placental HLA-G expression is restricted to differentiated cytotrophoblasts. J Immunol 1995;154:3771–8.

19. Kurman RJ, Young RH, Norris HJ, Main CS, Lawrence WD, Scully RE. Immunocytochemical localization of placental lactogen and chorionic gonadotopin in the normal placenta and trophoblastic tumors, with emphasis on intermediate trophoblast and the placental site trophoblastic tumor. Int J Gynecol Pathol 1984;3:101–21.

20. King RW, Jackson PK, Kirschner MW. Mitosis in transition [see comments]. Cell 1994;79:563–71.

21. Gartel AL, Serfas MS, Tyner AL. p21—negative regulator of the cell cycle. Proc Soc Exp Biol Med 1996;213:138–49.

22. Damsky Ch, Librach C, Lim KH, Fitzgerald ML, McMaster MT, Janatpour M et al. Integrin switching regulates normal trophoblast invasion. Development 1994;120: 3657–66.

23. Hertig AT. On the eleven-day pre-villous human ovum with special reference to the variations in its implantation site. Anat Rec 1942;82:420.

24. Graeber TG, Osmanian C, Jacks T, Housman DE, Koch CJ, Lowe SW et al. Hypoxia-mediated selection of cells with diminished apoptotic potential in solid tumours [see comments]. Nature 1996;379:88–91.

25. Boyd JD, Hamilton WJ. Development and structure of the human placenta from the end of the 3rd month of gestation. J Obstet Gynaecol Br Commonw 1967;74:161–226.
26. Stone J, Itin A, Alon T, Pe'er J, Gnessin H, Chan-Ling T et al. Development of retinal vasculature is mediated by hypoxia-induced vascular endothelial growth factor (VEGF) expression by neuroglia. J Neurosci 1995;15:4738–47.
27. Zhou YF, C.H., Fisher, S.J. Preeclampsia is associated with failure of human cytotrophoblasts to mimic a vascular adhesion phenotype: one cause of defective endovascular invasion in this syndrome? J Clin Invest 1997;99:2152–64.

5

Embryo–Maternal Interactions after Diapause in a Marsupial

MARILYN B. RENFREE AND GEOFFREY SHAW

In all mammals, development of the embryo depends on complex interactions with the uterus. In the most commonly used experimental animals, mice and rats, the development of the egg cylinder and the formation of the invasive placenta at implantation early in gestation complicate analysis, so that the signals passing between the uterus and mother in early pregnancy are not clearly defined. Marsupials, in contrast, remain free and unattached to the uterus for two thirds of gestation, surrounded by an acellular mucoid coat and keratinous shell that prevents direct cell–cell contact between the endometrium and trophoblast cells. Embryo development must therefore be controlled by soluble factors in the uterine secretions. This is seen very clearly in the control of embryonic diapause, which is characteristic of about 35 marsupial species (1). Almost all of these species belong to the family Macropodidae; the kangaroos and wallabies, but it is important to note that diapause does occur in at least two small possum families, the Burramyidae and Tarsipedidae (2).

The tammar is the best understood species, partly because of its highly seasonal reproductive pattern and its interesting dual control of diapause (Fig. 5.1). During the first half of the year, the sucking stimulus associated with lactation maintains the inhibition on the blastocyst, but in the second half of the year (after the winter solstice) photoperiod assumes the dominant control so the blastocysts remain in diapause after weaning. Reactivation occurs soon after the longest day on December 22, so births normally take place between the end of January and the beginning of February.

The tammar wallaby, like most macropodid marsupials, has a postpartum oestrus and normally mates within 1 hour of birth (3). Over the next 8 days the embryo develops into a unilaminar 80 to 100 cell blastocyst (4,5). If the female is still suckling a young in the pouch, the embryo will then enter diapause. During diapause the tammar blastocyst has no detectable mitotic activity, and there are no signs of growth Despite this suspended animation, the reproductive success rate is extremely high and all oocytes fertilized apparently survive as blastocysts through the normal 11 months of diapause (4). Removal of the sucking pouch

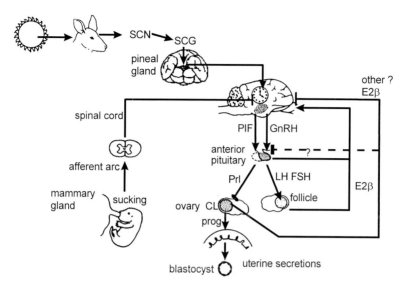

FIGURE 5.1. Hypothetical scheme showing the known and suggested pathways for the control of quiescence of *Macropus eugenii*. CL, corpus luteum; GnRH, gonadotrophin releasing hormone; LH, luteinizing hormone; E$_2$β, oestradiol-17β; FSH, follicle-stimulating hormone; Prog, progesterone; PIF, prolactin inhibiting factor; Prl, prolactin; SCG, superior cervical ganglion; SCN, suprachiasmatic nucleus. ↓ Stimulation; ⊥ inhibition. Redrawn from Renfree (2) and (7).

young during the breeding season induces reactivation of the embryo from diapause and birth occurs 26.5 days later (6).

Control of Embryonic Diapause and Subsequent Pregnancy

The endocrine control of diapause in the tammar is now well understood (Fig. 5.1) and has been extensively reviewed (6,7), so only a brief summary will be provided here. Prolactin has an unusual action in this species because it acts as a luteostatin during lactation (8–13), ensuring that the quiescent corpus luteum (CL) produces only basal concentrations of progesterone (14,15). Removal of the pouch young, denervating the teats, hypophysectomy, or treatment with the dopamine-agonist bromocriptine, which blocks pituitary prolactin release, all induce reactivation of the CL, with a concomitant increase in progesterone production (8,14,16,17). During seasonal quiescence, it is also possible to induce reactivation by denervating the pineal (18) or by melatonin implant or injection (19–21). Treatment with exogenous progesterone also induces reactivation, but gestation is shortened by 3 to 4 days (4,22,23) (Fig. 5.2). Blastocyst

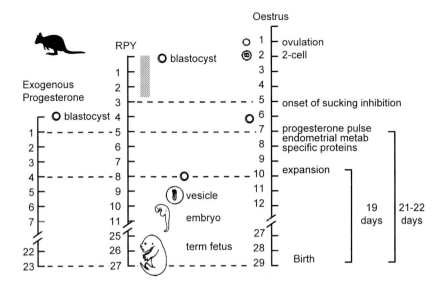

FIGURE 5.2. Intervals from either exogenous progesterone injection (left column), removal of pouch young (middle column) or oestrus (right column) to the withdrawal or onset of sucking inhibition, the early rise in progesterone (progesterone pulse), the increase in endometrial wet weight and metabolism (metab), the first measurable expansion of the blastocyst and birth. Although not shown, the progesterone pulse also coincides with an oestradiol-17β pulse after RPY. Note that, while the timing from injection, RPY or oestrus to the early progesterone pulse or to expansion is variable, the duration of pregnancy from the pulse is more or less constant and takes 21–22 days (6), and from expansion to birth 19 days. Based on data in Renfree (36); Renfree and Tyndale-Biscoe (4); Tyndale-Biscoe (5); Hinds and Tyndale-Biscoe (13); Shaw and Renfree (38); Fletcher and Renfree (22); Gordon et al. (50). Redrawn from Renfree (7).

transfer experiments demonstrate that the secretions of the CL do not stimulate the blastocyst directly (24), but act on the uterine endometrium to produce specific uterine secretions that allow embryo reactivation. It is therefore relatively easy to control reactivation of diapausing blastocysts in tammars for experimental purposes.

Implantation *sensu strictu* does not occur until the last third of gestation and occurs as an apposition or attachment of the chorio-vitelline placenta in the region of the bilaminar yolk sac. The *sinus terminalis* marks the boundary of the vascular trilaminar yolk sac and the attached region. The yolk sac placenta is fully functional and maintains significant concentration gradients across it. Despite its apparent simplicity, the tammar placenta is also a highly active endocrine organ. Although the tammar placenta produces only limited amounts of steroids (25,26), it synthesizes both prostaglandin-F2α and prostaglandin E$_2$ in increasing quantities near term, and this may be important for the process of birth (27,28). Similarly, the relaxin gene is expressed in the placenta in late pregnancy

(29) suggesting that the placenta may synthesize and release this peptide hormone. Further studies will no doubt discover other hormones.

Uterine Secretion and Endometrial Responses During Diapause and after Reactivation

Ovulation occurs about 42 h postpartum. The oocyte, surrounded by a zona pellucida secreted in the follicle, moves down the oviduct rapidly (30). Fertilization takes place in the oviduct (31). By the time the fertilized egg enters the uterus 24 h after ovulation, it is surrounded by the mucoid coat with histochemical properties of a highly sulphated glycoprotein. Outside the mucoid coat a disulphide rich ovokeratinous shell membrane forms from proteins which are secreted by the luminal epithelium of the uterotubal junction and the adjacent endometrial glands (30,32–34). By the blastocyst stage the shell is at its thickest. The blastocyst remains enclosed by this shell membrane throughout diapause.

The endometrium consists of a stroma of connective tissue through which run the secretory tubules of the endometrial glands lined by secretory epithelia continuous with the uterine luminal epithelium. There are junctional complexes between the epithelial cells (35) that provide a barrier between the blood and extracelluar fluid and the uterine luminal fluid. The uterine secretions are complex and change dramatically through pregnancy (4,36,37). However, although the endometrium enlarges greatly by hyperplasia and hypertrophy during gestation, it never produces copious quantities of uterine fluid (36).

In tammars it is possible to compare gravid and nongravid uterus in the same animal because although there are two uteri with separate cervices, they only have a single embryo. During diapause, both uteri appear alike and after embryo transfer both uteri are capable of supporting embryonic development (24). However, between days 11 and 15 after reactivation the endometrium from the gravid uterus is significantly heavier than the contralateral nongravid uterus, and has greater secretory activity (36). The hormone(s) responsible for this local stimulation is not identified. There is, however, a local circulation of progesterone from the corpus luteum via its ipslateral utero-ovarian vein as well as via shunts to the contralateral uterus, which could initiate the endometrial proliferation. After day 11 there is a continued increase only in the gravid endometrium (Fig. 5.3) which must be the result of stimulation from the developing embryo or the fetal membranes (36,37).

In tammars there are several uterine-specific prealbumins that appear after reactivation (36), but the identity of these has not yet been investigated using modern, molecular techniques. Both progesterone and oestradiol can stimulate rapid and dramatic changes in uterine protein secretion within 2 or 3 days (38,39). Oestradiol treatment increases progesterone receptor levels in uterine tissue of the brushtail possum (40,41), so it is possible that oestradiol

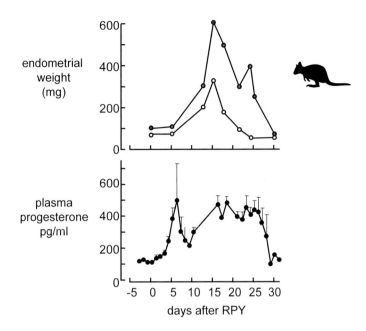

FIGURE 5.3. Endometrial wet weights (top) and plasma progesterone (bottom) in the tammar, *Macropus eugenii* during pregnancy. Gravid uteri (•) show a greater and more sustained response than contralateral, nongravid uteri (○). Plasma progesterone measured by radioimmunoassay after removal of pouch young. There is a marked pulse of progesterone 3–6 days after removal of their pouch young, and a sharp fall in progesterone at the time of parturition. Data from Cake et al., (64); redrawn from Renfree (7).

promotes a progesterone mediated response. In the tammar, progesterone and oestradiol cytosol receptors both approximately double between the day of RPY and days 5 to 7, but as peripheral plasma progesterone concentration steadily increases (see Fig. 5.3), both of these receptors are down regulated (Renfree & Blanden, unpublished manuscript). However, the profiles of secreted proteins differ quantitatively and qualitatively in response to treatment with these two steroids. The fact is that both hormones can trigger reactivation, but only progesterone can maintain development (4,23) suggests that each steroid may act differently to trigger secretory changes that induce mitosis and expansion, but a factor, or factors, needed later (from around day 5) to maintain the expanding embryo is induced only by progesterone, not oestradiol.

Cytokines and Growth Factors in the Uterus

There is virtually no data available for marsupials on cytokines and growth factors in the reproductive tract. One cytokine well studied in the mouse, platelet activating factor (PAF; 1-O-alkyl-2 acetyl-sn-glycero-3-phosphocholine), is produced by both uterine tissue and embryos, and may be important for implantation and maternal recognition of pregnancy (reviewed in (42)). PAF stimulates inflammatory-type responses in the uteri of eutherian mammals studied, thus altering the composition of the uterine secretions around the time of reactivation. PAF also stimulates mitosis in preimplantation mouse embryos (43).

The tammar endometrium in vitro has been assayed for the presence of PAF through gestation (44). During diapause female tammars produced low amounts of PAF, but production increased in half the animals on or after day 3 (44), just before metabolic reactivation of the blastocyst and the resumption of mitoses (see below). The increase in progesterone which occurs from day 3 to day 7 may induce the PAF. Thus again, the key time period for reactivation is after day 3 and before day 7.

In many eutherian mammals, embryonic diapause is maintained by the presence of inhibitory factors in the uterus (45). In mice, reactivation from diapause is associated with increased metabolic activity, a change in the ATP:ADP ratio and trophoblast outgrowth (reviewed in 45). Trophoblast outgrowth requires certain amino acids, serum factors or glucose, or reduced levels of certain ions, so that the uterus could control embryonic growth by regulating these components of uterine secretions. However, while trophoblast outgrowth is prevented, embryo metabolism is not reduced, suggesting that these two indices of blastocyst activation may be independently controlled by uterine factors (45,46).

One approach to quantifying the uterine changes that lead to reactivation is to use a bioassay system. O'Neill and Quinn (47) showed that mouse uterine fluids contain a factor that inhibits RNA synthesis by mouse blastocysts in vitro, which disappeared transiently from the uterine fluids of pregnant mice 6.5 h after injection of oestrogen, a treatment that terminates diapause. Thornber et al. (48) incubated mouse blastocysts in medium supplemented with a fixed concentration of protein from tammar uterine exudates collected from either quiescent (diapause) and day 10 reactivated uteri. Uptake and incorporation of uridine by these mouse blastocysts were significantly reduced compared to control blastocysts incubated with BSA, suggesting that an inhibitor could be present. However uridine uptake and incorporation were significantly higher in the presence of day 10 secretions than with secretions from quiescent tammar uteri, suggesting either a reduced level of inhibitor, or the presence of an additional stimulator.

We have recently extended these results using mouse blastocysts to assay growth and metabolism-regulating components of uterine secretions using higher concentration of exudates (2mg/ml) than in the earlier study (49). There is a stimulatory effect of d5 wallaby exudates on mouse blastocysts. Quiescent mouse blastocysts in d0 (quiescent) wallaby exudates did not achieve the same reduction in the ATP:ADP ratio as nondelayed mouse blastocysts, again suggesting there may be some inhibitory substance in tammar endometrial secretions. However, the result may be due equally to a species-specific response. Furthermore, diapause could not be induced in normally developing mouse blastocysts by quiescent tammar exuates, which argues against an inhibitor. Although it is still impossible to exclude the influence of an inhibitor (as distinct from the need for a stimulator) in the tammar, it remains unlikely because diapause can be maintained for up to two years in the *absence* of the corpus luteum whose secretions are necessary for reactivation (12,50). Nevertheless, it is clear that there are stimulatory factors in both d5 and d10 wallaby exudates. Further studies are needed to identify these substances.

Blastocyst Reactivation after Diapause

It takes at least 72 h after the cessation of sucking by the pouch young to irreversibly terminate diapause (50) (Fig. 5.4). Mitoses are first observed 4 days after reactivation induced by removal of the pouch young (Spindler et al., unpublished manuscript). By day 4 after RPY there is a substantial increase in oxidative metabolism of the blastocyst that provides a four-fold increase in ATP production (52). By day 5, RNA synthesis has increased (53,54). These changes are dependent on progesterone-induced changes in the composition and quantity of uterine secretions (36). Oestradiol can also initiate reactivation, but only progesterone can sustain it (23). It appears, therefore, that there is a sequence of changes that regulate different stages of reactivation and expansion. The nature of these uterine regulatory factors is still not known, although in early studies using gel-electrophoresis changes in uterine proteins, particularly in the prealbumin regions of the gel were seen (36,38).

Our recent studies have examined the metabolic changes that accompany reactivation in greater detail using noninvasive fluorimetric assays. Blastocysts were able to use both glucose and pyruvate as sources of energy at all stages (Spindler et al., unpublished manuscript). The first significant increase in glucose or pyruvate utilization was not seen until day 8 after RPY, at the start of embryo expansion (Fig. 5.3). By day 10 there is a more than ten-fold increase. While there was no significant increase in substrate uptake between days 3 and 5, there was a relative decline in lactate production suggesting a change to more complete oxidation with a corresponding increase in energy produced per mole of substrate. Spindler et al. (unpublished manuscript) assessed this by determining the metabolic products of embryos incubated with 6-[^{14}C]-glucose and 5-[^{3}H]-glucose to determine rates of conversion to $^{14}CO_2$ and $^{3}H_2O$. These experiments show that less than 5% glucose was oxidized to CO_2 during quiescence, but by day 4 after RPY almost 60% was oxidized fully (Spindler et al., 52, unpublished manuscript). This substantial increase in the full oxidation of glucose corresponds to a more than four-fold increase in energy production. Thus, a switch to more efficient carbohydrate metabolism occurs at the time of embryo reactivation.

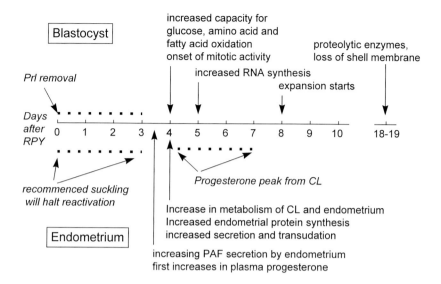

FIGURE 5.4. Diagrammatic representation of the timing of various maternal and embryo responses initiated by removal of the pouch young at day 0. The sucking stimulus must be withdrawn for 72 h to allow reactivation, and it appears that the ovaries must be present for all of this time. If they are removed at day 2, and probably day 3, reactivation is prevented, but at day 4 and day 6 reactivation occurs but pregnancy fails. The progesterone (and oestradiol) pulse occurs at days 5–6, after endometrial metabolism (day 4) and blastocyst metabolism (day 5) have already increased. The ovaries are necessary for a successful pregnancy only to day 8, as after removal between days 6 and 8 pregnancy can go to term in the absence of the ovary or the pituitary. Endometrial weight has significantly increased by day 6, and blastocyst diameter by day 8. Thus, the limit (earliest day 6; latest day 8) of the maternal influence on early pregnancy (stippling) is very brief, and the ovary and pituitary only become necessary again for the closing stages of pregnancy and parturition. See text for full references. Redrawn with additional data from Shaw (39).

Carbohydrates are not the only potential energy source for early embryos. Ruminant embryos may utilize fatty acids and amino acids (55), which are present in high levels in the maternal blood as a result of the ruminant digestion. Tammars are also fore-gut fermenters, their blastocysts may also depend on fatty acids and amino acids for energy. We tested this by assessing utilization of palmititate and glutamate. Tammar blastocysts metabolized both of these substrates. Glutamate uptake and ammonia production increased by day 4 RPY, as did oxidation of palmitate. These increases coincided with the onset of mitotic activity in the blastocysts (Spindler et al., unpublished manuscript).

The vesicle expands, as does the shell, for up to approximately 18 days after RPY, which is the end of the somite stage and the beginning of the head fold stage of development (4). During this time, additional secretion and shell protein deposition must occur as the shell increases its volume from about $0.001mm^3$ during diapause to $>0.250mm^3$ at day 18 (39). The disintegration of the shell membrane about day 18 RPY is therefore not the result of mere attenuation, but apparently is actively brought about by proteolytic activity (56). Low levels of an acidic protease, thought to be involved with protein transport from the endometrium into the yolk sac, was present in uterine slices throughout pregnancy. However, about day 18, an alkaline protease became detectable by gelatinase assays in the uterine lumen about day 18, but not before (56). Similar proteolytic activity was seen in both embryonic and uterine cells so it was unclear if the fetal or maternal tissues, or both secreted the protease, but as it coincides exactly with the shell breakdown it appears to play an important role in the process of attachment of the trophoblast to the uterine epithileum (56).

Conclusions and Future Directions

It is clear from work on eutherian mammals that there are many growth factors in the uterine secretions which may potentially regulate embryonic metabolism and development through paracrine and autocrine interactions (57,58). The clear separation of embryonic reactivation and implantation in the tammar provides an interesting contrast to the most studied species, the mouse. More work is in progress to characterize the uterine secretory factors that regulate metabolic reactivation of the embryo. Further studies are needed to define the action of PAF and the concentrations of key growth factors. Recent studies in several eutherian species implicate leucocyte-inhibiting factor (LIF), epidermal growth factor (EGF), transforming growth factor-β (TGFβ), colony stimulating factor 1 (CSF1), and insulin like growth factors I and II (IGF-I and IGF-II) in early development and implantation (59). By addition of purified growth factors to cultured embryos and gene knockout studies, both LIF and EGF have been shown to be essential for normal development of mouse embryos in the periimplantation period. In mice LIF is produced in the endometrial glands specifically on day 4 of pregnancy, and is essential for implantation in mice (60). Analysis of expression in pseudopregnant and delayed implanting mice indicates that LIF expression is maternally controlled, and its expression coincides with blastocyst formation and always precedes implantation (61). EGF is a potent mitogen, and EGF receptors are present on early mammalian embryos (reviewed in (59)). EGF also has important effects on the endometrium where it may mediate the effects of oestradiol on uterine growth and differentiation (62). Both these factors could affect the embryo directly, but they also act on the uterus to alter protease activity (59,63), which may be essential to allow implantation and continued development. Contrasting the timing of expression of these factors between mice and wallabies may help define the physiological role underlying the control of embryonic diapause, metabolic activation, mitosis, blastocyst expansion, and finally, implantation.

References

1. Renfree MB, Calaby JH. Background to delayed implantation and embryonic diapause. J Reprod Fertil 1981;29 (Suppl):1–9.
2. Renfree MB. Embryonic diapause in marsupials. J Reprod Fertil 1981;29(Suppl): 67–8.
3. Rudd CD. Sexual behaviour of male and female tammar wallabies (*Macropus eugenii*) at post-partum oestrus. J Zool (Lond) 1994;232:151–62.
4. Renfree MB, Tyndale-Biscoe CH. Intrauterine development after diapause in the marsupial *Macropus eugenii*. Devel Biol 1973;22:29–40.
5. Tyndale-Biscoe CH. Hormonal control of embryonic diapause and reactivation in the tammar wallaby. In: Maternal recognition of pregnancy, Ciba Found Symp 64 (new series). Amsterdam: Excerpta Medica, 1979;173–90.
6. Tyndale-Biscoe CH, Renfree MB. Reproductive physiology of marsupials. Cambridge: Cambridge University Press, 1987:476.
7. Renfree MB. Endocrinology of pregnancy, parturition and lactation of marsupials. In: Lamming GE, ed. Marshall's physiology of reproduction. London: Chapman and Hall, 1994;677–766.
8. Hearn JP. Pituitary inhibition of pregnancy. Nature 1973;241:207–8.
9. Hinds LA. Pregnancy deferred: an unusual role for prolactin in a marsupial. In: Yoshinaga K, ed. Blastocyst implantation. Boston: Serono Symposia USA, Adams Publishing Group, 1989:201–7.
10. Hinds LA. Morning pulse of prolactin maintains seasonal quiescence in the tammar, *Macropus eugenii*. J Reprod Fertil 1989;87:735–44.
11. Tyndale-Biscoe CH, Hawkins J. The corpora lutea of marsupials, aspects of function and control, In: Calaby JH, Tyndale-Biscoe CH, eds. Reproduction and evolution, Australian Academy of Sciences, 1977:245–52.
12. Tyndale-Biscoe CH, Hearn JP. Pituitary and ovarian factors associated with seasonal quiescence in the tammar wallaby *Macropus eugenii*. J Reprod Fertil 1981;63:225–30.
13. Hinds LA, Tyndale-Biscoe H. Plasma progesterone levels in the pregnant and nonpregnant tammar, *Macropus eugenii*. J Endocrinol 1982;93:99–107.
14. Renfree MB, Green SW, Young IR. Growth of the corpus luteum and its progesterone content during pregnancy in the tammar wallaby, *Macropus eugenii*. J Reprod Fertil 1979;57:131–6.
15. Hinds LA, Tyndale-Biscoe H. Prolactin in the marsupial, *Macropus eugenii* during the estrous cycle, pregnancy and lactation. Biol Reprod 1982;26:391–8.
16. Sharman GB. Delayed implantation in marsupials. In: Enders AC, ed. Delayed implantation. Chicago: University of Chicago Press, 1963:3–14.
17. Tyndale-Biscoe CH, Hinds LA. Seasonal patterns of circulating progesterone and prolactin and response to bromocriptine in the female tammar, *Macropus eugenii*. Gen Endocrinol 1984;53:58–68.
18. Renfree MB, Lincoln DW, Almeida OFX, Short RV. Abolition of seasonal embryonic diapause in the tammar wallaby by sympathetic denervation of the pineal gland. Nature (Lond) 1981;293:138–9.
19. Renfree MB, Short RV. Seasonal reproduction in marsupials. In: Labrie F, Proulx L, eds. Proceedings of the 7th International Congress of Endocrinology; Excerpta Medica International Congress Series. Amsterdam: Elsevier, 1984:789–92.
20. McConnell SJ, Hinds LA. Effect of pinealectomy on plasma melatonin, prolactin and progesterone concentrations during seasonal reproductive quiescence in the tammar. *Macropus eugenii*. J Reprod Fertil 1985;7:433–40.

21. McConnell SJ, Tyndale-Biscoe CH. Response to photoperiod in peripheral plasma melatonin and the effects of exogenous melatonin on seasonal quiescence in the tammar *Macropus eugenii.* J Reprod Fertil 1985;73:529–38.

22. Fletcher TP, Renfree MB. Effects of corpus luteum removal on progesterone, oestradiol-17β and LH in early pregnancy of the tammar wallaby *Macropus eugenii.* J Reprod Fertil 1988;83:185–91.

23. Fletcher TP, Jetton AE, Renfree MB. Influence of progesterone and oestradiol-17β on blastocysts of the tammar during seasonal diapause. J Reprod Fertil 1988;83:193–200.

24. Tyndale-Biscoe CH. Resumption of development by quiescent blastocysts transferred to primed, ovariectomised recipients, in the marsupial *Macropus eugenii.* J Reprod Fertil 1970;23:25–32.

25. Renfree MB, Heap RB. Steroid metabolism in the placenta, corpus luteum, and endometrium of the marsupial *Macropus eugenii.* Theriogenology 1977;8:164.

26. Heap RB, Renfree MB, Burton RD. Steroid metabolism in the yolk sac placenta and endometrium of the tammar wallaby, *Macropus eugenii.* J Endocrinol 1980;87:339–49.

27. Shaw G, Renfree MB, Fletcher TP. A role for glucocorticoids in parturition in a marsupial, *Macropus eugenii.* Biol Reprod 1995;54:728–33.

28. Renfree MB. Shaw G, Harry JL, Whitworth DJ. Sexual determination and differentiation in the marsupial *Macropus eugenii.* In: Saunders NA, Hinds LA, eds. Recent advances in marsupial biology. University of New South Wales Press, 1997:132–41.

29. Parry LJ, Rust W, Ivell R. Marsupial relaxin: complementary deoxyribonucleic acid sequence and gene expression in the female and male tammar wallaby, *Macropus eugenii.* Biol Reprod 1997;57:119–27.

30. Renfree MB, Lewis A. McD. Cleavage *in vivo* and *in vitro* in the marsupial *Macropus eugenii.* Reprod Fertil 1996;8:725–42.

31. Hughes RL. Morphological studies on implantation in marsupials. J Reprod Fertil 1974;39:173–86.

32. Tyndale-Biscoe CH, Hinds LA. The hormonal milieu during early development in marsupials, In: Yoshinaga K, ed. Development of preimplantation embryos and their environment. New York: Liss, 1989:237–46.

33. Roberts CT, Breed WG, Mayrhofer G. Origin of the oocyte shell membrane of a dasyurid marsupial: an immunohistochemical study. J Exp Zool 1994;270:321–31.

34. Roberts CT, Breed WG. The Marsupial shell membrane: an ultrastructural and immunogold localization study. Cell Tissue Res 1996;284:99–110.

35. Shaw G. Pregnancy after diapause in the tammar wallaby, *Macropus eugenii.* PhD thesis, Murdoch University, Western Australia, 1983.

36. Renfree MB. Proteins in the uterine secretion of the marsupial *Macropus eugenii.* Devel Biol 1973;32:41–9.

37. Renfree MB. Influence of the embryo on the marsupial uterus. Nature 1972;240:475–7.

38. Shaw G, Renfree MB. Uterine and embryonic metabolism after embryonic diapause in the tammar wallaby (*Macropus eugenii*). J Reprod Fertil 1986; 76:339–47.

39. Shaw G. The uterine environment in early pregnancy in the tammar wallaby. Reprod Fertil Devel 1996;8:811–8.

40. Young CE, McDonald IR. Oestrogen receptors in the genital tract of the Australian marsupial *Trichosurus vulpecula.* Gen Comp Endocrinol 1982;46:417–27.

41. Curlewis J, Stone GM. Effects of oestradiol, the oestrous cycle and pregnancy on weight, metabolism and cytosol receptors in the uterus of the brush-tail possum *(Trichosurus vulpecula)*. J Endocrinol 1986;108:201–10.

42. O'Neill C. A consideration of the factors which influence the viability and developmental potential of the preimplantation embryo. Bailliere's Clin Obstet Gynecol 1991;5: 159–78.

43. Roberts CC, Wright L. Platelet activating factor (PAF) enhances mitosis in preimplantation mouse embryos. Reprod Fertil Devel 1993;5:271–9.

44. Kojima T, Hinds LA, Muller WJ, O'Neill. C, Tyndale-Biscoe CH. Production and secretion of progesterone *in vitro* and presence of platelet activating factor (PAF) in early pregnancy of the marsupial, *Macropus eugenii*. Reprod Fertil Devel 1993;5: 15–25.

45. Weitlauf HM. (1994) Biology of implantation. In: Knobil E, O'Neill JD, eds. The physiology of reproduction, 2nd ed. New York: Raven, 1994:391–440.

46. Surani MAH, Fishel SB. Embryonic and uterine factors in delayed implantation in rodents. J Reprod Fertil 1981;29(Suppl):159–72.

47. O'Neill C, Quinn P. Inhibitory influence of uterine flushings on mouse blastocysts decreases at the time of blastocyst activation. J Reprod Fertil 1983;68:269–74.

48. Thornber EJ, Renfree MB, Wallace GI. Biochemical studies of intrauterine components of tammar wallaby *Macropus eugenii* during pregnancy. J Embryol Exp Morphol 1981;62:325–38.

49. Spindler RE, Renfree MB, Gardner DK. Mouse embryos used as a bioassay to determine the control of marsupial embryonic diapause. Biol Reprod 1997;56(Suppl):1:379.

50. Sharman GB, Berger PJ. Embryonic diapause in marsupials. Adv Reprod Physiol 1969;4:211–40.

51. Gordon K, Fletcher TP, Renfree MB. Reactivation of the quiescent corpus luteum and diapausing embryo after temporary removal of the sucking stimulus in the tammar wallaby *(Macropus eugenii)*. J Reprod Fertil 1988;83:401–6.

52. Spindler RE, Renfree MB, Gardner DK. Metabolic assessment of wallaby blastocysts during embryonic diapause and subsequent reactivation. Reprod Fertil Dev 1995;7:1157–62.

53. Moore GPM. Embryonic diapause in the marsupial *Macropus eugenii*. Stimulation of nuclear RNA polymerase activity during resumption of development. J Cell Physiol 1978;94:31–6.

54. Pike IL. Comparative studies of embryo metabolism in early pregnancy. J Reprod Fertil 1981;29(Suppl.):203–13.

55. Gardner DK, Lane M, Batt P. Uptake and metabolism of pyruvate and glucose by individual sheep preattachment embryos developed in vivo. Mol Reprod Devel 1993;36:313–9.

56. Denker HW, Tyndale-Biscoe CH. Embryo implantation and proteinase activities in a marsupial *(Macropus eugenii)*. Cell Tissue Res 1986;246:279–91.

57. Brigstock DR, Heap RB, Brown KD. Polypeptide growth factors in uterine tissues and secretions. J Reprod Fertil 1989;85:747–58.

58. Schultz GA, Heyner S. Growth factors in preimplantation mammalian embryos. Oxf Rev Reprod Biol 1993;15:43–81.

59. Harvey MB, Leco KJ, Arcellana-Panlilio MY, Zhang X, Edwards DR, Schultz GA. Roles of growth factors during peri-implantation development. Hum Reprod 1995;10:712-8.

60. Stewart CL, Kaspar P, Burnet L. Blastocyst implantation depends on natural expression of leukemia inhibitory factor. Nature 1992;359:76.

61. Bhatt H, Burnet L, Stewart C. Uterine expression of leukemia inhibitory factor coincides with the onset of blastocyst implantation. Proc Natl Acad Sci USA 1991;164:956–9.

62. Nelson KG, Takahasi T, Bossert NL. Epidermal growth factor replaces estrogen in the stimulation of female genital tract growth and differentiation. Proc Natl Acad Sci USA 1991;622:383.

63. Harvey MB, Leco KJ, Arcellana-Panlilio MY, Zhang X, Edwards DR, Schultz GA. Proteinase expression in early mouse embryos is regulated by leukaemia inhibitory factor and epidermal growth factor. Development 1995;121:1005–14.

64. Cake MH, Owen FJ, Bradshaw SD. Differences in concentration of progesterone in the plasma between pregnant and non-pregnant quokkas *(Setonix brachyurus)*. J Endocrinol 1980;84:153–8.

6

Cellular Interactions and the Cysteine Proteinases in the Process of Mouse Implantation

Bruce Babiarz, Suzanne Afonso, and Linda Romagnano

In the mouse, implantation and placentation require the invasion of the uterine stroma by trophoblast giant cells. Concurrent with this invasion, the uterine stroma undergoes the process of decidualization. Through changes in cell morphology and matrix remodeling, this tissue forms a barrier to invasion and much of the maternal vasculature associated with the placenta. Both uterine remodeling and trophoblast invasion are proteinase dependent events, requiring the synthesis and secretion of a number of different enzymes. The work summarized here focuses on the expression, localization, function, and possible control of the cysteine proteinases, cathepsins B and L, during mouse implantation and placentation.

Mouse Implantation and Placentation

When the mouse embryo enters the uterus it has developed to the blastocyst stage, consisting of an outer layer of trophectoderm surrounding an inner cell mass and fluid filled blastocoel cavity. Implantation is initiated when the blastocyst hatches from the zona pellucida and attaches to the uterine epithelium. After attachment on day 4.5 of development, the mural trophectoderm initiates uterine invasion by differentiating to primary trophoblast giant cells. These cells invade antimesometrially into the decidualizing stroma, phagocytosing cells and matrix. This creates space for the growing embryo and produces the initial contact between the trophoblast and maternal circulatory system (1). By day 7.5 of development, the implantation site is firmly established, with a surrounding shell of primary trophoblast giant cells in intimate contact with the decidua. During this time the polar trophectoderm has proliferated to form a cap-like structure, the ectoplacental cone (EPC), over the mesometrial (MZ) end of the embryo. These cells begin differentiation to invasive secondary trophoblast giant cells and, along with primary giant cells, invade into the uterine wall for the next three days of development. The primary trophoblast continue to invade the antimesometrial (AMZ) side of the uterus, while the secondary cells invade mesometrially as the leading edge of the placenta. During this second phase of invasion, apoptotic regression of the AMZ decidua begins (2) and, combined with continued trophoblast digestion and phagocytosis, allows for rapid expansion of the implantation chamber. By day 11.5 of development, the invasive period ends and by day 12 the placenta is fully developed and functional.

Proteolytic Involvement

The invasive and remodeling events of implantation and placentation have been shown to be dependent upon the synthesis and secretion of a number of different proteinases. One of the predominant proteinases expressed by trophectodermal derivatives of the implanting mouse embryo is matrix metalloproteinase-9 (MMP-9). MMP-9 is highly expressed and activated by primary trophoblast from mouse blastocysts in culture (3). The inclusion of MMP inhibitors in vitro prevents blastocyst lysis of the extracellular matrix (3,4). On day 7, MMP-9 is localized to primary and secondary trophoblast giant cells at the periphery of the egg cylinder staged embryo (2,5). By day 9.5, expression declines with only a few MMP-9 positive cells remaining within the secondary trophoblast at the leading edge of the placenta (5). Within the decidualizing stroma, a number of additional MMPs are expressed. These include stromelysin-1 and 3 and MMP-2, which all localize to the lateral differentiating stroma (2). Administration of MMP inhibitors to pregnant females in vivo retards decidual remodeling and growth suggesting an important role in stromal differentiation (2). MMP control is thought to be provided by the synthesis of tissue inhibitors of metalloproteinases (TIMPs). TIMP-1 and TIMP-2 are expressed in undifferentiated stroma, and TIMP-3 is detected from days 6 to 7 in the maternal decidua immediately adjacent to embryonic cells expressing MMP-9 (2,4). TIMP-3 declines as the decidual cells undergo apoptosis during the main period of MMP-9 expression and ectoplacental expansion (2).

A second class of proteinases, the plasminogen activators, has also been implicated in extracellular matrix degradation during tissue invasion and remodeling in mouse and rat implantation. Most activity present in preimplantation embryos appears to be urokinase-type plasminogen activator (uPA) (6). High levels of uPA mRNA are found in invasive trophoblast giant cells and zymography demonstrated the presence of active uPA in the ectoplacental cone region at days 7.5 and 8.5 (4,7). In the uterus, low levels of uPA are observed in the endometrium during the first 4 days of pregnancy. Levels increase until day 7 and uPA is localized to the decidua adjacent to the implanting embryo (8). With subsequent development and decidual regression, uPA expression declines. Control of uPA activity appears to be provided by the decidual synthesis of plasminogen activator inhibitor (PAI) (7,8). PAI, like the TIMPs, is not synthesized by the invasive trophoblast cells (7).

Until recently (9), a third family of proteinases, the cysteine proteinases, had received little attention for their role in implantation and placentation. These enzymes include cathepsin B (CB) and cathepsin L (CL), which have an acidic pH optimum and are normally localized to the lysosomal apparatus of phagocytic cells (10). CB has multiple transcripts ranging from 1.2kb to 5kb, with a 2.2 kb transcript representing the lysosomal form of the enzyme (11). CB is synthesized as a 42 kDa proenzyme that is proteolytically processed to an enzymatically active molecule in the 29 to 34 kDa range in a number of tissues and cell lines (11). The CL transcript is approximately 1.7kb and produces proteins of 43, 39, 29, and 20 kDa (12). The 39kDa protein is the secreted pro-CL form and is the precursor of the two lysosomal species whose molecular weights are 29 and 20 kDa (13). Elevated levels and secretion of CB and CL have been observed in a number of normal invasive processes. The secretion of CB and CL, and the upregulation within lysosomes, has been noted in osteoclasts during bone resorption (14) and endothelial cells during the early steps of angiogenesis (15). Additionally, increased levels of CB and CL are associated with tumor progression and aggressiveness in many types of cancers (16). In particular, the metastatic capability is often correlated with increased CB activity associated with the plasma membrane and secretion of precursor forms (17). CL is the major induced protein of *ras* transformed cells and the major excreted protein (MEP) of virally transformed cells (18). CL accumulates in the media as acid activated pro-CL (19). Inhibitors of CL suppress cancer cell invasion of amniotic membranes (20). The association of these enzymes with normal and metastatic cells involved in invasion and tissue remodeling make them attractive candidates as important molecules in implantation. We first became interested in this possibility after observing that cathepsin inhibitors prevented the invasion of EPC trophoblast into decidual monolayers in vitro (21).

Cathepsin Expression

Initial experiments analyzed CB and CL mRNA and protein expression in microdissected primary trophoblast and rudiments of the EPC/developing placenta from days 7 to 11. Northern blot analysis showed that message levels remained consistent for CB (9). CL message levels decreased after day 8, but increased again at the end of the invasive period (data not shown). Western blotting showed that CB protein was upregulated by primary trophoblast giant cells from days 7 to 11, and during placental formation and secondary giant cell differentiation (Fig. 6.1A and B). The low molecular weight (lysosomal) form of CL remained consistent in primary trophoblast, with a slight

Cathepsin protein expression

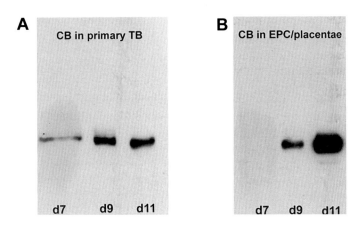

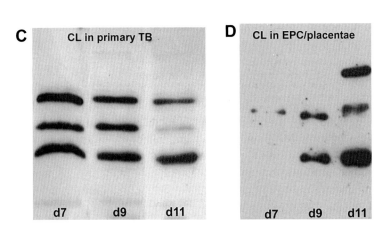

FIGURE 6.1. Western blot analysis of CB and CL synthesis in trophoblast cell lysates. (A) CB protein (31 kDa) is detected in primary giant cells and increases during invasion from days 7–11. (B) CB protein is barely detectable in day 7 EPCs, but increases dramatically with placental formation and secondary giant cell invasion from days 9–11. (C) CL antiserum detects three proteins in primary trophoblast (34, 26, 22 kDa). The low molecular weight lysosomal form remains consistent through days 7–11, with the high molecular weight form showing a slight decrease. (D) Within the developing EPC, CL is barely detectable at day 7, with increases in both lysosomal and proforms as invasion continues on days 9–11.

decrease observed in the high molecular weight pro- or secreted form (Fig. 6.1C). Within the developing EPC, CL is barely detectable on day 7, but increased throughout the period of secondary giant cell invasion and placental development (Fig. 6.1D). To localize both message and protein, in situ hybridization and immunohistochemistry were used. At day 7.5, both message (Fig. 6.2A,B) and protein for CB (Fig. 6.2C) and CL were localized to the trophoblast giant cells. While these cells labeled heavily, the core cells of the EPC, representing the noninvasive, proliferating trophoblast, remained negative. Within the decidua, both enzymes were expressed in the lateral decidualizing zone, with CL showing additional expression in the lateral sinuses and MZ decidua (Fig. 6.2A–C). By day 9.5 of development, primary and secondary giant cells remained positive for CB and CL message (Fig. 6.2D,F) and protein (Fig. 6.2E,G), with expression also seen within the developing spongiotrophoblast of the placenta. The labyrinthine trophoblast remained unlabeled. A distinct upregulation of CB message and protein were associated with the regressing AMZ (Fig. 6.2D,E). From days 7.5 to 9.5, both enzymes are present in the developing visceral endoderm/yolk sac (Fig. 6.2A–G).

Cathepsin Activity

These localization studies suggested that both mRNA and protein for CB and CL are upregulated by the invasive primary and secondary giant cells from days 7 to 9 of gestation. To determine if cathepsin activity could be detected in these tissues, substrate gel electrophoresis (zymography) was performed. Lysates of day 7.5 EPCs and primary trophoblast from days 7.5, 9.5, and 11.5 all possessed bands of 34kDa gelatinase activity at pH 5.2 (Fig. 6.3A, lanes 1–4). Increased levels of the 34 kDa zymogen were apparent in primary trophoblast tissue from days 7.5 and 9.5 compared to the undifferentiated day 7.5 EPC core. Primary trophoblast from day 11.5 showed a change in zymogen activity with most activity associated with a 62 kDa zymogen (Fig. 6.3A, lane 4). This suggested that at this stage of development, acidic proteinases were in an unprocessed (precursor) or aggregate form. Class specific proteinase inhibitors were used to identify the gelatinases showing activity at pH 5.2 (Fig. 6.3B). No inhibitory effect on activity was observed with an aspartic proteinase (pepstatin A), serine proteinase (PMSF), or metalloproteinase (EDTA) inhibitor. E-64, a specific inhibitor of CB and CL, completely inactivated proteinase activity as did the cysteine proteinase inhibitor, leupeptin (Fig. 6.3B, lanes 3,4). This indicated that the observed zymogens were members of the cysteine proteinase family. EPCs cultured for 48 h showed a zymogen intensity comparable to primary giant cells suggesting that secondary giant cell formation is also associated with an increased synthesis of enzyme (Fig. 6.3C, lane 1). In EPC conditioned media, secreted

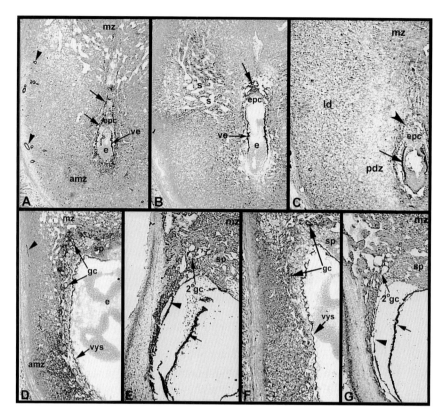

FIGURE 6.2. Localization of CB and CL message and protein within implantation site on days 7.5 (A–C) and 9.5 (D–G). (A,B) In situ hybridization of CB (A) and CL (B) on day 7.5. Message for both is localized to primary and secondary giant cells (*arrows*), but lacking in the core of the EPC. Within the embryo, expression is restricted to the visceral endoderm (ve). CB decidual message expression remains low with high signal in the uterine glands (arrowheads). CL message shows a specific localization to the developing lateral sinuses (s). (C) A similar localization of CB (C) and CL (not shown) protein was observed by immunohistochemistry. Both primary and secondary giant cells (*arrowhead*), and visceral endoderm (*arrow*) stain positive. Within the decidua, the primary decidual zone (pdz) showed no expression, while the lateral decidual (ld) zone stains for CB and CL. (D and F) In situ hybridization for CB (D) and CL (F) at day 9.5 shows continued expression in giant cells (gc) and visceral yolk sac (vys), and in the developing spongiotrophoblast (sp). Upregulation of CB is associated with the regression of the AMZ decidua. (E,G) Immunohistochemistry showed a similar localization of CB (E) and CL (G) protein, with the AMZ showing a distinct upregulation of CB. All photos at ×6.

forms of proteinases with molecular masses 31 and 32 kDa were observed (Fig. 6.3C, lane 2) suggesting that further processing occurred. Western blotting will be used to further identify these secreted cathepsins. Our preliminary studies, using CL antiserum, has detected bands at 35 and 36 kDa in EPC conditioned media (Fig. 6.3C, lane 3).

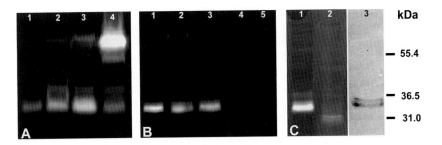

FIGURE 6.3. Substrate gel electrophoresis of trophoblast tissues. (A) Gelatin zymogram of acidic proteinase activity from day 7.5 EPCs (lane 1) and primary trophoblast from days 7.5, 9.5, and 11.5 (lanes 2, 3 and 4, respectively). A major 34 kDa band is observed in EPCs which is upregulated in primary trophoblast giant cells. By day 11.5, high zymogen activity is detected at 62 kDa with decreased activity of the 34 kDa and 37/38 kDa species. (B) Class specific inhibitors pepstatin A (lane 1), PMSF (lane 2), and EDTA (lane 3) do not inhibit proteinase activity of day 9.5 primary trophoblast samples. Complete inactivation of proteinase activity is seen in the presence of cathepsin inhibitors E-64 and leupeptin (lanes 4 and 5, respectively). (C) Zymography of lysates of in vitro differentiating EPCs show the synthesis of the 34 kDa and 37/38 kDa forms of cysteine proteinases (lane 1). Faint bands at 31 and 32 kDa are detected from EPC conditioned media (lane 2). CL antiserum detected bands at 35 and 36 kDa in a Western blot of EPC conditioned media (lane 3).

Cathepsin Perturbation

To determine a functional role for cathepsins, E-64 was injected into pregnant females. Since cysteine proteinase inhibitors have been shown to inhibit blastocyst hatching (22), intraperitoneal injections were made after blastocyst attachment (days 4.5 and 5.5) to determine the effects of cysteine proteinase inhibition on implantation. Females were sacrificed on day 7.5 and a dose dependent effect on development was observed (Table 6.1). At 10mg/kg of E-64, decidualization and embryonic development were unaffected. Significant differences were observed when animals treated with 30 mg/kg of E-64 were compared to the controls (Table 6.1). More than one third of the capsules contained resorbed embryos and 53% were stunted at the egg cylinder stage showing no mesoderm formation. Effects were also observed on stromal decidualization, with abnormalities in the size and shape of the decidual capsule. When measured through the midplane, the treated decidual capsules were significantly shorter in length (77% of the control) and the capsule area was decreased to 69% of the controls. Contributing to the observed size and shape differences was the lack of lateral sinus development in the MZ region of E-64 treated capsules. Light microscopic analysis of treated capsules showed that all expected layers were present, but reduced in size, when compared to controls (9). No evidence of abnormal cell death or invasion of lymphatic cells was observed in nonresorbing capsules. When animals were treated with 50 mg/kg of E-64, total resorption of all implantation sites was observed (Table 6.1).

TABLE 6.1. Analysis of day 7.5 decidual capsules from mice treated with the cysteine proteinase inhibitor, E-64.

| Treatment (# of mice) | # of capsules | Embryonic stage | | | Decidua | | | |
		Prim. streak¶	Stunted EC*	Resorbed	Width (mm)	Length‡ (mm)	Area (mm²)	Shape§ (w/l)
Control (4)	45	45	0	0	2.48 ± 0.11	3.32 ± 0.02	6.46 ± 0.92	0.74 ± 0.01
E64 (10mg/kg) (2)	11	11	0	0	2.46 ± 0.005 ($p > 0.9$)ƒ	3.13 ± 0.01 ($p < 0.02$)ƒ	6.07 ± 0.14	0.78 ± 0.01
E64 (30mg/kg) (4)	38	5	20	13	2.18 ± 0.06 ($p > 0.015$)ƒ	2.57 ± 0.11 ($p << 0.001$)ƒ	4.46 ± 0.98 ($p << 0.001$)ƒ	0.85 ± 0.01 ($p < 0.006$)ƒ
E64 (50mg/kg) (4)	34	—	—	34				

¶Primitive streak stages embryos with mesoderm formation.

*Stunted egg cylinder staged embryos lacking mesoderm.

‡Mean length in millimeters (mm) ± the standard deviation calculated from serial longitudinal sections measured through the center of 6–9 capsules/treatment.

§Shape determined by the ratio of capsule width to length (w/l) measured from longitudinal sections through the center of 6–9 capsules/treatment.

ƒSignificance was determined using the student's t-test where $p < 0.01$.

Possible Roles for Cathepsin Proteinases in Implantation

The observed upregulation of CB and CL during the differentiation of invasive trophoblast giant cells correlated with the period of maximal trophoblast phagocytosis (days 7–11). Zymographic analysis further suggested that, following the invasive period, trophoblast cells alter cathepsin processing with the precursor or aggregate form predominating. In addition, giant cells also secrete cathepsin enzymes, which could have a number of roles during implantation. Both CB and CL are capable of digesting matrix molecules at a neutral pH, including laminin, collagen IV, and fibronectin (23,24). CB and CL also activate other proteinases involved in matrix degradation. CL activates pro-uPA (25) and CB activates the metalloproteinase, stromelysin (26). It has been reported that soluble cysteine proteinase digests liberated 3 proteolytically active fibronectin fragments, suggesting that these enzymes can activate latent proteinase activity from the basement membrane and thus initiate a novel proteolytic cascade (24). In summary, cysteine proteinases may contribute to invasion by the digestion of matrix molecules, the extracellular activation of other proenzymes, and the intracellular breakdown of phagocytosed molecules.

Inhibition of the cathepsins in vivo produced stunted embryos. This could result from decreased phagocytosis and macromolecular breakdown by both the giant cells and the developing visceral yolk sac. In particular, the visceral endoderm, which begins CB and CL expression as early as day 5.5 (9), has an absorptive function beginning as early as day 6.5 of development (27). In vitro perturbation of yolk sacs with E-64 or leupeptin resulted in decreased protein processing and embryo growth retardation (28), suggesting that enzyme activity is required for normal breakdown of proteins during embryogenesis (29).

Perturbation of cathepsin activity also retarded decidualization producing small, abnormally shaped capsules. One of the hallmarks of stromal differentiation is the remodeling of the extracellular matrix, mediated in part by the phagocytosis of collagen type I by stromal cells (30). The expression of CB and CL seen within the lateral decidualizing zone on day 7.5 is most likely critical to this phagocytic process. Disruptions of the matrix remodeling process by inhibiting cysteine proteinase activity could prevent normal expansion and architectural changes of the decidual tissue. This possibility was supported by the observed decrease in thickness of the primary decidual zone and lateral decidualizing zone in treated capsules, and the lack of lateral sinus development. Decidua showed a second burst of CB synthesis associated with the onset of apoptotic regression. Electron microscopy of regressing decidua showed an accumulation of autophagosomes and lysosomes (31) suggesting increased lysosomal CB may play a role in their apoptotic program.

Control of Cathepsins

If CB and CL play numerous roles during implantation and placentation, then one would assume that these enzymes are tightly controlled. Like the MMPs and PAs, cysteine proteinases are controlled by physiological inhibitors. These are members of the cystatin superfamily which include both intracellular (stefins A and B) and secreted (cystatin C) forms. Cystatin C is a low molecular weight protein (14 kDa) that is expressed in several tissues and is present in high concentrations in a number of biological fluids (32). It is known to be an inhibitor of cathepsin B and cathepsin L (33) and is also the principle cathepsin inhibitor regulated in chronic inflammatory diseases (34) and tissue remodeling events (35). Therefore, the expression of cystatin C was analyzed during implantation and placentation.

Northern analysis showed that a 0.7 kb cystatin C transcript was upregulated by a factor of 5 during stromal decidualization, with Western analysis showing a 20-fold increase of protein (9). In situ hybridization showed no upregulation of cystatin C at the site of blastocyst attachment. By day 5.5, with the formation of distinct decidual swellings, cystatin C message localized to the peripheral decidualizing cells of the AMZ and MZ decidua (Fig. 6.4A). At day 7.5, message levels remained high in the lateral zones and were also localized to decidual cells in contact with the primary trophoblast (Fig. 6.4B). No expression was observed in trophoblast giant cells. Cystatin C message was also upregulated in the regressing decidua on days 9 to 11 and appeared for the first time in primary giant cells on day 11 (Fig. 6.4C). Although highest message levels were found in the lateral decidualizing zone on day 7.5, cystatin C protein was localized to the primary decidual zone surrounding the embryo (Fig. 6.4D). Within the MZ region, cystatin C was localized to the decidua surrounding the EPC and in the endothelial cells lining the sinuses (Fig. 6.4E). This localization suggested that cystatin C regulate trophoblast cathepsins and decidual cathepsins, associated with angiogenesis in the MZ region. Cystatin C upregulation is not dependent upon the presence of the embryo, since cystatin C protein showed a similar pattern of expression in oil induced deciduomas (9). The onset of decidual regression was also associated with an upregulation of cystatin C. It is possible that cystatin C contributes to decidual apoptosis by protecting the extracellular matrix from aberrant cysteine proteinase activity and/or preventing untimely cysteine proteinase activation of other pro-enzymes that are involved in tissue destruction. The lack of expression by trophoblast until late in the invasive period suggested that endogenous cystatin C is not upregulated in the invasive program.

The events surrounding implantation and placentation are dependent on the regulation of metalloproteinases, plasminogen activators, and their inhibitors (2,4,7). The work presented here provides strong evidence that the cysteine proteinases CB and CL, and their inhibitor cystatin C, also play an important role in these processes. Future directions will focus on determining the regulation of the proteolytic cascade, including the interactions between multiple families of enzymes and inhibitors, growth factors, and matrix interactions.

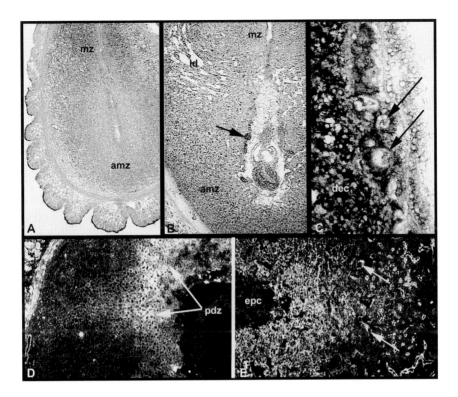

FIGURE 6.4. Localization of cystatin C message and protein within the implantation site. (A) In situ hybridization of day 5.5 decidual capsules localized cystatin C message to lateral decidual zones. ×6 (B) At day 7.5, cystatin C message is expressed throughout the AMZ decidua with the highest expression in cells immediately adjacent to the invading trophoblast (*arrow*). ×6. (C) At day 11.5, heavy expression is associated with the regressing decidua and is observed for the first time in giant cells (*arrows*). ×40 (D) Immunofluorescent localization of cystatin C at day 7.5 shows the protein accumulates within the primary decidual zone (pdz) within the AMZ decidua. ×10. (E) Within the MZ decidua, cystatin C accumulates around the EPC and is expressed by endothelial cells lining the decidual sinuses (*arrows*). ×10.

References

1. Cross J, Werb Z, Fisher S. Implantation and the placenta: key pieces of the development puzzle. Science 1994;266:1508–18.
2. Alexander CM, Hansell EJ, Behrendtsen O, Flannery ML, Kishnani NS, Hawkes SP et al. Expression and function of matrix metalloproteinases and their inhibitors at the maternal-embryonic boundary during mouse embryo implantation. Development 1996;122:1723–36.
3. Behrendtsen O, Alexander C, Werb Z. Metalloproteinases mediate extracellular matrix degradation by cells from mouse blastocyst outgrowths. Development 1992;114:447–56.

4. Harvey MB, Leco KJ, Arcellana-Panlilio MY, Zhang X, Edwards DR, Schultz GA. Proteinase expression in early mouse embryos is regulated by leukaemia inhibitory factor and epidermal growth factor. Development 1995;121:1005–14.

5. Leco KJ, Edwards DR, Schultz GA. Tissue inhibitor of metalloproteinase-3 is the major metalloproteinase inhibitor in the decidualizing murine uterus. Mol Reprod Devel 1996;45:458–65.

6. Zhang X, Kidder GM, Zhang C, Khamsi F, Armstrong DT. Expression of plasminogen activator genes and enzymatic activities in rat preimplantation embryos. J Reprod Fertil 1994;101:235–40.

7. Teesalu T, Blasi F, Talarico D. Embryo implantation in mouse: fetomaternal coordination in the pattern of expression of uPA, uPAR, PAI-1 and alpha 2MR/LRP genes. Mechanisms Devel 1996;56:103–16.

8. Wang S, Kennedy TG, Zhang X. Presence of urokinase plasminogen activator and plasminogen activator inhibitor-1 messenger ribonucleic acids in rat endometrium during decidualization in vivo. Biol Reprod 1966;55:493–7.

9. Afonso S, Romagnano L, Babiarz B. The expression and function of cystatin C and cathepsin B and cathepsin L during mouse embryo implantation and placentation. Development 1997;124:3415–25.

10. Everts V, van der Zee E, Creemers L, Beertsen W. Phagocytosis and intracellular digestion of collagen, its role in turnover and remodeling. Histochem J 1996;28: 229–45.

11. Berquin IM, Sloane BF. Cathepsin B expression in human tumors. Adv Exp Med Biol 1996;389:281–94.

12. Hamilton RT, Bruns KA, Delgado MA, Shim J, Fang Y, Denhardt DT. et al. Developmental expression of cathepsin L and c-ras[Ha] in the mouse placenta. Mol Reprod Devel 1991;30:285–92.

13. Gal S, Willingham M, Gottesmann M. Processing and lysosomal localization of a glycoprotein whose secretion is transformation stimulated. J Cell Biol 1985;100: 535–44.

14. Kakegawa H, Tagami K, Ohba Y, Sumitani K, Kawata T, Katunuma N. Secretion and processing mechanisms of procathepsin L in bone resorption. FEBS Lett 1995;370: 78–82.

15. Sinha AA, Gleason DF, Staley NA, Wilson MJ, Sameni M, Sloane BF. Cathepsin B in angiogenesis of human prostate: an immunohistochemical and immunoelectron microscopic analysis. Anatl Rec 1995;241:353–62.

16. Gottesman MM. Do proteases play a role in cancer? Semi Cancer Biol 1990;1:97–9.

17. Ryan RE, Sloane B, Sameni M, Wood PL. Microglial cathepsin B: an immunological examination of cellular and secreted species. J Neurochem 1995;65:1035–45.

18. Sloane BF, Rozhin J, Hatfield JS, Crissman JD, Honn KV. Plasma membrane-associated cysteine proteinase in human and animal tumors. Exp Cell Biol 1987;55:209–24.

19. Troen BR, Gal S, Gottesman MM. Sequence and expression of the cDNA for MEP, a transformation-regulated secreted cathepsin. Biochem J 1987;246:731–5.

20. Yagel S, Warner AD, Nellens HN, Lala PK, Waghorne C, Denhardt DT. Suppression by cathepsin L inhibitors of the invasion of amniotic membranes by murine cancer cells. Cancer Res 1989;49:3553–7.

21. Babiarz B, Romagnano L, Kurilla G. The interaction of mouse ectoplacental cone trophoblast and uterine decidua in vitro. In Vitro Cell Devel Biol 1992;8A:500–8.

22. Ichikawa S, Shibata T, Takehara Y, Tamada H, Oda K, Murao S. Effects of proteinase inhibitors on preimplantation embryos in the rat. J Reprod Fertil 1985:73:385–90.

23. Lah TT, Buck MR, Honn KV, Crissman JD, Rao NC, Liotta AL et al. Degradation of laminin by human tumor cathepsin B. Clin Exp Metastasis 1989;7:461–9.

24. Guinec N, Dalet-Fumeron V, Pagano M. In vitro study of basement membrane degradation by the cysteine proteinases, cathepsins B, B-like and L. Biol Chem Hoppe-Seyler 1993:374:1135–46.

25. Goretzki L, Schmitt M, Mann K, Calvete J, Chucholowski N, Kramer M, et al. Effective activation of the proenzyme form of the urokinase-type plasminogen activator (pro-uPA) by the cysteine protease cathepsin L. FEBS Lett 1992;297:112–8.

26. Murphy G, Ward R, Gavrilovic J, Atkinson S. Physiological mechanisms for metalloproteinase activation. Matrix 1992;1(Suppl):224–30.

27. Palis G, Kingsley PD. Differential gene expression during murine yolk sac development. Mol Reprod Devel 1995;42:19–27.

28. Daston GP, Baines D, Yonker JE, Lehman-McKeeman L. Effects of lysosomal proteinase inhibition on the development of the rat embryo in vitro. Teratology 1991;43: 253–61.

29. Grubb JD, Koszalk TR, Drabick JJ, Metrione RM. The activities of thiol proteases in the rat visceral yolk sac increase during late gestation. Placenta 1991;12:143–51.

30. Zorn T, Bevilacqua E, Abrahamsohn PA. Collagen remodeling during decidualization in the mouse. Cell Tissue Res 1986;244:443–8.

31. Abrahamsohn PA. Ultrastructural study of the mouse antimesometrial decidua. Anatomy and Embryology 1983;166:263–74.

32. Huh C, Nagle J, Kozak C, Abrahamson M, Karlsson S. Structural organization, expression and chromosomal mapping of mouse cystatin C encoding gene (Cyst 3). Gene 1995;152:221–6.

33. Abrahamson M, Barrett AJ, Salvensen G, Grubb A. Isolation of six cysteine proteinase inhibitors from human urine. J Biol Chem 1986;261:11282–9.

34. Henskens YM, Veerman EC, Mantel MS, Van der Veldem U. Nieuw-Amerongen AV. Cystatins S and C in human whole saliva and in glandular salivas in periodontal health and disease. J Dental Res 1994;73:1606–14.

35. Lerner UH, Grubb A. Human cystatin C, a cysteine proteinase inhibitor, inhibits bone resorption in vitro stimulated by parathyroid hormone and parathyroid hormone-related peptide malignancy. J Bone Miner Res 1992;7:433–40.

Part III

Hormonal Regulation

7

Novel Steroid-Regulated Markers of Implantation

INDRANI C. BAGCHI

The process of implantation involves a series of complex interactions between the embryo and the uterus (1–4). In humans and rodents, implantation occurs 4 to 6 days after fertilization, when the blastocyst reaches the uterus (1–4). The initial adherence of the blastocyst to the uterine epithelium is followed by intimate interaction of the blastocyst trophectoderm with epithelial cells that leads to the progressive phases of implantation. The uterus simultaneously undergoes certain hormone-dependent changes that prepare it to be receptive to invasion by the embryo. The specific modifications leading to acquisition of the receptive state of the uterus are regulated by a timely interplay of the maternal steroid hormones, estrogen and progesterone (1–4). Estrogen initiates hypertrophy and hyperplasia of endometrial epithelia. Progesterone transforms this prepared endometrium into a secretory tissue and creates an environment within the uterine milieu that is conducive to embryo attachment. Although previous research has established that estrogen and progesterone regulate the events leading to implantation, relatively little is known of the molecular mechanisms through which these hormones promote uterine receptivity. Steroid hormones act through their intracellular receptors, which are ligand-inducible gene regulatory factors (5–7). It is therefore likely that steroids trigger the expression of a unique set of genes during the early stages of pregnancy and that these eventually lead to synthesis of new proteins that prepare the uterus to accept the invading blastocyst.

To investigate the molecular basis of the hormonal regulation of implantation, identification of the genes whose expression in the uterus temporally coincides with the steroid hormone surge at the onset of implantation was undertaken. By employing the gene expression screen method of Wang and Brown (8) and the mRNA differential display technique of Liang and Pardee (9), several cDNA clones representing genes that are either up- or down-regulated during the implantation stage of pregnancy were isolated. Table 7.1 shows a list of genes that have been characterized so far. These include calcitonin, ferritin heavy chain (FHC), uterine estrogen-regulated gene (UEG), interferon-α-inducible gene p27,

TABLE 7.1. Genes that are regulated in the uterus during pregnancy.

Clone	Identity	Expression	Steroid regulation	Function
#70	Calcitonin	↑	P, E	Peptide hormone, controls calcium homeostatis
#39	Ferritin heavy chain	↑	P	Iron homeostasis
#77	Kidney androgen regulated protein	↓	E	Glycoprotein, unknown
#4	β-Tropomyosin 1	↑	none	Muscle contraction
#7	RY-1	↑	none	RNA binding protein
#13	Interferon-α-inducible gene (p27)	↑	E	Unkown
#20	UEG	↓	E	Unknown
#28	Angiotensin-binding protein	↑	?	Metalloendopeptidase

and kidney androgen-regulated protein (KAP). As shown in Table 7.1, some of these genes are regulated by estrogen and/or progesterone, while others are not under steroid regulation. This chapter describes the spatiotemporal expression and possible functional roles of three of the steroid-regulated genes, FHC, UEG, and calcitonin, during early pregnancy.

Ferritin Heavy Chain (FHC) Is Regulated by Progesterone in the Uterus

The gene encoding ferritin heavy chain (FHC), a component of the multisubunit iron-binding protein ferritin, is induced in response to progesterone in the uterus. As shown in Figure 7.1, the uterine expression of the FHC mRNAs rises dramatically at the onset of pregnancy, coincident with the surge of progesterone. The FHC expression continues at this elevated level after implantation and throughout gestation when the progesterone concentration remains high (10). At term, FHC expression declines sharply as the progesterone concentration drops. By immunocytochemistry FHC proteins are localized exclusively in the uterine stromal cells, a major site of action of progesterone during pregnancy (10). Administration of mifepristone, an antiprogestin, during early stages of pregnancy abolishes both FHC mRNA and protein expression, clearly suggesting a primary role of progesterone in the regulation of this gene. Consistent with this scenario, administration of progesterone to ovariectomized animals after a brief estrogen priming leads to a marked (25-fold) induction of FHC mRNA in the uterus, whereas estrogen alone or dexamethazone or dihydrotestosterone have no effect. Based on

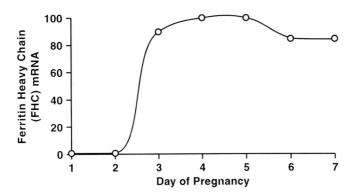

FIGURE 7.1. Profile of expression of FHC mRNA in rat uterus at different stages of early pregnancy. Poly (A)⁺ RNA isolated from uteri of animals at 1, 2, 3, 4, 5, and 7 days of gestation, respectively, were analyzed by Northern blotting. Hybridization was performed with ³²P-labeled FHC cDNA probes. The intensities of the FHC mRNA signals were quantified by densitometric scanning and normalized with respect to the GAPDH signals in the same blot. The relative intensities representing FHC mRNA levels at different days of gestation were plotted. Appearance of a vaginal plug after mating was considered day 1 of pregnancy.

these results, we propose that FHC is a novel and useful marker to study progesterone-regulated events in the uterine stroma during pregnancy. Although the precise functional role of FHC during pregnancy remains unclear, it is likely that this protein plays an important role in maintaining proper iron homeostasis within the uterus, which may be crucial for maintenance of gestation.

Expression of Uterine Estrogen-Regulated Gene (UEG) During Early Pregnancy

UEG is expressed in response to estrogen in the uterus and is therefore termed uterine estrogen-regulated gene. Although very little UEG is expressed in heart, brain, kidney, skeletal muscle, or testis, a high level of this mRNA is observed in the uteri of nonpregnant rats at proestrus and estrus stages of the reproductive cycle. In the pregnant animals the level of this mRNA remains high on day 1 of gestation, but starts to decline with the progression of pregnancy, falling to almost undetectable levels on day 5 of gestation, the day of implantation (Fig. 7.2). In situ hybridization with a UEG cDNA fragment reveals the luminal epithelium as the uterine site of synthesis of UEG mRNA. Known antagonists of estrogen, such as 4-hydroxy tamoxifen and ICI 182,780, strongly inhibit the synthesis of this mRNA in the uterus, suggesting a regu-

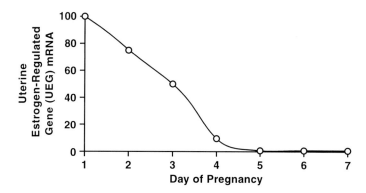

FIGURE 7.2. Profile of expression of UEG mRNA in rat uterus at 1, 2, 3, 4, 5, and 7 days of gestation. Quantitation of UEG mRNA was performed by densitometric scanning as described in the legend to Figure 7.1.

latory role of estrogen in this process. Consistent with this observation, estrogen significantly stimulates UEG mRNA in the uteri of ovariectomized rats within 8 h of administration. Nucleotide sequence analysis of a partial cDNA clone of UEG reveals that it codes for a putative membrane protein with distinct structural motifs. These motifs include the zona pellucida binding domain (ZP) that is present in several zona pellucida binding proteins and multiple CUB motifs that are present in several genes involved in cell growth and differentiation (11,12). The nucleotide sequence analysis of a full-length cDNA clone is under way. The precise cellular function of UEG remains unknown. In light of its stage- and site-specific expression in the uterus during early pregnancy, it is possible that it plays an important regulatory role during the reproductive cycle and implantation.

Progesterone and Estrogen Regulate Calcitonin Gene Expression in the Uterus

Calcitonin, a peptide hormone that regulates calcium homeostasis, is transiently expressed in the uterus during early pregnancy. The level of uterine calcitonin mRNA in cycling rats is low (less than 1% of the mRNA present in the thyroid gland) but rises dramatically (to about 10%-20% of that synthesized by the thyroid gland) during the implantation phase of gestation. As shown in Figure 7.3, the expression of calcitonin mRNA increases by day 2 (postfertilization) of gestation and reaches a peak on day 4, the day before implantation (13). On day 5, the day implantation occurs, the expression of the gene starts to decline and by day 6, when implantation is completed, the calcitonin level falls to below detection limits. The immunocytochemical experiments and in situ hybridization analyses indicate that the burst of cal-

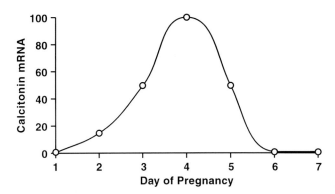

FIGURE 7.3. Profile of expression of calcitonin mRNA in rat uterus at 1, 2, 3, 4, 5, and 7 days of gestation. Quantitation of calcitonin mRNA was performed by densitometric scanning as described in the legend to Figure 7.1.

citonin expression at the time of implantation is restricted predominantly to the glandular epithelial cells of the endometrium (13). The timing and location of its synthesis in the glandular epithelium raise the possibility that calcitonin is secreted by the glands into the uterine lumen, and its principal function may be to regulate blastocyst implantation in an autocrine or paracrine manner.

Calcitonin expression in the uterus is regulated by progesterone. Treatment of ovariectomized rats with progesterone leads to a 20-fold increase in the synthesis of calcitonin (13). In pregnant rats, the rise in calcitonin expression on day 2 of gestation coincides with the surge in circulating progesterone level following fertilization. Previous studies indicated that serum progesterone concentration increases at least three fold on day 2 of pregnancy (14,15). The level of progesterone rises further on day 4 and remains high until term (15). The fact that progesterone is indeed an inducer of calcitonin gene expression in the uterus during pregnancy is confirmed by experiments employing the antiprogestin drug RU486 (13). In rodents and humans, treatment with RU486 during early pregnancy disrupts progestational action and terminates pregnancy (16,17). Treatment of pregnant rats during the preimplantation stage (day 3) with a single dose of RU486, which is known to block implantation, abolishes calcitonin expression within 24 h. It is believed that RU486 exerts its inhibitory effects by impairing the gene regulatory activity of the progesterone receptor (18,19). It is therefore likely that progesterone influences calcitonin gene transcription. Consistent with this prediction, it is observed that cotransfection of progesterone receptor and a reporter gene linked to a 1.3-kb fragment of calcitonin promoter into human endometrial Ishikawa cells, leads to a significant progesterone-dependent enhancement of reporter gene expression (K.C. Bove and I.C. Bagchi, unpublished observation). This result indicates that the regulatory effects of progesterone are indeed exerted at the level of transcription of the calcitonin gene.

Estrogen has no significant effect on calcitonin gene expression when administered alone to ovariectomized rats. In ovariectomized animals it has been shown that administration of estrogen together with progesterone inhibits progesterone-mediated calcitonin gene induction (13). Such antagonistic interactions between estrogen and progesterone pathways have been documented previously in breast and uterine cells (21,22). It has been proposed that these phenomena reflect transcriptional cross-talk occurring between estrogen and progesterone receptors coexpressed in the same target tissue (21,22). During pregnancy in the rat, the circulating levels of estrogen do not change on day 2 after fertilization, increase sharply on the evening of day 4, decline again by day 5 of pregnancy, and remain low throughout gestation until term (23). It is interesting to note that the transient surge of estrogen on the evening of day 4 of pregnancy is coincident with the decline in calcitonin expression. To understand how the interplay of progesterone and estrogen through their respective nuclear receptors may regulate calcitonin promoter function, the expression of calcitonin in a delayed implantation model is analyzed. It is observed that in the absence of estrogen, progesterone alone stimulates calcitonin mRNA synthesis. Continued administration of this hormone maintains calcitonin expression in the glands, while the embryo remains free-floating but viable. Administration of estrogen, which triggers implantation, also reduces the progesterone-mediated enhancement of calcitonin expression. These events, therefore, mimic the physiological pattern of calcitonin expression during early pregnancy. These results suggest that a complex interplay of the two ovarian hormones, progesterone and estrogen, in the uterine milieu is critical for optimal calcitonin gene expression.

Possible Role of Calcitonin During Implantation

One way of investigating the biological role of calcitonin during implantation is by analyzing a calcitonin-deficient mutant mouse model system; however, such a system is currently not available. A calcitonin antagonist that functions effectively in vivo is also not available Therefore, an alternative approach of blocking calcitonin gene expression by using antisense ODNs targeted against calcitonin mRNA is taken. Administration of antisense oligodeoxynucleotides (ODNs), targeted specifically against calcitonin mRNAs, into the lumen of the preimplantation phase uterus results in a dramatic reduction in the number of implanted embryos (24). Similar treatment with the corresponding sense ODNs exhibits no effect on implantation. The antisense ODN intervention also markedly suppresses the steady-state level of the calcitonin mRNA and protein in the uterus, without affecting the expression of unrelated genes. These results collectively suggest that the block in embryonic implantation upon administration of the antisense ODNs into the uterus is a direct phenotypic consequence of the suppression of calcitonin gene expression in the implantation phase of gestation.

The mechanism of action of calcitonin in the uterus during implantation is unclear. Implantation is the culmination of a sequence of discrete functional events, such as successful attachment of the blastocysts to the appropriate sites on the luminal epithelium and proper embryonic development. Calcitonin might be involved in the preparation of the endometrium for implantation. If this is the case then attenuation of calcitonin expression following treatment with antisense ODNs may prevent the acquisition of the receptive state of the endometrium, leading to a failure of implantation. Alternatively, calcitonin may play a role in early embryogenesis. In this scenario, attenuation of its expression during development by antisense ODN may hinder the proper growth and differentiation of the embryos and these abnormal embryos might fail to implant. Studies are currently in progress to distinguish these possibilities.

Recent studies in my laboratory show that the expression of calcitonin is induced in the glandular epithelium of human endometrium around the midsecretory phase of the menstrual cycle but is undetectable in the proliferative phase. In the human, the fertilized ovum arrives in the uterine cavity around day 18 (day 14 is considered as the day of ovulation of a 28-day cycle), and remains there as a free-floating embryo until about day 19; implantation then occurs between days 19 and 22 (25–28). To evaluate the possibility that calcitonin may function as a potential marker of implantation in the human, the profile of calcitonin mRNA expression in human endometrium during the menstrual cycle was analyzed by RT-PCR analysis. The results show that calcitonin mRNA is not detected either in the proliferative or in the late secretory endometrium. However, an intense signal corresponding to calcitonin mRNA was observed during the mid-secretory phase of the cycle. These studies indicate that calcitonin is expressed in the human endometrium in a stage-specific manner and its expression coincides with the putative implantation phase of the menstrual cycle. Calcitonin therefore may play a crucial role in the uterus during blastocyst implantation.

Calcitonin Is a Potential Marker of Uterine Receptivity

An ideal marker of the uterus receptive for blastocyst implantation must fulfill a number of important criteria. It should be present in the endometrium preferably at or near the site of implantation. It should appear within the window of implantation or precede it by a certain amount of time and disappear with the termination of the receptive phase. Studies in my laboratory demonstrate that calcitonin fulfills a large number of criteria to be an appropriate marker that forecasts uterine receptivity for implantation in the rat. There is an urgent need to identify biochemical markers that are faithful and sensitive predictors or indicators of the receptive state of human endometrium during blastocyst implantation. This knowledge in the long run will assist in the diagnosis and treatment of female infertility caused by lack of uterine receptivity. Future studies involving an extensive analysis of spatio-temporal expression of calcitonin in human endometrium will determine whether this peptide hormone emerges as a bonafide marker of uterine receptivity in the human.

Acknowledgments. The research summarized in this article was supported in part by research grants HD-34527 and HD-34760 (National Cooperative Program on Markers of Uterine Receptivity for Blastocyst Implantation) from NIH. The data presented in this article were collected by my colleagues to whom I owe a great deal of gratitude. These individuals are Li-Ji Zhu, Ying Qing Ding, Kathleen Bove, Sushma Kumar, Maarit Angervo, and Mary Polihronis. I also thank Dr. M.K. Bagchi for his valuable comments and criticisms of the work. Finally I thank Evan Reed for the artwork and Jean Schweis for carefully reading the manuscript.

References

1. Psychoyos A. Endocrine control of egg implantation. In: Greep RO, Astwood EG, eds. Handbook of Physiology. Washington, DC: American Physiological Society, 1973:187–215.
2. Yoshinaga K. Uterine receptivity for blastocyst implantation. Ann NY Acad Sci 1988;541:424–31.
3. Parr MB, Parr EL. The implantation reaction. In: Wynn RM, Jollie WP, eds. Biology of the Uterus. New York: Plenum, 1989:233–77.
4. Weitlauf HM. Biology of implantation. In: Knobil E, Neill JD, eds. The Physiology of Reproduction, New York: Raven, 1994:391–440.
5. Evans RM. The steroid and thyroid hormone receptor superfamily. Science 1988;240:889–95.
6. Beato M. Gene regulation by steroid hormones. Cell 1989;56:335–44.
7. Tsai MJ, O'Malley BW. Molecular mechanisms of action of steroid/thyroid receptor superfamily members. Annu Rev Biochem 1994;63:451–86.
8. Wang Z, Brown DD. A gene expression screen. Proc Natl Acad Sci USA 1991;88:11505–9.
9. Liang P, Pardee AB. Differential display of eukaryotic messenger RNA by means of polymerase chain reaction. Science 1992;257:967–71.
10. Zhu L-Z, Bagchi MK, Bagchi IC. Ferritin heavy chain is a progesterone-inducible marker in the uterus during pregnancy. Endocrinology 1995;136:4106–15.
11. Epifano O, Liang LF, Familari M, Moos MC, Dean J. Coordinate expression of the three zona pellucida genes during mouse oogenesis. Development 1995;121(7): 1947–56.
12. Bork P, Beckmann G. The CUB domain a widespread module in developmentally regulated proteins J Mol Biol 1993;231:539–45.
13. Ding YQ, Zhu LJ, Bagchi MK, Bagchi IC. Progesterone stimulates calcitonin gene expression in the uterus during implantation. Endocrinology 1994;135:2265–74.
14. Kalra SP, Kalra PS. Temporal interrelationships among circulating levels of estradiol, progesterone and LH during the rat estrous cycle: effects of exogenous progesterone. Endocrinology 1974;95:1711–8.

15. Wiest WG. Progesterone and 20 α-hydroxypregn-4-en-3-one in plasma, ovaries and uteri during pregnancy in the rat. Endocrinology 1970;87:43–8.

16. Philibert D, Moguilewsky M, Mary I, Lecaque D, Tournemine C, Secchi J et al. Pharmacological profile of RU 486 in animals. In: Baulieu EE, Segal SJ, eds. The antiprogestin steroid RU 486 and human fertility control. New York: Plenum, 1985: 49–68.

17. Sitruk-Ware R, Billaud L, Mowszowica I, Yaneva H, Mauvais-Jarvais P, Bardin CW et al. The use of RU 486 as an abortifacient in early pregnancy. In: Baulieu EE, Segal SJ, eds. The antiprogestin steroid RU 486 and human fertility control. New York: Plenum, 1985:243–8.

18. Baulieu EE. Contragestion and other clinical applications of RU 486, an antiprogesterone at the receptor. Science 1989;245:1351–7.

19. Baulieu EE. The antisteroid RU 486. Its cellular and molecular mode of action. Trends Endocrinol Metab 1991;2:233–9.

20. Kirkland JL, Murthy L, Stancel GM. Progesterone inhibits the estrogen-induced expression of c-fos messenger ribonucleic acid in the uterus. Endocrinology 1992;130:322–30.

21. Kraus WL, Katzenellenbogen. Regulation of progesterone receptor gene expression and growth in the rat uterus: modulation of estrogen action by progesterone and sex steroid hormone antagonists. Endocrinology 1993;132:2371–9.

22. Yoshinaga K, Hawkins RA, Stocker JF. Estrogen secretion by the rat ovary in vivo during the estrous cycle and pregnancy. Endocrinology 1969;85:103–12.

23. Zhu L-J, Bagchi MK, Bagchi IC. Attenuation of calcitonin gene expression in pregnant rat uterus leads to a block in embryonic implantation. Endocrinology 1998;139: 330–9.

24. Hertig AT, Rock J, Adams EC. A description of 34 human ova within the first 17 days of development. Am J Anat 1956;98:435–93.

25. Formigli L, Formigli G, Roccio C. Donation of fertilized uterine ova to infertile women. Fertil Steril 1987;47:62–5.

26. Rogers PAW, Murphy CR. Uterine receptivity for implantation: human studies. In: Yoshinaga K, ed. Blastocyst implantation. Boston: Serono Symposia, 1989:231–8.

27. Navot DM, Anderson TL, Droesch K, Scott RT, Kreiner RT, Kreiner D et al. Hormonal manipulation of endometrial maturation. J Clin Endocrinol Metab 1989;68:801–7.

28. Navot DM, Scott RT, Droesch K, Veeck LL, Liu H-C, Rosenwaks Z. The window of embryo transfer and the efficiency of human conception in vitro. Fertil Steril 1991;55:114–7.

8

Molecular Signaling in Implantation

Sanjoy K. Das, Bibhash C. Paria, and Sudhansu K. Dey

The synchronized development of the preimplantation embryo to the blastocyst stage is essential to the process of implantation (1,2). The establishment of a differentiated uterus for supporting embryo development and implantation is primarily dependent on the coordinated effects of progesterone (P_4) and estrogen (1,2). In the rodent, the first conspicuous sign that the implantation process has been initiated is an increased endometrial vascular permeability at the sites of blastocysts. This can be visualized as discrete blue bands along the uterus after an intravenous injection of a blue dye (1,2). This increased vascular permeability coincides with the initial attachment reaction between the blastocyst trophecto-derm and uterine luminal epithelium (3). In the mouse, the attachment reaction occurs in the evening (2200-2400 h) on day 4 of pregnancy (4) and is preceded by uterine luminal closure which in turn results in an intimate apposition of the trophectoderm with the luminal epithelium (1,3,5). The attachment reaction is followed by localized stromal decidualization and luminal epithelial apoptosis at the sites of blastocyst implantation (6).

The heterogeneous uterine cell types respond uniquely to P_4 and/or estrogen. In the adult ovariectomized mouse uterus, estrogen stimulates proliferation of epithelial cells, while this process in the stroma requires both P_4 and estrogen (7). Similar steroid hormonal regulation occurs during the periimplantation period. On days 1 and 2, preovulatory ovarian estrogen directs epithelial cell proliferation. On day 3, P_4 from newly formed corpora lutea initiates stromal cell proliferation, which is further potentiated by preimplantation ovarian estrogen secretion on day 4. In contrast, epithelial cells cease to proliferate and become differentiated on this day. With the initiation of implantation, stromal cells at sites of blastocysts undergo extensive proliferation and differentiation into decidual cells (7).

In the mouse, the receptive state of the uterus for implantation occurs only for a limited period during pregnancy or pseudopregnancy. Thus, the uterus be-comes receptive on day 4 (the day of implantation) and by day 5, it becomes nonreceptive for blastocyst implantation. This conclusion is derived from results of blastocyst transfer in pseudopregnant recipients (2). Ovariectomy in the morn-ing of day 4 of pregnancy, prior to preimplantation ovarian estrogen secretion, results in blastocyst dormancy and failure of implantation, a condition known as delayed implantation. Delayed implantation can be terminated with blastocyst activation and attainment of uterine receptivity for implantation by an injection of estrogen only when the uterus is primed with progesterone (P_4) for 24 to 48 h (2,8,9). As determined by blastocyst transfer experiments in pseudopregnant mice, once the uterus achieves the receptive phase, it automatically proceeds to the nonreceptive (refractory) phase (2). The mechanism(s) by which P_4 differentiates the uterus for estrogen to initiate the process of implantation is not known. It is also not known how the receptive uterus spontaneously becomes nonreceptive. It is likely that these P_4- and/or estrogen-mediated events are accomplished by the expression of a unique set of genes in target tissues.

An emerging concept is that polypeptide growth factors could be involved in preimplantation embryo development and implantation. Indeed the expression of several growth factors and their receptors in the uterus and/or embryo suggests that these factors could be involved in these processes (4,9,10, and reviewed in (11)). Recent observations suggest the possibility of ligand-receptor signaling with the EGF family of growth factors in implantation. In the mouse, the EGF receptor (EGF-R) is expressed both in the blastocyst and uterus, and this expression is tightly regulated by the maternal steroid hormonal status at the time of implantation (9,10). The EGF family includes EGF, transforming growth factor-α (TGF-α), heparin binding-EGF (HB-EGF), amphiregulin (AR), betacellulin, epiregulin and neu differentiation factors (NDFs) (12–18). These ligands can interact with the receptor subtypes of the erbB gene family via homodimerization and heterodimerization (19–24). This family is comprised of four receptor tyrosine kinases: ErbB1 (EGF-R), ErbB2, ErbB3, and ErbB4. They share a common structural feature, but differ in their ligand specificity and kinase activity (19–21). Thus, "cross-talk" between the receptor subtypes with various ligands can serve as a potential signaling mechanism (25,26).

This chapter describes the differential regulation and expression of heparin-binding EGF-like growth factor (HB-EGF) and amphiregulin (AR) in the periimplantation and delayed implantation uterus, as well as the differential effects of HB-EGF and AR on ligand-induced autophosphorylation of EGF-R in uterus/blastocysts. Both HB-EGF and AR are synthesized as transmembrane precursor proteins, which are proteolytically processed to release the mature forms. Although both HB-EGF and AR are heparin-binding growth factors, the effects of HB-EGF are potentiated while those of AR are inhibited by heparin (27–29).

Expression of HB-EGF and AR in the Mouse Uterus

Northern Blot Analysis of HB-EGF and AR mRNA in the Periimplantation Uterus

Steady state levels of HB-EGF and AR mRNA in the uterus during periimplantation period (days 1–8) were examined by Northern blot hybridization (Fig. 8.1). A 2.5

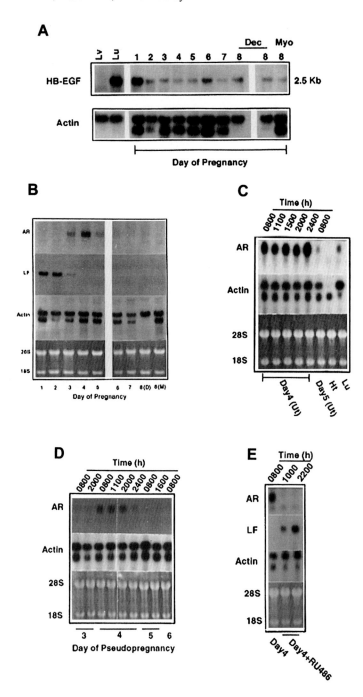

FIGURE 8.1. (A) Northern blot hybridization of HB-EGF mRNA in the mouse uterus. The mRNA levels were assessed on days 1–7 of pregnancy or from the separated deciduum (Dec) and myometrium (Myo) on day 8 as indicated. RNAs isolated from

kb transcript of HB-EGF mRNA, similar to that identified in other tissues (10,30), was detected in the uterus (Fig. 8.1.A). Levels of HB-EGF mRNA in whole uterine poly (A)$^+$ RNA samples were higher on day 1 of pregnancy, but remained virtually unaltered during the rest of the periimplantation period.

Interestingly, in contrast, a 1.4 kb transcript for AR mRNA in whole uterine total RNA samples was primarily detected on day 4 preceded or followed by little or no detectable AR mRNA on other days of pregnancy (Fig. 8.1B). The accumulation of AR mRNA was maintained at elevated levels throughout day 4 of pregnancy (the day of implantation), but remarkably dropped to very low levels by the morning of day 5 when the implantation process is well underway (Fig. 8.1C). In contrast, lactoferrin (LF), an estrogen responsive gene, was expressed in the uterus on days 1 and 2 of pregnancy when the uterus is under the influence of preovulatory estrogen surge, but not later when plasma P_4 levels are rising, as reported here (Fig. 8.1B) and previously (31). We assessed AR mRNA levels in pseudopregnant mice to evaluate whether the expression is influenced by the presence of the blastocyst. Similar to the day 4 pregnant uterus, AR mRNA accumulated primarily in the day 4 pseudopregnant uterus with the exception of very low levels at 2400 h, the time of attachment reaction in the pregnant animal (Fig. 8.1D). These results provide evidence that the "surge" in AR mRNA levels on day 4 is correlated first with rising P_4 levels and then with the attachment reaction. An injection of RU-486, a P_4 receptor antagonist (32), on day 3 interfered with implantation and the uterine induction of AR mRNA on day 4 of pregnancy. However, this treatment induced LF mRNA, which under normal conditions is not induced on this day (31) (Fig. 8.1E). Since LF is induced by estrogen but antagonized by P_4 (31,33), the induction of this gene suggests that P_4 effects were neutralized by RU-486.

---

lung (Lu) or liver (Lv) tissues were used as positive and negative controls, respectively. Poly (A)$^+$ RNA (2 µg) samples were separated by formaldehyde-agarose gel electrophoresis, transferred and UV cross-linked to nylon membranes and hybridized sequentially to ^{32}P-labeled HB-EGF and β-actin probes. Autoradiographic exposures were 2 h for HB-EGF and 0.5 h for β-actin. The two species of β-actin transcripts present in whole uterine RNA samples reflects the abundance of muscle-specific actin mRNA contributed by the myometrium. Reprinted with permission from Das et al (4). (B–E). Northern blot hybridization of AR mRNA in the mouse uterus. (B) Samples from the whole uterus on days 1–7 of pregnancy, or from the separated deciduum (D) and myometrium (M) on day 8 as indicated. (C) Samples from day 4 and day 5 uteri (Ut) at various times, and from heart (Ht) or lung (Lu) tissue. (D) Uterine samples from days 3–6 of pseudopregnancy at various times. (E) Samples from day 4 uterus at the indicated times after an injection of RU-486 (400 µg/mouse) on day 3 at 1000 h. Total RNA (6 µg) samples were separated by formaldehyde-agarose gel electrophoresis, transferred and UV cross-linked to nylon membranes and hybridized sequentially to ^{32}P-labeled AR, LF and β-actin probes as indicated. Autoradiographic exposures were 18 h for AR, 2 h for LF and 0.5 h for β-actin. Reprinted with permission from Das et al. (11).

In Situ Hybridization of HB-EGF and
AR mRNA in the Periimplantation Uterus

The above observation suggested that, if HB-EGF and AR expression is important for implantation, it would be through localized cell type-specific expression
in the uterus. Thus we examined the distribution of HB-EGF and AR mRNA in the

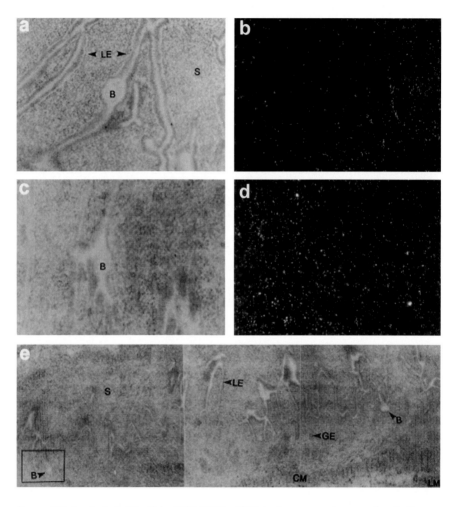

FIGURE 8.2. In situ hybridization of HB-EGF mRNA in the mouse uterus on day 4 of pregnancy and pseudopregnancy. Brightfield and darkfield photomicrographs of longitudinal
sections of uteri collected at 0900 h (a,b), 1400 h (c,d), and 1600 h (e,f) on day 4 of pregnancy
are shown. Note distinct hybridization signals in luminal epithelial cells surrounding two
blastocysts (e,f). Microphotographs in g and h represent higher magnification of one of the two
areas containing a blastocyst. Panels in the bottom row (i,j) represent brightfield and darkfield
photomicrographs of day 4 pseudopregnant uterine sections at 1600 h showing no hybridization signals. b, blastocyst; le, luminal epithelium; ge, glandular epithelium; cm, circular muscle;
lm, longitudinal muscle; s, stroma; icm, inner cell mass; and tr, trophectoderm. Reprinted with
permission from Das et al. (4).

uterus by in situ hybridization. On day 1 of pregnancy, autoradiographic signals for HB-EGF mRNA showed heterogeneous distribution in the luminal (LE) and glandular (GE) epithelia (data not shown). The signals for HB-EGF mRNA are virtually absent on days 2 and 3 of pregnancy (data not shown). However, HB-EGF mRNA was again detected in a specific cell-type and at a specific time on day 4 of pregnancy. Autoradiographic signals of HB-EGF hybrids were detected in the LE surrounding the blastocyst at 1600 h (Fig. 8.2e-h), but not at 0900 h (Fig. 8.2a,b) or 1400 h (Fig. 8.2c,d). Furthermore, no autoradiographic signals could be detected in LE in between sites of blastocysts (Fig. 8.2e,f), or in uterine cells of pseudopregnant mice at 1600 h on day 4 (Fig. 8.2i,j), as well as at morning and afternoon of day 5 (data not shown). With the initiation of attachment reaction (blue reaction) at 2300 h on day 4 or with the progression of the implantation process through day 6 of pregnancy, the distribution of the mRNA extended along the LE above the implantation chamber towards the mesometrial pole of the uterus (data not shown).

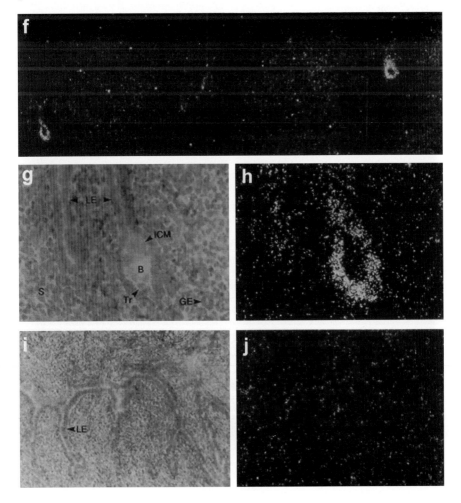

Figure 8.2. (*continued*)

In case of AR mRNA, no specific autoradiographic signals could be detected on days 1 to 3 or days 6 to 8 of pregnancy (representative data from day 1 shown in Fig. 8.3, parts 1–7). The induction of AR mRNA was primarily limited to the day 4

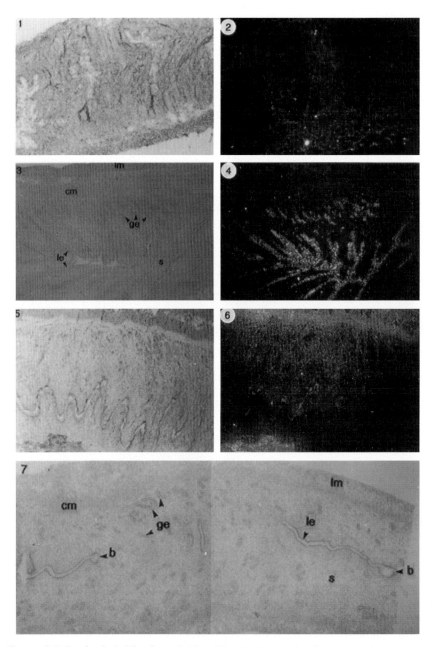

Figure 8.3. In situ hybridization of AR mRNA in the periimplantation mouse uterus. Brightfield and darkfield photomicrographs of representative longitudinal uterine sections

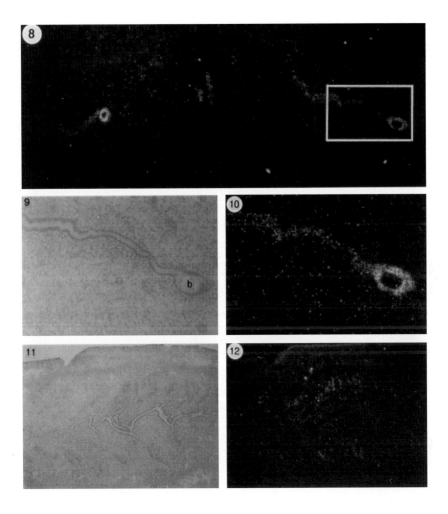

collected at 0900 h on day 1 (panels 1 and 2), and at 1800 h on day 4 (panels 3 and 4) are shown. Note that there are no hybridization signals in any cell types in the day 1 uterine section, while distinct hybridization signals are present in epithelial cells in the day 4 uterine section. Panels 5 and 6 show brightfield and darkfield photomicrographs of a representative longitudinal uterine section at 1800 h on day 4 hybridized to a sense probe showing no hybridization signal. Brightfield and darkfield photomicrographs of a representative longitudinal uterine section collected at 2400 h on day 4 (panels 7 and 8) are shown. Note distinct hybridization signals in luminal epithelial cells surrounding the two blastocysts in this section. Panels 9 and 10 represent higher magnification of one of the two areas containing a blastocyst (rectangle in panel 8). Panels 11 and 12 show brightfield and darkfield photomicrographs of a representative uterine section from a sterile horn (ligated at the utero-tubal junction on day 1) at 2400 h on day 4 showing very little hybridization signal in epithelial cells. b, blastocyst; le, luminal epithelium; ge, glandular epithelium; cm, circular muscle; lm, longitudinal muscle; s, stroma. Magnification: panels 1–8, 11, and 12, ×100; panels 9 and 10, ×200. Reprinted with permission from Das et al. (11).

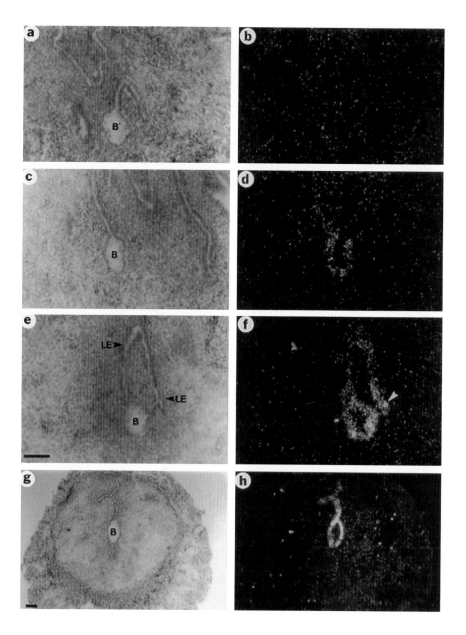

FIGURE 8.4. In situ hybridization of HB-EGF in uterine sections obtained from P_4-treated delayed implanting mice before and after E_2 treatment. Brightfield and darkfield photomicrographs of uterine sections are shown. The top row of panels (a,b) represents a longitudinal section from a delayed implanting mouse treated with P_4 from days 5–7 and killed 24 h after the last injection. The second (c,d) and third (e,f) row of panels represent longitudinal sections of uteri from P_4-treated delayed implanting mice killed 12 and 24 h after an E_2 injection, respectively. The bottom row of panels (g,h) represents a cross-section from a P_4-treated delayed

uterus, and exclusively to the glandular and luminal epithelial cells (Fig. 8.3, parts 3 and 4). Although AR mRNA was distributed indiscriminately throughout the glandular and luminal epithelial cells until 1800 h on day 4, with the onset of attachment reaction (2400 h), the levels of AR mRNA were high in the luminal epithelium surrounding the blastocyst in the implantation chamber, while epithelial cells away from the implantation chamber showed greatly reduced levels (Fig. 8.3, parts 7–10). The reduced levels of AR mRNA in epithelial cells in sterile uterine horns (ligated at the uterotubal junction on day 1) of pregnant mice (Fig. 8.3, parts 11 and 12), as well as in pseudopregnant uteri at 2400 h (data not shown) support the observation of embryonic influence on AR induction around the time of the attachment reaction. On day 5, the levels of AR mRNA in the luminal epithelium surrounding the blastocyst were greatly reduced and no mRNA could be detected in epithelial cells away from the implantation chamber (data not shown).

Expression of HB-EGF and AR mRNA in the Delayed Implantation Uterus

To further examine whether the expression of HB-EGF or AR gene in the LE requires the presence of an active blastocyst, in situ hybridization was performed on uterine sections obtained from P_4-treated delayed implanting mice, or after the initiation of blastocyst activation and implantation by an E_2 injection (Fig. 8.4). No hybridization signals were detected in luminal epithelial cells surrounding dormant blastocysts that had been in close apposition with luminal epithelial cells for 3 days during P_4 treatment (Fig. 8.4a,b). In contrast, with the E_2-induced termination of delayed implantation and onset of blastocyst activation, temporal and cell type-specific expression of uterine HB-EGF mRNA again became evident. The intensity of signals increased at sites of each blastocyst at 12 h (Fig. 8.4c,d) followed by a further increase at 24 h (Fig. 8.4e–h) after an E_2 injection. Because P_4 priming is essential for the preparation of the uterus for estrogen to initiate implantation, we analyzed the expression of AR in the P_4-primed delayed implanting uterus before and after an injection of an implantation-initiating dose of E_2 (25 ng/mouse). Levels of AR mRNA under these treatment conditions were comparable to those of day 4 pregnant mice (data not shown), again suggesting implantation-specific regulation of AR under the direction of P_4. Although, the expression of the AR gene in the uterus is primarily regulated by P_4 and localized expression of this gene in the uterine LE at the sites of blastocyst apposition persists during the termination of P_4-treated delayed implantation (unpublished).

←

implanting mouse killed 24 h after an E_2 injection. Note that there are no hybridization signals in the luminal epithelium at the site of the blastocyst in the P_4-treated delayed implanting uterus (a,b) as compared to clear hybridization signals in the luminal epithelium surrounding the blastocysts 12 or 24 h after termination of delayed implantation by E_2 injection (c-h). Also note the presence of hybridization signals (*the white arrow* in f) in the luminal epithelium outside the implantation chamber around the blastocyst. b, blastocyst and le, luminal epithelium. Bars, 100 μm. Reprinted with permission from Das et al. (4).

Differential Autophosphorylation of EGF-R in the Uterus and Blastocyst by HB-EGF and AR

In the present investigation, we provide evidence that the same concentration of AR or HB-EGF (10 nM) can activate phosphorylation of the EGF-R in ovariectomized P_4-treated uterine membrane preparations, while an approximately 10-fold higher concentration of EGF was required to obtain the same effect (Fig. 8.5A,B). Thus, AR, HB-EGF, and EGF appear to be equipotent in the autophosphorylation of EGF-R in the E_2-treated uterus, whereas AR and HB-EGF are more potent than EGF in inducing this phosphorylation in the P_4-treated uterus. In contrast, AR was less potent than HB-EGF or EGF in inducing autophosphorylation of the EGF-R in day 4 blastocysts (Fig. 8.5C) (4,34).

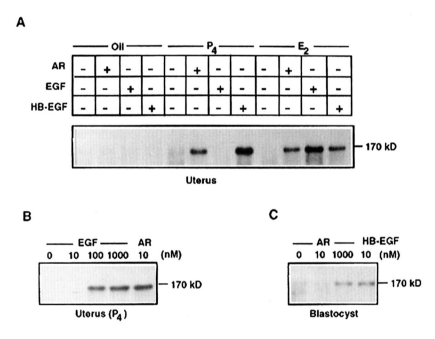

FIGURE 8.5. HB-EGF- and AR-induced autophosphorylation of EGF-R in the uterus and blastocyst. Autophosphorylation of the EGF-R was determined in uterine membranes and blastocyst homogenate after preincubation with (+) or without (–) HB-EGF, AR and EGF. The labeling reaction was initiated by the addition of γ-^{32}P-ATP. After 2 min of labeling, immunoprecipitations were performed with antibodies to EGF-R. Precipitates were separated by SDS-PAGE and detected by autoradiography for 1 to 2 days. (A) Ovariectomized mice were injected with oil, P_4 (1 mg/mouse), or E_2 (250 ng/mouse), and killed 18 h later. The ligand concentration used was 10 nM. (B) Ovariectomized mice were treated with an injection of P_4 (1 mg/mouse) and killed 18 h later. (C) Blastocysts collected at 1000 h on day 4 of pregnancy. Reprinted with permission from Das et al. (11).

Comments

The highlights of the present investigation are (1) that the expression of HB-EGF is induced in the LE by the blastocyst at the site of its apposition and at a specific time very early in the process of implantation, and (2) that the expression of AR is occurred throughout the LE for most of the day 4 of pregnancy, with the onset of blastocyst attachment reaction late on day 4, AR expression becomes restricted in the LE at the sites of blastocyst apposition followed by its downregulation by the morning of day 5.

An interesting structural feature of EGF-like growth factors is that they all appear to be synthesized as membrane-associated precursors that are processed by proteases to release mature growth factors (14,35–37). In the case of TGF-α, membrane-associated forms have been shown to signal neighboring cells via ligand-receptor interactions in a manner that has been termed juxtacrine regulation (35,37). The precursor form of HB-EGF is also active as a juxtacrine factor and is capable of stimulating the phosphorylation of EGF-R in target cells in coculture (38). Thus, both membrane-associated precursor and mature forms of this family of growth factors are likely to be operative in influencing biological functions (37). Although HB-EGF and AR can bind heparin, the biological effects of HB-EGF are potentiated by this interaction, whereas those of AR are inhibited. Therefore, luminal epithelial cell expression of HB-EGF at the site of the blastocyst coincident with the expression of heparan sulphate proteoglycans on the attachment-competent blastocyst is consistent with an interaction between epithelial HB-EGF and the blastocyst EGF-R (4,9,39). HB-EGF induced autophosphorylation of blastocyst EGF-R is consistent with a potential role of this growth factor in receptor mediated blastocyst functions associated with implantation.

The differential expression and regulation of HB-EGF and AR genes in the mouse uterus during pregnancy suggest specific roles for these two ligands in uterine biology and implantation. We propose a preferential role of AR in the differentiation of the uterus under the direction of P_4, while the expression of HB-EGF in the differentiated uterus by the blastocyst is more likely to be involved in interacting with blastocyst EGF-R in the process of implantation. AR can stimulate or inhibit cell proliferation depending upon the environment (40). In this respect, induction of AR in epithelial cells on day 4 of pregnancy or pseudopregnancy is closely associated with cessation of epithelial cell proliferation and onset of stromal cell proliferation. Thus, AR may function as an autocrine (41) and/or intracrine (42) factor in epithelial cells, while as a paracrine factor in stromal cells. Although it has not been established clearly, nuclear localization of AR in uterine epithelial cells is consistent with the speculation of an intracrine mode of action.

Interestingly, HB-EGF and AR are as potent as EGF in inducing autophosphorylation of the EGF-R in the E_2-treated uterus. Moreover, AR was more potent than EGF in the phosphorylation of uterine EGF-R in the P_4-treated ovariectomized mouse. In contrast, HB-EGF was more potent than AR in phosphorylating blastocyst EGF-R. These results have raised interesting questions. The differential effects of various ligands on the phosphorylation of uterine or blastocyst EGF-R under specific conditions suggest that the functions of the EGF family of growth factors in the uterus or embryo are regulated either at the levels of the ligands or by the expression of other known or unknown members of the type-1 receptor tyrosine kinase family.

Acknowledgments. This research was supported in part by grants from NIH (HD 12304) and National Cooperative Program on Markers of Uterine Receptivity for Nonhuman Blastocyst Implantation (HD 29968) to S.K. Dey. A center grant (HD 02528) provided access to various core facilities. We thank X.-N. Wang for in situ hybridization studies.

References

1. Psychoyos A. Endocrine control of egg implantation. In: Handbook of Physiology, Greep RO, Astwood EG, Geiger SR, eds. Washington, DC: American Physiological Society, 1973:87–215.
2. Paria BC, Huet-Hudson YM, Dey SK. Blastocyst's state of activity determines the "window" of implantation in the mouse receptive uterus. Proc Natl Acad Sci USA 1993;90:10159–62.
3. Enders AC, Schlafke S. A morphological analysis of the early implantation stages in the rat. Am J Anat 1967;120:185–226.
4. Das SK, Wang X-N, Paria BC, Damm D, Abraham JA, Klagsbrun M, et al. Heparin-binding EGF-like growth factor gene is induced in the mouse uterus temporally by the blastocyst solely at the site of its apposition: a possible ligand for interaction with blastocyst EGF-receptor in implantation. Development 1994;120:1071–83.
5. Enders AC. Anatomical aspects of implantation. J Reprod Fertil 1976;2:1–15.
6. Parr EL, Tung HN, Parr MB. Apoptosis as the mode of uterine epithelial cell death during embryo implantation in mice and rats. Biol Reprod 1987;36:211–5.
7. Huet-Hudson YM, Andrews GK, Dey SK. Cell type-specific localization of c-myc protein in the mouse uterus: modulation by steroid hormones and analysis of the periimplantation period. Endocrinology 1989;125:1683–90.
8. Yoshinaga K, Adams CE. Delayed implantation in the spayed, progesterone-treated adult mouse. J Reprod Fertil 1966;12:593–5.
9. Paria BC, Das SK, Andrews GK, Dey SK. Expression of the epidermal growth factor receptor gene is regulated in mouse blastocysts during delayed implantation. Proc Natl Acad Sci USA 1993;90:55–9.
10. Das SK, Tsukamura H, Paria BC, Andrews GK, Dey SK. Differential expression of epidermal growth factor receptor (EGF-R) gene and regulation of EGF-R bioactivity by progesterone and estrogen in the adult mouse uterus. Endocrinology 1994;134:971–81.
11. Das SK, Chakraborty I, Paria BC, Wang X-N, Plowman GD, Dey SK. Amphiregulin is an implantation-specific and progesterone-regulated gene in the mouse uterus. Mol Endocrinol 1995;9:691–705.

12. Cohen S. Isolation of a mouse submaxillary gland protein accelerating incisor eruption and eyelid opening in the mouse newborn. J Biol Chem 1962;237:1555–62.

13. Derynck R, Roberts AB, Winkler ME, Chen YE, Goeddel DV Human transforming growth factor-alpha: precursor structure and expression in E. coli. Cell 1984;38: 287–97.

14. Higashiyama S, Abraham JA, Miller J, Fiddes JC, Klagsbrun M. A heparin-binding growth factor secreted by macrophage-like cells that is related to EGF. Science 1991;251:936–9.

15. Holmes WE, Sliwkowski MX, Akita RW, Henzel WJ, Lee J, Park JW, et al. Identification of heregulin, a specific activator of p185^{erbB2}. Science 1992;256:1205–10.

16. Shoyab M, McDonald VL, Bradley JG, Todaro GJ. Amphiregulin: a bifunctional growth-modulating glycoprotein produced by the phorbol 12-myristate 13-acetate-treated human breast adenocarcinoma cell line MCF-7. Proc Natl Acad Sci USA 1988;85:6528–32.

17. Toyoda H, Komurasaki T, Uchida D, Takayama Y, Isobe T, Okuyama T, et al. Epiregulin: A novel EGF with mitogenic activity for rat primary hepatocytes. J Biol Chem 1995;270:7459–500.

18. Shing Y, Christofori G, Hanahan D, Ono Y, Sasada R, Igarashi K, et al. Betacellulin: a mitogen from pancreatic β cell tumors. Science 1993;259:1604–7.

19. Heldin CH. Dimerization of cell surface receptors in signal transduction. Cell 1995;80:13.

20. Prigent SA, Lemoine NR. The type I(EGFR-related) family of growth factor receptors and their ligands. Progr Growth Factor Res 1992;4:1–24.

21. Peles E, Yarden Y. Neu and its ligands: from an oncogene to neural factors. BioEssays 1993;15:815–24.

22. Riese II DJ, Bermingham Y, van Raaij TM, Buckley S, Plowman GD, Stern DF. Betacellulin activates the epidermal growth factor receptor and erbB-4, and induces cellular response patterns distinct from those stimulated by epidermal growth factor or neuregulin-BETA. Oncogene 1996;12:345–53.

23. Lim H, Dey SK, Das SK. Differential expression of the erbB2 gene in the periimplantation mouse uterus: potential mediator of signaling by epidermal growth factor-like growth factors. Endocrinology 1997;138:1328–37.

24. Elenius K, Paul S, Allison G, Sun J, Klagsbrun M. Activation of HER4 by heparin-binding EGF-like growth factor stimulates chemotaxis but not proliferation. EMBO J 1997;16:1268–78.

25. Earp HS, Dawson TL, Li X, Yu H. Heterodimerization and functional interaction between EGF receptor family members: a new signaling paradigm with implications for breast cancer research. Breast Cancer Res Treat 1995;35:115–32.

26. Hynes NE, Stern DF. The biology of erbB2/neu/HER2 and its role in cancer. Biochim Biophys Acta 1994;1198:165–84.

27. Cook PW, Mattox PA, Keeble WW, Pittelkow MR, Plowman GD, Shoyab M, et al. A heparin sulfate-regulated human keratinocyte autocrine factor is similar or identical to amphiregulin. Mol Cell Biol 1991;11:2547–57.

28. Higashiyama S, Abraham JA, Klagsbrun M. Heparin-binding EGF-like growth factor stimulation of smooth muscle cell migration: Dependence on interactions with cell surface heparan sulfate. J Cell Biol 1993;122:933–40.

29. Thompson SA, Higashiyama S, Wood K, Pollitt NS, Damm D, McEnroe G, et al. Characterization of sequences within heparin-binding EGF-like growth factor that mediate interaction with heparin. J Biol Chem 1994;269:2541–9.

30. Abraham JA, Damm D, Bajardi A, Miller J, Klagsbrun M, Ezekowitz RAB. Heparin-binding EGF-like growth factor: Characterization of rat and mouse cDNA clones, protein domain conservation across species, and transcript expression in tissues. Biochem Biophys Res Comm 1993;190:125–33.

31. McMaster MT, Teng CT, Dey SK, Andrews GK. Lactoferrin in the mouse uterus: analyses of the preimplantation period and regulation by ovarian steroids. Mol Endocrinol 1991;6:101–11.

32. Vegeto E, Allan GF, Schrader WT, Tsai MJ, McDonnell DP, O'Malley BW. The mechanism of RU-486 antagonism is dependent on the conformation of the carboxy-terminal tail of the human progesterone receptor. Cell 1992;69:703–13.

33. Wang X-N, Das SK, Damm D, Klagsbrun M, Abraham JA, Dey SK. Endocrinology 1994;135:1264–71.

34. Paria BC, Tsukamura H, Dey SK. Epidermal growth factor-specific protein tyrosine phosphorylation in preimplantation embryo development. Biol Reprod 1991;45: 711–8.

35. Derynck R. Transforming growth factor-α. Mol Reprod Devel 1990;27:3–9.

36. Plowman GD, Green JM, McDonald VL, Neubauer MG, Disteche CM, Todaro GJ, Shoyab M. The amphiregulin gene encodes a novel epidermal growth factor-related protein with tumor inhibitory activity. Mol Cell Biol 1990;10:1969–81.

37. Massague J, Pandiella A. Membrane-anchored growth factors. Annu Rev Biochem 1993;62:515–41.

38. Raab G, Kover K, Paria BC, Dey SK, Ezzell RM, Klagsbrun M. Mouse preimplantation blastocysts adhere to cells expressing the transmembrane form of heparin-binding EGF-like growth factor. Development 1996;122:637–45.

39. Carson DD, Tang J-P, Julian J. Heparan sulphate proteoglycan (perlecan) expression by mouse embryos during acquisition of attachment competence. Devel Biol 1993;155: 97–106.

40. Plowman GD, Green JM, McDonald VL, Neubauer MG, Disteche CM, Todaro GJ, et al. The amphiregulin gene encodes a novel epidermal growth factor-related protein with tumor inhibitory activity. Mol Cell Biol 1990;10:1969–81.

41. Normanno N, Selvam MP, Qi C-F, Saeki T, Johnson G, Kim N, Ciardiello F, et al. Amphiregulin as an autocrine growth factor for c-Ha-*ras*- and c-*erb*B-2-transformed human mammary epithelial cells. Proc Natl Acad Sci USA 1994;91:2790–4.

42. Modrell B, McDonald VL, Shoyab M. The interaction of amphiregulin with nuclei and putative nuclear localization sequence binding proteins. Growth Factors 1992;7: 305–14.

9

Identification of Progesterone-Regulated Genes in the Uterus

CINDEE R. FUNK, BERT W. O'MALLEY, AND FRANCESCO J. DEMAYO

Progesterone plays a critical role in transforming the nonpregnant uterus into an enriched environment specifically suited for the developing embryo. Its role in inducing and maintaining the pregnant state is paramount in mammalian systems and to a large extent, determines the success of any given pregnancy in the steps following fertilization. For years, reproductive biologists have tried to elucidate the actual mechanisms and the signaling pathways involved in mediating progesterone's activity. Yet little is currently known about the cascade of events which initiate and communicate the inductive effects of this uterine steroid. It has only been in the past few years that molecular targets of progesterone regulation have really been identified and characterized with respect to mediating pregnancy (1). Although this area of research is clearly burgeoning forward with the advances of gene knock out techniques and the identification of essential "pregnancy" genes, the small handful of genes known to be essential for pregnancy lends only suggestive information as to what signaling pathways are essential mediators of a successful pregnancy.

This chapter first presents a brief review of the importance of progesterone during the early stages of pregnancy, traditionally exemplified by the use of RU486 as a progesterone antagonist, but more convincingly demonstrated by the pleiotrophic reproductive phenotype of the progesterone receptor knock-out mouse. Then, it presents an overview of some of the currently available methodology utilizing steroid receptor mutant mice to isolate, identify, and characterize new targets of progesterone action with the ultimate goal of understanding the signaling pathways involved in the establishment of pregnancy.

Overview and Importance of Progesterone

Immediately following implantation and prior to development of the fetoplacenta unit, the growing embryo is completely dependent on the maternal uterine environment for both protection and nourishment. Later, the placenta makes a direct link between the fetal unit and the maternal blood supply, which is maintained until parturition. In most species, the placenta takes on an endocrine role, by which it assumes the role of steroid biosynthesis and assures the maintenance of pregnancy throughout birth. The uterine environment is therefore a crucial player in determining the success rate of a given pregnancy, and this in turn is critically dependent on the intricate interplay between the two female steroid hormones—estrogen and progesterone. After estrogen initiates the uterine transformation, progesterone is absolutely required to further sensitize the endometrial component through a series of steps that in the rodent requires about two days. Progesterone has been traditionally regarded as the "pregnancy" hormone because of its roles during both implantation and placental maintenance which is continued throughout birth. Following fertilization, progesterone induced responses ultimately determine the success of a given pregnancy (2).

The importance of progesterone is further exemplified in clinical situations in which progesterone antagonists have been used to both prevent implantation of a fertilized ovum, and to prematurely terminate an already established pregnancy (3). The aging uterus also underscores the importance of progesterone with respect to embryo implantation, whereby the natural decline of circulating hormone in aging women negatively influences the success rates associated with in vitro fertilizations. These poor rates have been drastically improved by administering a two-fold increase in the dose of progesterone in these older recipients whereby they slightly exceeded the success rates observed in younger women (4).

Regulation of Progesterone Activity

In the uterus, progesterone mediates its effects through the progesterone receptor which, when activated, migrates to the nucleus and initiates transcription of progesterone target genes. The gene encoding progesterone receptor is thought to be in single copy, producing at least nine independent transcripts through differential splicing (5). Although as many as four different protein isoforms of the receptor have been reported in various species (6,7), the two largest forms, PR-A (81-83 kDa), and PR-B (116-120 kDa) are the most abundant forms found in human, chick, and rodent tissue. They are thought to regulate gene transcription either by transcriptional activation through PR-B or by repression through the dominant repression of PR-B by the PR-A isoform. Consequently, the relative proportion of the PR isoforms in any given target cell will ultimately determine if a specific gene will be expressed in the cell upon hormonal stimulation (6). In general, the level of available progesterone receptor is induced in most reproductive tissue by estrogens, growth factors and cAMP, but the level of available receptor decreases in response to progesterone, and may therefore explain the continued need for estrogen in order to maintain efficient induction of the progesterone receptor throughout pregnancy (8).

In the absence of hormone, the human and avian progesterone receptors exist as inactive multiprotein complexes. The inactive avian receptor complex is primarily located in the cytosol and is comprised of the heat shock proteins, hsp90 and hsp70 (in some cases), a combination of at least two of the three immunophilins, FKBP52, FKBP54, or cyclophilin-40, and a critically important receptor associated protein, p23, which has been shown to be absolutely essential for receptor complex assembly and activation by ligand. Upon binding of the hormone, however, these complexes completely dissociate and undergo a series of conformational changes and modifications that ultimately result in activation of the receptor complex, translocation to the nucleus, and binding of the receptor as an active dimer to target DNA sequences (9).

Progesterone responsive genes contain specific sequences known as progesterone response elements (PREs) upstream of their promoters which mediate binding of the activated receptor dimer to the DNA target. However, a given progesterone response may be altered if other steroid response elements (SREs) are located near the PRE. Many target genes can be regulated by several different hormones in a time or tissue specific manner, and often have more than one SRE upstream of their promoters. Binding of different transcriptional units to these SREs can induce an interaction between different hormonal regulators resulting in either a synergistic or antagonistic response. This coordinate induction is common in estrogen and progesterone responsive genes (10,11). Consequently, steroid hormones can act either independently by binding of activated receptor to only its specific SRE, or coordinately, by cooperative binding of two different activated complexes to adjacent SREs.

Additional transcriptional "coactivators" and "corepressors" are also involved which help mediate conformational changes of the transcriptional complex (10,12). Even though the molecular mechanisms governing cooperative interaction of dual receptor complexes have not yet been clearly explained, both estrogen and progesterone play critical roles during pregnancy and can mediate their regulatory effects either independently, synergistically or antagonistically. Thus, progesterone mediated events are complex, involving one or more levels of regulation including hormone synthesis, receptor synthesis, receptor activation, and receptor–receptor interaction.

Receptor Deficient Mice as Tools for Understanding Hormone Action

Construction of the progesterone receptor mutant provided the essential information that implicates the critical role of progesterone in "all" aspects of female reproduction, including lordosis, ovulation, uterine development, and development of the mammary gland. The knock-out mouse was constructed by insertionally inactivating the two primary forms of the progesterone receptor (PR-A and PR-B) by insertion of a neoR gene downstream of the second ATG initiation codon, effectively disrupting transcription from both start sites (13). In a predictable manner, the PR mutants carried little or no observable phenotype and both the male and female offspring were able to grow normally into adulthood.

Northern analysis demonstrated the total loss of transcription from the mutated gene in the homozygote female, suggesting successful ablation of the only gene encoding PR. Similarly, binding assays of uterine tissue confirmed that the ability to bind titrated-progestin in vitro was compromised in a dose dependent manner. The heterozygote mutant predictably retained about 50% of the wild type activity, whereas the homozygote mutant had no detectable activity, supporting the success of ablating a single gene encoding PR (13).

The homozygote female is infertile, although the heterozygotes of both sexes as well as the homozygote male retain the ability to sire normal (although somewhat smaller size) litters. The lordodic response of the homozygote females was completely abolished in experiments where their ovariectomized wild type littermates elicited a normal response after injection of estrogen and progesterone. Likewise, ovarian function was compromised upon superovulation with PMSG and hCG. Unlike the wild type controls, superovulation of the PR mutant did not elicit the appearance of oocytes in the oviduct or upper uterus; rather, histological examination showed that the mature oocytes were trapped within the mature follicle, apparently able to develop properly, but unable to be released in an appropriate manner. Mammary gland development, normally induced with prolonged exposure to pregnancy levels of estrogen and progesterone, showed no ductile branch development in the mutant female as compared to wild type, and clearly emphasizes the importance of progesterone in mammary gland development (13).

The mice used for these experiments (long exposure to high dose of estrogen and progesterone) also demonstrated distinct uterine phenotypes with unusual fluid retention, hyperplastic growth of the luminal epithelium, and an unexpected infiltration of polymorphonuclear leukocytes. These observations are not only in agreement with a theory of unopposed estrogen activity, but are also indicative of an acute inflammatory response, which suggests a role for progesterone in mediating pregnancy related immunity as well. Subsequent analysis of the uterine decidual response showed that the mutant uterus was unable to stimulate stromal cell differentiation, which in wild type females elicits a 20-fold increase in uterine weight (13,14). Clearly, this latter finding emphasizes the importance of progesterone during the early stages of pregnancy, primarily in the uterine stroma, at a time when stromal–epithelial cell interactions are critical for mediation of blastocyst attachment and trophoblast invasion.

The PR mutant is a very powerful tool for looking specifically at differentially expressed genes regulated by progesterone, and can be used to identify new gene targets that play crucial roles in pregnancy. Identification of new downstream targets should therefore facilitate the elucidation of progesterone-specific signaling pathways which should in turn, aid in the development of effective clinical treatments for the promotion and prevention of human pregnancy as well as for the diagnosis and treatment of diseased states including endometriosis and cancer.

Targets of Progesterone Regulation During Early Pregnancy

As the "pregnancy" hormone, progesterone clearly mediates specific expression of numerous genes in a coordinated manner, and in many cases is dependent upon estrogen mediated responses. This becomes apparent with the opening and closing of the "window of uterine receptivity" that requires progesterone sensitization as well as "triggering" by nidatory estrogen (15). The sensitization by progesterone requires a minimum of 48 h in the rodent, which clearly suggests that progesterone triggers a "cascade" of gene induction, undoubtedly involving multiple pathways that are cell type specific and temporally regulated to coordinate the transition of the multiple endometrial cell types. Following sensitization by progesterone, estrogen-dependent signaling processes must then be induced within a few h to transform the "sensitized" rodent endometrium to a "receptive" endometrium that can then facilitate attachment of an approaching blastocyst. This transformation involves signaling events both within the individual endometrial cellular compartments, as well as between the endometrium and the approaching embryo (16,17), but these individual mechanisms have not yet been coherently linked through a sequential gene induction pathway.

Some of the known targets of progesterone regulation in pregnancy include cytokines, growth factors, proteinases, proteinase inhibitors, angiogenic factors, and extracellular matrix components (for a comprehensive review, see (1)). Of these, it is likely that the growth factors and cytokines transmit more of the intracellular signaling between the different cell types in a cell specific paracrine manner. An example of such paracrine signaling would be typified by multiple activators of the receptor for epidermal growth factor (EGF-R). The existence of both estrogen-induced activators of EGF-R (epidermal growth factor) in the endometrial epithelium (18), and progesterone-induced activators (amphiregulin) in the epithelium (19), as well as activators that are induced either by estrogen in the epithelium or by progesterone in the stroma (heparin binding-growth factor like growth factor (HB-EGF) (20), clearly demonstrates the diversity of signaling with only a single membrane bound receptor. Such intricate regulation emphasizes the complexity of communication within the uterine milieu during the early stages of pregnancy. Another example is typified by the hormone dependent production of leukemia inhibitory factor (LIF) in the glandular epithelium and its receptor in the luminal epithelium just prior to implantation of the approaching blastocyst. Although it has been clearly demonstrated that blocking activation of the LIF receptor prevents implantation (21), the signaling mechanisms that mediate induction of LIF activity remain elusive.

Techniques for Identifying Downstream Targets of Progesterone Regulation In Vivo

It is clear that understanding the pathways of progesterone-induced signal transduction during pregnancy depends on the identification of more downstream targets, and their subsequent characterization both in terms of their independent regulation and their interrelationship with other mediators of pregnancy. An ideal approach would be to mechanically visualize differentially expressed genes dependent on the presence of hormone. Once target genes are identified, then the method should allow for easy isolation and subsequent molecular characterization. Below is an overview of some of the more popular techniques currently available for the identification and isolation of differentially expressed genes and a discussion of some of the advantages and limitations associated with each technique. The following section presents current work that utilizes some of this technology for identifying new targets of progesterone regulation.

Animal Treatments to Evaluate Progesterone Induction

The choice of animal treatments should be based on how the investigator wants to evaluate a particular physiological response. The most physiologically relevant way to identify genes involved in mediating the pregnant response would be to compare the natural pregnant state to the nonpregnant state. However, because of the highly complex nature of these states, many genes would be identified which could easily turn out to be down-regulated by estrogen rather than up-regulated by progesterone, or may be turned on by the embryo while having nothing to do with the maternal aspects of mediating uterine receptivity. This is clearly the most relevant system to study, but it is also the most complex and may result in identifying genes that are not necessarily involved in progesterone mediated events in the uterus.

To focus more on progesterone specific targets, one can simplify the system by isolating the uterine environment from the interactive interplay between the uterus and the approaching blastocyst by ovariectomizing the animals and hormonally inducing with the hormone(s) of choice. A regimen consisting solely of progesterone would also isolate the uterus from any interference from estrogenic effects. However, since in most pregnancy-related responses, expression of the progesterone receptor is dependent on induction by estrogen, this potentiates the possibility that many physiologically relevant progesterone targets may not be detectable in this system.

A more direct and effective system would be to use ovariectomized mice comparing wild type and PR mutant females which are subjected to a hormone regimen that mimics pregnancy (14). Theoretically in the PR mutant, estrogen would exert its normal effects, inducing all the respective estrogen-dependent precursor pathways, but the subsequent progesterone signaling pathways would be turned off even in the presence of progesterone. Several classes of progesterone targets would be differentially expressed: those that are solely regulated by progesterone (up or down in the mutant), those that normally interact with estrogen in a synergistic manner (down-regulated in the mutant), and those that normally interact with estrogen in an antagonistic manner (up-regulated in the mutant). The limitation of this system is that unopposed estrogen induction would resemble the latter category of genes and such induction would require subsequent characterization in terms of estrogen mediated effects.

Screening Techniques for Differentially Expressed Genes In Vivo

Upon isolation of the tissue from the various treatment groups, RNA would then be isolated and examined for differential expression using any one of several different methods. The method of choice will ultimately be dependent upon the availability of resources, time, and technical expertise. What is presented here is not at all a comprehensive review, rather just an overview of some of the popular alternative approaches for identifying differentially expressed genes that are regulated by progesterone. A brief comparison of these are presented in Table 9.1.

TABLE 9.1. Approaches for identification of differentially expressed genes.

Technique	Considerations
Direct screening	Hypothesis driven; limited to only a few probes at one time.
Chip technology	Many sequences screened simultaneously; limited to only known sequences; limited accessibility.
Differential screening	Direct approach; limited to abundantly expressed genes.
Subtracted libraries	Enriches for unique sequences; one directional; loss of less abundant sequences; requires substantial amount of time and starting material.
Differential display RNA fingerprinting	Straightforward; comparison of multiple samples simultaneously; yields distinct profiles of gene expression; very sensitive; minimal starting material needed; redundant; time consuming verification; high frequency of false positives.

Direct Evaluation

This approach, in which suspected targets are directly evaluated based upon previously published work, is hypothesis driven. For this, one simply needs to attain the probe(s) suspected to be involved and simply evaluate them for differential expression using either Northern analysis, RNase protection analysis, or even quantitative RT-PCR. Screening by this approach is straightforward and could easily produce quick results but is limited to evaluation of only a few genes at a time. This screening approach is clearly limited since it does not have the ability to identify alternative candidates.

Chip Technology

A recently developed robotic-based system used to quickly and mechanically screen large numbers of samples for specific gene expression has been modified to monitor and identify differentially expressed genes in two populations of RNA (22). Samples of individual cDNAs are initially amplified by PCR in microtiter plates and are then transferred in nl amounts by robotic pinheads to glass microscope slides. In preparation for subsequent hybridizations, these cDNAs are chemically linked to the glass surface and denatured by heat. In differential screenings of two different populations of RNA, each RNA population is labeled with a fluorescently labeled form of dCTP in a single round of reverse transcription. One population is labeled with fluorescein, while the other population is labeled with lissamine. After labeling, the fluorescently labeled probes are mixed and hybridized to a single microarray. Hybridizations and washing steps typically utilize high stringency conditions and therefore is very specific for the cDNAs tested. Following washing, the array is then scanned at two wavelengths following excitation of the two fluors. This method facilitates the quantitative and direct comparison of the levels of expression in each of the two samples, facilitating the identification of differentially expressed genes. Although set-up is expensive, the ability to both identify specific expression of any known cDNA and to simultaneously screen for differential expression between two populations makes this a technique of high value for laboratories that screen numerous samples continuously. The major limitation is that the arrays are imprinted with only known sequences although these sequences may only represent partial cDNAs such as ESTs, and therefore circumvents the possibility of identifying unique sequences.

Differential Screening

Another straightforward approach is to differentially screen a library containing the target genes. Duplicate sets of filters are used to lift representative lambda plaques infected with the library of interest. One set is then hybridized with total cDNA probes made from one tissue type, the other set probed with total cDNA from the other tissue type. Clones that only hybridize with one or the other tissue specific probes represent genes that are specifically expressed in one of the treatment groups. This approach has the advantages of being straightforward, not requiring detailed molecular strategies, and is useful in identifying unique genes in either population. However, the major drawbacks are that screening depends on the loss of a signal that can be easily camouflaged by neighboring positive signals and is better for abundantly expressed transcripts because rare sequences will have very low specific concentrations in the cDNA probes. In some screens for pregnancy related targets, differential screening yielded 40 potential clones which ultimately resulted in representing only two independent transcripts (23). Although useful, there is a clear preference for abundantly expressed transcripts. Also, this method is dependent upon the construction of a good cDNA library which is often difficult, and requires a large amount of cDNA for the screening steps.

Subtracted Libraries

A way to enrich for unique sequences in one of two populations is to eliminate the transcripts common to both populations through the construction of a subtracted library. This procedure is time consuming, entailing the synthesis of cDNA from tissue containing the unique transcripts and hybridizing it to the poly(A)+RNA from the tissue lacking the transcripts of interest. Separation of the remaining single stranded cDNAs from the cDNA-mRNA hybrids with hydroxy-lapatite column chromatography leaves a pool of nonhybridized cDNAs enriched for unique sequences. A purification step includes the rehybridization of the enriched cDNA to the original pool of poly(A)+RNA and the double stranded hybrids are then isolated and subjected to second strand cDNA synthesis. The enriched cDNA is then cloned into a vector such as lambda bacteriophage and differentially screened as described above. Usually, such libraries enrich the population so that 20% to 50% of the resulting clones are unique to the tissue of interest.

Unfortunately, such subtraction will eliminate sequences that have either a high degree of homology to other subtracted sequences or which contain repetitive sequences (such as Alu repeats in the 3' untranslated region), and it has a high potential for eliminating sequences with small differences in expression. Not only is this method limited because of a single direction of differential expression, but a substantial amount of initial starting tissue must be acquired for both treatments just to have enough useful poly(A)+RNA for the hybridization-subtraction step and then again for the subsequent differential screening of the library. Although this can be somewhat offset by PCR amplification after each of the subtraction steps, such amplification results in preferential cloning of smaller cDNAs. In a tissue like mouse uterine endometrium, it can be quite time consuming just to acquire sufficient tissue for these steps. This has however, been successfully accomplished using rat endometrial tissue to identify HB-EGF as a progesterone regulated target in endometrial stroma (20).

Differential Display or RNA Fingerprinting

Differential display (DDRT-PCR) is RNA fingerprinting using sets of arbitrary primers for PCR amplification, and is useful in quickly identifying and isolating differentially expressed RNAs in multiple samples simultaneously. Comparisons are done using reverse transcription and PCR amplification of the different cDNA pools (24,25). A strong advantage of this technique is that for a given set of arbitrary upstream primers, it gives a fingerprint of the amplified RNA's and allows comparison of multiple fingerprints on a single sequencing gel. In a clinical setting, such fingerprints of diseased tissue can be used for quick preliminary diagnostic applications (26). From these RNA fingerprints, differentially expressed bands can be isolated and cloned for further identification and evaluation in mediating the physiological response. Quantitative amplification of the RNA samples is based on the fidelity of a single round of reverse transcription within each sample and consistency of simultaneous PCR amplifications using different combinations of upstream primers. A high degree of reproducibility and therefore a high yield of true positives, can be achieved through the simultaneous comparison of different pools of RNA and duplicate RT reactions for each treatment group. Although the initial RNA fingerprint is quick and can be optimized with minimal expertise, this method entails visualization of low abundant as well as abundantly expressed PCR amplified products. This warrants that very sensitive assays (i.e., quantitative RT-PCR) may be required for the subsequent verification of differential expression, and in such cases may require timely optimization of the assay system for each of the individual candidates.

Variations of this method include Molecular Indexing (27) and Gene Expression Indexing (28), which both rely upon the restriction enzyme cleavage of the cDNA and ligation to tagged linkers for PCR amplification. These methods theoretically reduce redundancy and can allow for amplification of upstream regions of the cDNAs, but these are not yet popular methods of choice probably since they require more technical handling. A major drawback of early attempts with this technique had been that only short PCR amplified products usually representing the 3' untranslated regions of the genes would be isolated, making it necessary to screen cDNA libraries to attain full length clones for characterization. Differential display is becoming more popular as systems using improved primers and better PCR amplification systems are being developed to increase the size of the PCR amplified products and to minimize false priming, thus improving the frequency of isolating true positives and also reducing the need to isolate larger cDNAs in subsequent characterizations. Because of its straightforward methodology, its sensitivity and the ability to evaluate numerous sets of RNAs simultaneously, differential display is becoming one of the strongest methods for the identification of differentially regulated genes.

Isolation of Progesterone Targets Using the PR Mutant Mouse and Differential Display RT-PCR

We currently have screens in progress for the identification of differentially expressed genes during the early stages of pregnancy using the PR mutant mouse line and differential display RT-PCR. These screens are designed to target the identification of new progesterone-dependent genes during receptivity and the very early stages of progesterone signaling without regulatory interference from estrogen. Such identification and characterization of a panel of genes should enable the compilation of an interactive signaling pathway for progesterone mediated responses during the periimplantation period.

In a screen for identification of markers of receptivity, total uterine RNA was taken from either wild type or PR mutant mice which had been ovariectomized, allowed to recover for two weeks, and artificially induced with hormones to mimic the sensitization of the pregnant uterus. After resting, the mice were subjected to three daily injections of estrogen (100 ng, for priming of the uterine compartments) and after two days, injected with a single dose of progesterone (1 mg) in the presence of nidatory estrogen (6.7 ng) (15). Following exposure to progesterone for 24 h in both the wild type and PR mutant, the uteri were harvested and used for RNA isolation. The RNAs were then reverse transcribed and PCR amplified in accordance with the manufacturers of the GeneHunter RNA-Image kit.

Duplicate animals for each treatment group and duplicate RT reactions for each batch of RNA were run simultaneously on the same sequencing gels. Only those bands that showed reproducible differential expression were cut from the gels, PCR amplified, cloned and subsequently sequenced and verified for differential expression. A total of 27 independent sequences were identified in this screen, where the PCR amplified products ranged between 100 and 750 bp. Only eight sequences were detectable by Northern analysis, but of these, five were verified for having differential expression (Table 9.2). One of the five inducible genes had homology for alcohol dehydrogenase-Type III, which is thought to be involved in free radical metabolism. The remaining four clones represent unique sequences with no known homology to GenBank sequences. Two of the unique sequences show at least a five fold induction by progesterone in the wild type uterus after 24 h and one of these seems to be preferentially expressed in reproductive tissue. Full length cDNAs are currently being isolated for each clone to further characterize their roles in mediating pregnancy.

This screen is only at the early stages of identifying a panel of progesterone regulated genes, but offers the potential of clearly implicating new bio-

TABLE 9.2. Differential display screen for markers of receptivity.

	Number of isolated clones
Total independent sequences	27
Detectable by Northern analysis	8
Verified positives by Northern analysis	5(63%)
Known sequences	1 (Alchohol dehydrogenase, Type III)
Unique sequences	4

chemical information in mediating the progesterone mediated response in the pregnant uterus. Detailed characterization of the expression of each gene will include hormone induction in vivo, induction during pregnancy, timing of induction, and characterization of secondary effects on downstream targets. It should be noted that at this point, our screen has identified numerous candidates for hormonal regulation of which just a small handful have been analyzed for verified differential expression—with a high degree of success. The remaining clones that were not effectively detected by Northerns are still awaiting verification and remain viable candidates for hormone regulated gene targets. Although our initial focus is to characterize the genes we have already verified, the next step will be to work out more sensitive assays to verify differential expression and identify additional targets from the clones we have already isolated. The genes identified by these techniques could be used to discern the regulatory mechanisms involved in the biology of the uterus as well as provide tools to identify the factors regulating uterine gene expression. Once fully characterized in the mouse, the panel of genes identified can then be evaluated in terms of mediating the human pregnant state. It would certainly be of interest if some of the markers of receptivity in the mouse could be used as clinical tools to help identify optimal times and/or conditions for mediating conception in humans. As tools, these markers may also prove to be useful in identifying and treating molecular abnormalities in diseased or cancerous uterine tissue as well.

References

1. Funk CR, DeMayo FJ. The role of progesterone in the uterus. In: Knobil E, Neil JD eds. Encyclopedia of reproduction. San Diego: Academic Press, 1998.
2. Baulieu EE. Contraception and other clinical applications of RU 486, an antiprogesterone at the receptor. Science 1989;245:1351–7.
3. Baulieu EE. RU 486 as an antiprogesterone steroid: from receptor to contraception and beyond. JAMA 1989;262:1808–14.
4. Meldrum DR. Female reproductive aging–ovarian and uterine factors. Fertil Steril 1993;59(1):1–5.
5. Kraus WL, Monano MM, Katzenellenbogen BS. Cloning of the rat progesterone receptor gene 5'-region and identification of two functionally distinct promoters. Mol Endocrinol 1993;7:1603–16.
6. Graham JD, Yeates C, Balleine RL, et al. Progesterone receptor A and B protein expression in human breast cancer. J Steroid Biochem Mol Biol 1996;56(1–6):93–98.
7. Wei LL, Miner R. Evidence for the existence of a third progesterone receptor protein in human breast cancer cell line T47D. Cancer Res 1994;54:340–3.
8. Kraus WL, Kazenellenbogen BS. Regulation of progesterone receptor gene expression and growth in the rat uterus: modulation of estrogen actions by progesterone and sex steroid hormone antagonists. Endocrinology 1993;132:2371–9.
9. Johnson JL, Toft DO. A novel chaperone complex for steroid receptors involving heat shock proteins, immunophilins, and p23. J Biol Chem 1994;269(40):24989–93.
10. Beato M, Herrlich P, Schutz G. Steroid hormone receptors: many actors in search of a plot. Cell 1995;83:851–7.

11. Bradshaw MS, Tsai SY, Leng X, et al. Studies on the mechanism of functional cooperativity between progesterone and estrogen receptors. J Biol Chem 1991;266(25): 16684–90.

12. Oñate SA, Tsai SY, Tsai M-J, O'Malley BW. Sequence and characterization of a coactivator for the steroid hormone receptor superfamily. Science 1995;270:1354–7.

13. Lydon JP, DeMayo FJ, Funk CR, et al. Mice lacking progesterone receptor exhibit pleiotropic reproductive abnormalities. Genes Devel 1995;9:2266–78.

14. Ledford BE, Rankin JC, Markwald RR, Baggett B. Biochemical and morphological changes following artificially stimulated decidualization in the mouse uterus. Biol Reprod 1976;15:529–35.

15. Finn CA, Martin L. The role of the oestrogen secreted before oestrus in the preparation of the uterus for implalntation in the mouse. J Endocrinol 1970;47:431–8.

16. Pollard JW. Regulation of polypeptide growth factor synthesis and growth factor-related gene expression in the rat and mouse uterus before and after implantation. J Reprod Fertil 1990;88:721–31.

17. Weitlauf HM. Biology of implantation. In: Knobil E, Neill J, eds. The physiology of reproduction. New York: Raven, 1988:231–62.

18. Huet-Hudson YM, Chakraborty C, De SK, Suzuki Y, Andrews GK, Dey SK. Estrogen regulates the synthesis of epidermal growth factor in mouse uterine epithelial cells. Mol Endocrinol 1990;4:510–23.

19. Das SK, Chakraborty I, Paria BC, Wang X-N, Plowman G, Dey SK. Amphiregulin is an implantation-specific and progesterone-regulated gene in the mouse uterus. Mol Endocrinol 1995;9:691–705.

20. Zhang Z, Funk C, Roy D, Glasser S, Mulholland J. Heparin-binding epidermal growth factor-like growth factor is differentially regulated by progesterone and estradiol in rat uterine epithelial and stromal cells. Endocrinology 1994;134(3):1089–94.

21. Cullinan EB, Abbondanzo SJ, Anderson PS, Pollard JW, Lessey BA, Stewart CL. Leukemia inhibitory factor (LIF) and LIF receptor expression in human endometrium suggests a potential autocrine/paracrine function in regulating embryo implantation. Proc Natl Acad Sci USA 1996;93:3115–20.

22. Schena M. Genome analysis with gene expression microarrays. BioEssays 1996;18(5): 427–31.

23. Kasik J, Rice E. A novel complementary deoxyribonucleic acid is abundantly and specifically expressed in the uterus during pregnancy. Am J Obstet Gynecol 1997;176(2):452–6.

24. Liang P, Pardee A. Differential display of eukaryotic messenger RNA by means of the polymerase chain reaction. Science 1992;257:976–7.

25. Welsh J, Chada K, Dalal SS, Ralph D, Chang R, McClelland M. Arbitrarily primed PCR fingerprinting of RNA. Nucl Acids Res 1992;20:4965–70.

26. Mok SC, Wong K-K, Chan RKW, et al. Molecular cloning of differentially expressed genes in human epithelial ovarian cancer. Oncology 1994;52:247–52.

27. Kato K. RNA fingerprinting by molecular indexing. Nucl Acids Res 1996;24(2): 394–5.

28. Ivanova NB, Belyavsky AV. Identification of differentially expressed genes by restriction endonuclease-based gene expression fingerprinting. Nucl Acids Res 1995;23(15): 2954–8.

Part IV

Molecular Markers of Receptivity

10

Mucins Provide a Barrier
to Embryo Implantation

MARY M. DESOUZA, GULNAR A. SURVEYOR, XINHUI ZHOU,
JOANNE JULIAN, AND DANIEL D. CARSON

Implantation Is a Multistep Process
and Hormonally Regulated

The process of embryo implantation is in actuality a multistep event. The initial phase involves the interaction or attachment of the embryonic trophectoderm with the uterine lumenal epithelia. Subsequently, a more intimate contact forms between the embryo and the uterus with ultimate placental formation. The secondary processes of implantation are classified into several categories based on whether the trophectoderm/trophoblast cells invade or fuse with the uterine epithelia (UE). In contrast, although there are differences in these secondary processes, the initial phase of implantation, that is, the attachment stage, is a universal phenomenon among species (reviewed in (1)). On the gross anatomical and histological scale, the process appears identical in all species examined. Yet, it is still unclear at the molecular level whether these different mammalian species utilize common factors to facilitate this initial event in implantation.

Uterine Environment: Nonreceptive Versus Receptive

The ovarian steroid hormones, estrogen (E) and progesterone (P), are critical for implantation. These hormones, when presented at appropriate ratios and temporal program create a discrete interval of time in the uterus during which implantation can take place. This period is referred to as the receptive phase. Prior to and after this phase the uterus is nonreceptive, and embryos are not able to attach and implant. Although the seminal discovery of the importance of steroid hormones in implantation was made approximately 40 years ago, little is know about the critical cell surface molecules regulated by these hormones that mediate attachment (For review (1,2)). Criteria for positively acting factors are that they are expressed during the receptive phase of pregnancy, that the expression must occur on the apical surface of UE, and, lastly, that complementary ligands or receptors must be expressed on the apical trophectodermal surface of the attachment competent embryo. There are few proteins put forth as mediating implantation that meet these criteria (1). Furthermore, the universality of these specific molecules in facilitating attachment is questionable. It remains possible that different species use different cell adhesion systems during the attachment phase.

Similarly, little is known about the factors present in the nonreceptive uterus that prevent embryo attachment. A universal characteristic of the uterine epithelium (UE) is the presence of a glycocalyx covering of the apical surface of these cells. One class of molecules found in the glycocalyx are mucin glycoproteins. Mucins are extremely large glycoproteins categorized into two classes, secreted and transmembrane mucins. O-linked carbohydrate moieties typically represent greater than 50% of the total molecular mass of these glycoproteins. The secreted forms of mucin are responsible for the gel-like mucus found lining the lumens of multiple organs systems (e.g., stomach, colon, trachea). Eight different secreted mucin genes have been cloned in the human; of these, only one gene is a transmembrane mucin, Mucin-1 (MUC1).

MUC1 Structure

MUC1 is organized into three regions (reviewed in (3)). The extracellular or ectodomain region contains a tandem repeat region largely consisting of serine, threonine, and proline residues. The serine and threonine residues provide a multitude of potential O-linked glycosylation sites, and the prolines are theorized to lend rigidity to the peptide core of the protein. This rigidity creates a structure that extends 200 to 500 nm from the epithelial cell surface (Fig. 10.1). This is in dramatic comparison to other glycocalyx components which extend no more than 30 to 35 nm (4). The transmembrane domain of 31 amino acids spans the plasma membrane once, thus making MUC1 a type-I membrane glycoprotein. Lastly, the cytoplasmic tail is approximately 69 amino acids long and contains several tyrosine residues that can be phosphorylated (5). Evolutionarily, the transmembrane and cytoplasmic (CT) regions of MUC1 are highly conserved. In fact, antibodies raised against a specific 17 amino acid peptide sequence within the CT region is found to cross react with multiple species (6). In contrast, the ectodomain sequence varies greatly among species. A conserved feature of the ectodomain sequence is the presence of multiple tandem repeat regions containing abundant serine, threonine, and proline residues rather than specific primary amino acid sequence. The tandem repeat region differs among species and in humans genetic polymorphisms within this region cause the number of repeats to vary (7). This large structure creates a steric barrier such that adhesive

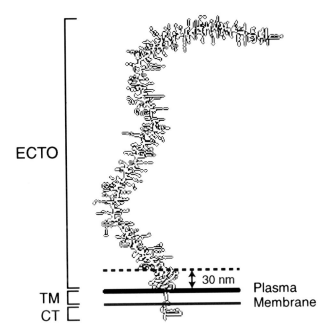

ECTO

30 nm

TM

CT

Plasma
Membrane

FIGURE 10.1. Structure of MUC1 molecule. MUC1 is a type-I transmembrane glycoprotein organized into 3 domains. The extracellular or ectodomain (ECTO), transmembrane
(TM) domain, and cytoplasmic tail region (CT). The ectodomain can extend 200–500nm
above the cell surface (4) and contains a large number of O-linked carbohydrate chains.

molecules are not able to interact with their targets (4,8,9). Given the abundance of MUC1 in the nonreceptive uterus and its nonadhesive nature, it is
proposed that MUC1 represents a barrier to attachment.

Expression of MUC1 in Nonhuman Species

Allowing that MUC1 is expressed in the uterus and creates a barrier to embryo
attachment, how then can implantation proceed? Examination of the expression
pattern of murine uterine Muc1 (lowercase letters indicate nonhuman ortholog)
revealed that Muc1 decreases in the estrous cycle at diestrus and also decreases
at the time of receptivity (i.e., day 4.5 of pregnancy) (10). Furthermore, Muc1
expression also is diminished during the receptive phase in other mammalian
species (11,12, DeSouza and Carson, unpublished observation). In species such
as mouse, rat, baboon, and pig, there is a loss of Muc1 expression on the entire
lumenal surface of the uterus (10–12, DeSouza and Carson, unpublished observation). In contrast, the rabbit exhibits a local loss of Muc1 only at embryo
implantation sites (Hoffman, Olson, Chilton, and Carson, unpublished observa-

tion). In the mouse and rat there is a coordinate loss of the transcript which encodes Muc1(10). While strategies for removing Muc1 may vary among species, loss of Muc1 during the receptive phase appears to be a general principle. As discussed below, humans may be an important exception to this rule.

Steroid Hormone Regulation of Muc1

Ovarian steroids regulate the timing of receptivity in the uterus and are responsible for regulating the expression pattern of Muc1. In the mouse, E stimulates the expression of Muc1 and P opposes the E-stimulation (10). Steroid hormone replacement studies in the pig and baboon also have shown that Muc1 expression is altered by exogenous steroidal regimens (11,12). Thus, it is apparent that there is a hormonal regulation of the expression of Muc1 in several mammalian species. However, it is not clear if this regulation occurs at the transcriptional or translational levels. Studies in the mouse and rat indicate that the steady state level of mRNA encoding Muc1 are reduced during the receptive phase of pregnancy (10, DeSouza and Carson, unpublished observation). In addition, steroid hormone receptor antagonists are able to block the steroid-mediated responses in the mouse uterus demonstrating that the changes are controlled through the respective steroid hormone receptors, estrogen receptor (ER) and progesterone receptor (PR) (10). While the increase in response to E is likely to be the result of increased transcription, loss of Muc1 mRNA could be the result of a decrease in transcription rate, increase in mRNA degradation rate, or a combination of both processes. Classically, transcriptional changes in steroid-regulated genes occur through the interaction of the liganded hormone receptors with steroid response elements (SRE) located in the gene promoter. Examination of the mouse Muc1 promoter revealed several potential SREs in the 5' promoter sequence (Fig. 10.2). Results from tran-

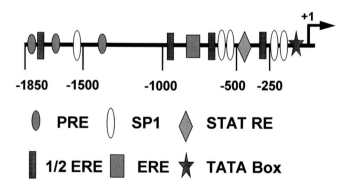

FIGURE 10.2. Schematic representation of mouse Muc1 promoter. Sequence analysis of 1.85 kb of the 5' mouse Muc1 promoter revealed several cis-DNA elements for potential regulation of the mouse Muc1 gene. Putative PRE elements are assigned according to the criteria of von der Ahe et al. (25).

sient transfection assays performed in both normal murine breast and uterine epithelial cells indicate that the potential estrogen response elements (ERE) do not function to activate transcription of the mouse Muc1 gene. This is true either in the context of the 1.8kb mouse promoter, in the presence of the first intron of the Muc1 gene or heterologous promoter constructs. It remains possible that sequences outside the 1.8 kb promoter are necessary to cooperate with these potential EREs to produce E-responsiveness (Zhou and Carson, unpublished observation). Alternatively, it is plausible that in ovariectomized mice, E acts at the level of the uterine stroma which, in turn, elicits a signal or factor that stimulates Muc1 transcription in UE. Such "cross-talk" between UE and stromal cells has been demonstrated for mitogenesis and lactoferrin gene activation in response to E (13). Muc1 gene regulation in response to P also may be complex. Three potential P response elements (PRE) exist in the distal region of the mouse Muc1 promoter (Fig. 10.2); however, the modest repression of transcription seen (35%–50%) in response to P and PR does not account for the large (90%–95%) reduction of Muc1 observed in response in vivo (10). Linkage of the first intronic sequence to the promoter to provide additional gene sequence does not alter the minimal changes seen in promoter activity (DeSouza and Carson, unpublished observation). Again, the possibility remains that there are Muc1 gene sequences outside of these regions that are necessary to synergize with the promoter. Alternatively, liganded PR may not act directly on the mouse Muc1 promoter, but rather act upstream on other genes that regulate Muc1 within UE cells. In addition, the reduction in relative levels of Muc1 mRNA in response to P administration could, at least in part, reflect increased Muc1 mRNA degradation. These possibilities currently are being examined. It also will be of interest to utilize tissue recombinant models (13) with UE or uterine stroma derived from ER null and PR null mice to determine which uterine cell types mediate the ER and PR driven effects on Muc1 expression. Regardless of the steps involved in the molecular regulation of the Muc1 gene, it is clear that steroid hormones are key regulators of uterine Muc1 expression in multiple species.

Human MUC1 Expression and Regulation

In contrast to the expression pattern seen in many animals, humans do not display a general loss in MUC1 expression during the receptive (midluteal) phase (14). MUC1 is expressed throughout the menstrual cycle and actually appears to increase during the secretory phase correlating with the time of receptivity in the pregnant uterus (14–16). This increase in MUC1 expression in the human during the secretory phase correlates with changes in the hormonal environment, but no published studies have shown a direct regulation by steroid hormones. In spite of the lack of such data, it seems clear that neither E nor P appreciably decreases MUC1 expression in the human. Thus regulation of MUC1 expression in human uteri has some features distinct from laboratory or domestic species.

MUC1 Function in the Human Uterus

Given that MUC1 is maintained in the human uterus, how is it possible for the human embryo to implant during the receptive phase? Two possibilities exist: (1) The first is that MUC1 is lost focally at implantation sites as occurs in rabbits (Hoffman, Olson, Chilton, and Carson, unpublished observation). It has been suggested that MUC1 is proteolytically processed and released into the uterine lumen. In fact, ELISA assays of uterine flushings readily detect MUC1 (16). Furthermore, the form of MUC1 seen in these flushings lacks the cytoplasmic tail, suggesting that it is cleaved by a protease. It is possible that the MUC1 protein is released from the lumenal surface by a protease activity though no such protease has been isolated from the same flushings. Potentially, the blastocyst could produce such an enzyme or signal the UE to activate an endogenous cell surface mucin-releasing protease. A protease of blastocyst origin was postulated to function in rabbit implantation. This protein, dubbed "blastolemmase," was proposed to digest the mucin coat surrounding rabbit blastocysts (17). Given that the rabbit has a focal loss of Muc1 during implantation, it is possible that a "blastolemmase" also may degrade uterine Muc1. A similar mechanism could function in the human, though mucin-degrading activities have not been described in either human UE or blastocyst cultures.

The second possibility is that MUC1 might be converted from an antiadhesive to an adhesive molecule during the receptive phase. Changes in the carbohydrate structures on the MUC1 core protein could mediate such a switch in function and have been reported in glandular UE and in uterine flushings of women (14,18). In addition, evidence from our lab indicates that the luminal UE of women also undergoes a switch in glycoform expression from day 9 to day 21 of the menstrual cycle although this does not parallel the changes seen in glandular UE (Julian, DeSouza, Babaknia, and Carson, unpublished observation). Certain carbohydrate groups, that is, sialyl-Lewis[x] and sialyl-Lewis[a], are found on forms of MUC1 in secretory phase uterine flushings (18). These sugar epitopes are known to function as ligands for a class of cell adhesion molecules called selectins. Selectin molecules are proteins usually expressed on cells of the immune system and mediate inflammatory and wound responses (reviewed in (19)). In theory, initial attachment of human embryos could be mediated via selectin molecules on the apical surface of the trophectoderm and if UE switch MUC1 glycoforms to selectin ligands. Previous studies suggest that the sialyl-Le[x] and sialyl-Le[a] epitopes are expressed by both glandular UE at the proliferative and secretory phase, indicating that no glycoform "switching" occurs (18). Nonetheless, patterns of expression in lumenal and glandular UE can be distinct (11, Julian et al., unpublished observation). Thus, it remains unclear whether selectin ligands appear at the lumenal UE surface at the time of receptivity and if MUC1 bears these epitopes at this site. Furthermore, it is not known if human blastocysts express selectin molecules on their exterior surface although human oocytes do express L-selectin (20).

MUC1 Antiadhesive Behavior

Given the pattern of MUC1 expression, can it truly prevent embryo attachment to UE? In mice, in vitro embryo attachment assays indicate that mucins, in general, and particularly Muc1 can prevent mouse embryo attachment to polarized UE. Polarized UE normally express abundant amounts of mucins (21) and are functionally nonreceptive (22,23). Digestion of polarized UE with an enzyme that specifically degrades mucins increases the percentage of embryos that attach to more than 50% (Surveyor and Carson, unpublished observation). Thus, general removal of mucins facilitates embryo:UE attachment. A similar enhancement in embryo attachment is seen when comparing polarized UE from wildtype mice and mice that have a targeted disruption in the Muc1 gene (24). These data suggest that the loss of Muc1 alone creates an environment receptive to embryo attachment in vitro. Is the antiadhesive behavior of Muc1 to embryo interaction unique to UE? To answer this question, in vitro aggregation assays of human cell lines that were stably transfected with the full length form of human MUC1 (4,8,9) were tested for their ability to interact with attachment competent mouse blastocysts. These studies revealed that cells which did not express MUC1 readily bind to mouse embryos, while expression of MUC1 alone severely reduced this activity (Julian, DeSouza, and Carson, unpublished observation). Collectively, these data indicate that MUC1 is a critical molecule in the maintenance of a nonreceptive uterus.

Summary

In conclusion, while it is evident that steroid hormones are critical in the regulation of uterine receptivity, there is little known about the steroid-regulated target proteins in the uterus during the periimplantation period. The mucin glycoprotein, MUC1, proposed to provide a barrier to embryo implantation, is down-regulated in multiple species at the time of receptivity. Uterine Muc1 expression in several species is regulated by E and P and this response is mediated by the respective steroid hormone receptors, ER and PR. The critical Muc1 gene elements responsible for modulating changes in Muc1 expression are an active area of investigation. The expression pattern of human MUC1 differs from that found in several other mammalian species. MUC1 in human glandular and lumenal UE is not down-regulated in the midluteal phase of the menstrual cycle. It remains to be determined whether human MUC1 is lost focally at implantation sites or undergoes a change in glycosylation to become an adhesive molecule. Clearly, understanding the regulation of MUC1 during the peri-implantation period will enhance our knowledge of how steroid hormones control uterine receptivity.

Acknowledgments. This work was supported in part by NIH grant HD29963 (to D.D.C.) as part of the National Cooperative Program for Markers of Uterine Receptivity and a Lalor Foundation Fellowship (to M.M.D.)

References

1. Tabibzadeh S, Babaknia A. The signals and molecular pathways involved in implantation, a symbiotic interaction between blastocyst and endometrium involving adhesion and tissue invasion. Mol Hum Reprod 1995;10:1579–602.
2. Psychoyos A. Nidation window: from basic to clinic. In: Dey SK, ed. Molecular and Cellular Aspects of Periimplantation Processes. New York: Springer-Verlag, 1995:1–14.
3. Gendler SJ, Spicer AP. Epithelial mucin genes. Annu Rev Physiol 1995;57:607–34.
4. Wesseling J, van der Valk SW, Hilkens J. A mechanism for inhibition of E-cadherin-mediated cell–cell adhesion by the membrane-associated mucin episialin/MUC1. Mol Biol Cell 1996;7:565–77.
5. Zrihan-Licht S, Baruch A, Elroy-Stein O, Keydar I, Wreschner DH. Tyrosine phosphorylation of the MUC1 breast cancer membrane protein: cytokine receptor-like molecules. FEBS Let 1994;356:130–6.
6. Pemberton L, Taylor-Papadimitriou J, Gendler SJ. Antibodies to the cytoplasmic domain of the MUC1 mucin show conservation throughout mammals. Biochem Biophys Res Comm 1992;185:167–85.
7. Lancaster CA, Peat N, Duhig T, Wilson D, Taylor-Papadimitriou J, Gendler SJ. Structure and expression of the human polymorphic epithelial mucin gene: an expressed VNTR Unit. Biochem Biophys Res Comm 1990;173:1019–29.
8. Ligtenberg MJL, Buijs F, Vos HL, Hilkens J. Suppression of cellular aggregation by high levels of episialin. Cancer Res 1992;52:2318–24.
9. Wesseling J, van der Valk SW, Vos HL, Sonnenberg A, Hilkens J. Episialin (MUC1) Overexpression inhibits integrin-mediated cell adhesion to extracellular matrix components. J Cell Biol 1995;129:255–65.
10. Surveyor GA, Gendler SJ, Pemberton L, Das SK, Chakraborty I, Julian J, et al. Expression and steroidal hormonal control of Muc-1 in the mouse uterus. Endocrinology 1995;136:3639–47.
11. Hild-Petito S, Fazleabas AT, Julian J, Carson DD. Mucin (Muc-1) expression is differentially regulated in uterine luminal and glandular epithelia of the baboon (Papio anubis). Biol Reprod 1996;54:939–47.
12. Bowen JA, Bazer FW, Burghardt RC. Spacial and temporal analyses of integrin and Muc-1 expression in porcine uterine epithelium and trophectoderm in vivo. Biol Reprod 1996;55:1098–106.
13. Cooke PS, Buchanan DL, Young P, Setiawan T, Brody J, Korach KS, et al. Stromal estrogen receptors mediate mitogenic effects of estradiol on uterine epithelium. Proc Natl Acad Sci 1997;94:6535–40.
14. Hey NA, Graham RA, Seif MW, Aplin JD. The polymorphic epithelial mucin muc1 in human endometrium is regulated with maximal expression in the implantation phase. J Clin Endocrinol Metab 1994;78:337–42.
15. Rye PD, Bell SC, Walker RA. Immunohistochemical expression of tumor-associated glycoprotein and polymorphic epithelial mucin in the human endometrium during the menstrual cycle. J Reprod Fertil 1993;97:551–6.
16. Hey NA, Li TC, Devine PL, Graham RA, Saravelos H, Aplin JD. MUC1 in secretory phase endometrium: expression in precisely dated biopsies and flushings from normal and recurrent miscarriage patients. Human Reprod 1995;10:2655–62.

17. Denker HW. Basic Aspects of ovoimplantation. Obstet Gynecol Annu 1983;12:1542.
18. Hey NA, Aplin JD. Sialyl-lewis x and sialyl-lewis a are associated with MUC1 in human endometrium. Glycoconjugate J 1996;13:769–79.
19. Lasky L. Selectin-carbohydrate interactions and the initiation of the inflammatory response. Ann Rev Biochem 1995;64:113–39.
20. Campbell S, Swann HR, Seif MW, Kimber SJ, Aplin JD. Cell adhesion molecules on the oocyte and preimplantation human embryo. Mol Human Reprod 1995;10:1571–8.
21. Pimental RA, Julian J, Gendler SJ, Carson DD. Synthesis and intracellular trafficking of MUC1 and mucins by polarized mouse uterine epithelial cells. J Biol Chem 1996;271:28128–37.
22. Valdizan M, Julian J, Carson DD. WGA-binding, mucin glycoproteins protect the apical cell surface of mouse uterine epithelial cells. J Cell Physiol 1992;151: 451–65.
23. Julian J, Carson DD, Glasser SR. Polarized rat uterine epithelium in vitro: responses to estrogen in defined medium. Endocrinology 1992;130:240–8.
24. Spicer AP, Rowse GJ, Lidner TK, Gendler SJ. Delayed mammary tumor progression in Muc-1 null mice. J Biol Chem 1995;270:30093–101.
25. von der Ahe D, Janich S, Scheidereit C, Renkawitz R, Schutz G, Beato M. Glucocorticoid and progesterone receptors bind to the same sites in two hormonally regulated promoters. Nature 1985;313:706–9.

11

Potential Involvement of Trophinin, Bystin, and Tastin in Embryo Implantation

MICHIKO N. FUKUDA, DAITA NADANO, NAO SUZUKI, AND JUN NAKAYAMA

Human Cell Lines Useful for Studying Implantation

Defining the cellular and molecular bases of embryo implantation is an important yet extremely difficult problem in developmental biology because of the lack of an appropriate in vitro model for implantation. In this regard two human cell lines, HT-H and SNG-M, are noteworthy, as these cells appear to mimic some, if not all, of the mechanisms involved in implantation. In particular, their unique manner of initial attachment at their respective apical cell surfaces and subsequent morphological changes leading to stronger adhesive interactions resemble the trophectoderm cells of blastocyst and endometrial epithelial cells at the implantation stage (1).

HT-H is a cell line established from a testicular teratocarcinoma tumor. HT-H cells spontaneously differentiate into syncytiotrophoblastic cells (2). Differentiated HT-H cells synthesize and secrete progesterone and human chorionic gonadotrophin. They also express cytokeratin, but not vimentin, which is indicative of the epithelial nature of this cell line.

The SNG-M line has been established from a metastatic region of an endometrial tumor. SNG-M cells respond to progesterone and estrogen and exhibit epithelial cell characteristics (3).

Both HT-H cells and SNG-M cells grow as adherent cells in culture. When HT-H cells are detached from a culture dish by trypsinization and added to a monolayer of SNG-M cells, the HT-H cells instantly attach to the upper or apical surfaces of SNG-M cells (Fig. 11.1A,B). HT-H cells also attach to the upper cell surfaces of each other, as do SNG-M cells. However, neither HT-H nor SNG-M cells attach to other types of human epithelial cells, such as HeLa, SW480, A431, and HepG2. Thus adhesion between HT-H and SNG-M cells are cell type specific and may be homotypic. EDTA has no effects on the initial attachment between HT-H and SNG-M cells, excluding the involvement of calcium dependent cell adhesion molecules, such as cadherins and integrins.

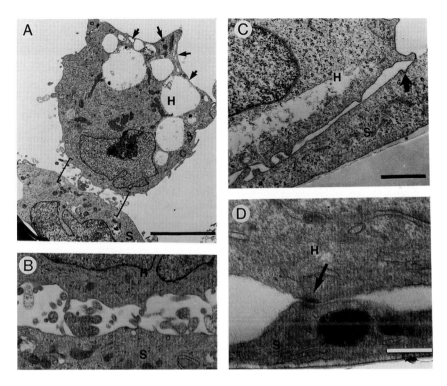

FIGURE 11.1. Electron micrographs of the HT-H cells cocultured on a SNG-M cell mono-layer. HT-H cells were added to a monolayer of SNG-M cells and both cell types were cocultured for up to four days. (A) An HT-H cell (marked as H, upper cell) after 10 minutes of attachment on a SNG-M cell (marked as S). The HT-H cell has microvilli on the lower side (presumably an apical surface originally) facing the upper surface of the SNG-M cell. The basal surface of the HT-H cell is indicated by short arrows. (B) Higher magnification of the area shown by a parenthesis in panel (A). Note that these two cell types contact via microvilli. H, HT-H cell; S, SNG-M cell. (C) Contact between the two cell types after 6 hours of attachment. Note that the microvilli are flattened in both cell types. Tips of microvilli extended from one cell type appear to attach directly to the plasma membrane of the other cell type. The SNG-M cells at this stage of contact often show invagination activity (shown by an arrow). (D) An HT-H cell cocultured on a monolayer of the SNG-M cells for 4 days. Note the absence of microvilli on the surface of both the HT-H (H, upper) and SNG-M (S, lower) cells. The contact between these two cell types are mostly focal, and occasional development of an adherent junction (shown by an *arrow*) is detected (1). Scale bars; 5 (A), 1 (B), and 0.5 (C and D) microns.

Electron micrographs of HT-H and SNG-M cells taken ten minutes after adhe-sion show that these two cell types attach at their respective apical surfaces, since numerous microvilli are present between the cells (Fig. 11.1A,B). At six hours after initial attachment, the numbers of these microvilli are significantly reduced, and the remaining microvilli are flattened and short (Fig. 11.1C). The apical surfaces of the endometrial SNG-M cells at this stage exhibit invagination activity resembling that of surface endometrium several hours after implantation. After 20 h of attachment, adhesion between HT-H and SNG-M becomes stronger and adherent junctions appear between these cells (not shown). After 4 days of coculture, microvilli completely disappear and desmosomes develop between the two cell types. Desmosomes, which in general are characteristic of lateral surfaces between epithelial cells, now appear at the apical surfaces of HT-H and SNG-M cells (Fig. 11.1D). Thus the initial attachment of HT-H and SNG-M cells leads to drastic rearrangements of the cytoskeleton and changes in cell polarity.

Therefore, the unique initial attachment at their respective apical cell surfaces and subsequent morphological changes seen in HT-H and SNG-M cells resembles trophoblasts and endometrial epithelial cells at implantation sites in vivo and suggests that these cell lines can be used to identify molecules involved in embryo implantation.

Identification of Trophinin, Bystin, and Tastin by Expression Cloning

Because we did not know the identity of adhesion molecules present in HT-H and SNG-M cells, we undertook an expression cDNA cloning strategy. Thus a mammalian expression cDNA library was constructed from HT-H cell mRNA using the pcDNAI vector. COS cells were chosen as a recipient line because they do not attach to the upper surface of SNG-M cells. Another advantage of COS cell is that they express SV40 T antigen for replication, allowing the pcDNAI plasmid containing an SV40 replication origin to be amplified upon transfection. COS cells were transfected with the HT-H cell library, and cells that adhered to SNG-M cells were selected (Fig. 11.2). The plasmid cDNA was rescued from the adherent COS cells and amplified in bacteria. This method allowed us to identify three novel molecules: trophinin, tastin, and bystin. We subsequently showed that COS cells transfected with either trophinin and tastin or trophinin and bystin adhere to the SNG-M cells (1,4).

Among these proteins, trophinin, which is predicted to be an intrinsic membrane protein, may be primarily responsible for initial attachment between HT-H and SNG-M cells. The most striking structural feature of trophinin is that more than 90% of this protein consists of tandem repeats of a decapeptide which may be the structural element required for self-binding. As described below, tastin and bystin may play an accessory role in trophinin-mediated cell adhesion.

A Cytoplasmic Protein, Bystin, Interacts with Trophinin and Tastin

Both bystin and tastin are cytoplasmic proteins. When trophinin is expressed alone in COS cells, it is seen as a regularly distributed antigen on the cell

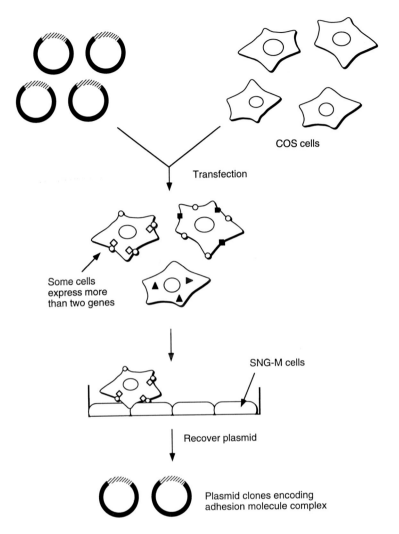

COS cells

Transfection

Some cells
express more
than two genes

SNG-M cells

Recover plasmid

Plasmid clones encoding
adhesion molecule complex

FIGURE 11.2. Expression cloning of molecules mediating an initial attachment between HT-H and SNG-M cells. A cDNA library of the HT-H cells was constructed in the mammalian expression vector pcDNAI. COS cells were transfected with the library. Because untransfected COS cells do not adhere to a monolayer of SNG-M cells, it was expected that if COS cells were transfected by cDNAs encoding an appropriate adhesion molecule, they would acquire the ability to adhere to a SNG-M cell monolayer. Transfected COS cells which adhered to a monolayer of the SNG-M cells were then selected and plasmid clones involved in cell adhesion were identified. The adhesion assay showed that a mixture of two cDNAs (either trophinin and tastin, or trophinin and bystin) was necessary for COS cells to adhere to SNG-M cells (1).

surface. In contrast, when trophinin and tastin are expressed together, trophinin is seen as a clustered patch on the cell surface. Thus tastin appears to induce clustering of trophinin. As tastin apparently associates with the cytoskeleton in both HT-H and SNG-M cells, association of trophinin with tastin would restrict the distribution of trophinin, creating multivalent and efficient cell adhesion sites in the plasma membrane.

The yeast two hybrid assay of protein–protein interactions showed, however, that trophinin and tastin do not directly bind to each other. We subsequently found another cytoplasmic protein, bystin, which binds trophinin and tastin. Thus a series of yeast two hybrid assays revealed that trophinin and tastin interact with each other through bystin (4).

The results obtained by the yeast two hybrid assay were confirmed by an in vitro protein binding assay. Thus recombinant bystin produced by in vitro translation using reticulocyte lysates binds to a fusion protein, glutathione-S-transferase (GST)-trophinin, produced in bacteria. Recombinant trophinin binds to GST-tastin when bystin is present. Thus bystin appears to be a key molecule bridging trophinin and tastin (Fig. 11.3).

Association of trophinin and cytoplasmic proteins may be important for regulating cell adhesion activity, as association of trophinin to the cytoskel-

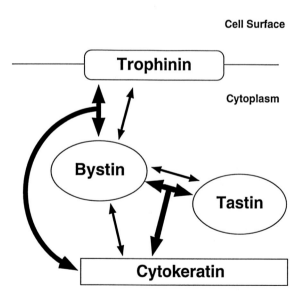

FIGURE 11.3. Moleculr interactions of trophinin, bystin, tastin, and cytokeratins Each trophinin, tastin, and cytokeratin independently binds to bystin as shown by the thin arrows. Interaction among three or trophinin, bystin, and cytokeratin (*thick arrow*) is stronger than that of the two. Similarly, interaction among bystin, tastin, and cytokeratin (*thick arrow*) is stronger than that of any two of these components (4).

eton may restrict its distribution on the cell surface and create potent adhesion foci. Bystin and tastin contain many potential phosphorylation sites, suggesting that these molecules are involved in signal transduction triggered by trophinin-mediated cell attachment. Future studies will address the molecular mechanism of the initial attachment between HT-H and SNG-M cells, leads to the morphological changes described above (Fig. 11.1).

After an initial attachment of the blastocyst to the endometrial epithelium, the trophoblasts at contact proliferate rapidly and invade endometrial tissues. It is likely that the initial contact sends signals to the cytoplasm and further to the nuclei, which induce gene expression involved in cell proliferation. Future studies will address the roles of cytoplasmic proteins in signal transduction and the in vivo role of the cytoplasmic proteins in implantation and trophoblast invasion.

Trophinin, Bystin, and Tastin Are Expressed in Cells Involved in Implantation

Immunohistology and Northern analysis of various human tissues revealed that trophinin, bystin, and tastin are either not expressed or expressed weakly in normal adult human cells. Trophinin and tastin are not detected in the human endometrium at the proliferation stage and at the ovulation stage. Strong expression of trophinin is seen in a restricted region of the apical plasma membranes of the surface epithelium at the early secretory phase (Fig. 11.4C). Tastin was also detected in the endometrial epithelial cells, which express trophinin.

Strong expression of trophinin is detected at the apical plasma membranes of trophectoderm of monkey blastocysts (Fig. 11.4E). Trophinins are elevated at the embryonic pole and are relatively weakly expressed at the mural pole. Such polarized distribution of trophinin is consistent with observations that in primates, including humans, a blastocyst attaches to endometrial epithelium at its embryonic pole (6).

Immunohistology and in situ hybridization show that trophinin, bystin, and tastin are coexpressed in trophoblasts and in endometrial epithelial cells at the implantation site in monkeys (Fig. 11.4F) and humans (Nakayama, unpublished data). Unique expression patterns of trophinin, bystin, and tastin in primate implantation site suggest that these molecules play an important role in human embryo implantation.

Testing the In Vivo Role of Trophinin by Creating Trophinin Gene Knock-Out Mice

Analysis of transgenic mice in which the gene of interest is knocked-out by homologous recombination is a reliable way to examine the in vivo function

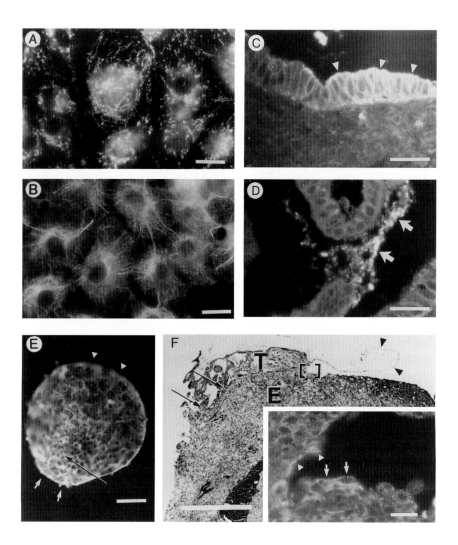

FIGURE 11.4. Immunofluorescence micrographs of trophinin and tastin in SNG-M cells and cells involved in implantation. (A) Trophinin expressed in SNG-M cells. (B) Tastin expressed in SNG-M cells. (C) A surface epithelium of human endometrium at early secretory phase. Trophinins are detected on the apical plasma membranes (*arrowheads*). (D) Presence of trophinin in mucus in human endometrium at the late secretary phase. (E) Immunofluorescence micrograph of rhesus monkey blastocyst stained with antitrophinin antibodies. Inner cell mass is shown (*long arrow*). Note that cells at the embryonic pole (*short arrows*) were stained more intensely than those at the mural pole (*arrowheads*). (F) A light micrograph of a macaque monkey uterus tissue with an implanted and approximately 15 day blastocyst. Arrowheads show cytotrophoblasts of blastocyst. Long arrows show anchoring villi (trophoblasts penetrating the endometrial epithelium). T, trophoblasts; E, hypertrophic endometrial epithelium. Inset shows an immunofluorescence micrograph of higher magnification of the area marked by a parenthesis. Both trophoblast (*arrowheads*) and endometrial epithelium cells (arrows) are stained by antitrophinin antibodies. Scale bars: 10 (A,B,C,D, and F inset), 25 (E), and 200 (F) microns.

of that gene. Although there are significant morphological differences in embryo implantation between humans and mice, creating trophinin null mice should provide an excellent animal model for studying the role of trophinin in vivo.

Because the trophinin gene maps to the X chromosome, heterozygous female mice in which one trophinin alle is replaced with the neo gene have been created. A cross between heterozygous females (+/−) and wild type males (+/) is expected to produce female (+/+, +/−) and male (+/) pups at a ratio of 2 to 1 if trophinin null male blastocysts (−/) fail to implant (Fig. 11.5).

Crosses between G-1 females (+/−) and wild type males (+/), however, resulted in the survival of many trophinin null (−/) male pups (G-2). Interestingly, when G-2 heterozygous females (+/−) were further crossed with wild type males (+/), G-3 pups resulting from these crosses showed female and

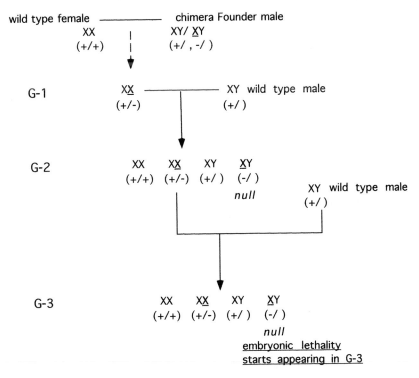

FIGURE 11.5. Examining the in vivo role of trophinin by creating trophinin gene knockout mice. Because trophinin gene maps to X chromosome, a cross between heterozygous female (+/−) and wild type male (+/) will produce wild type female (+/+) heterozygous female (+/−), wild type male (+/) and null male (−/) pups. If trophinin null male blastocysts fail to implant, then the ratio of female and male offsprings will be 2 to 1. As described in text, trophinin null male pups were born in early generation (G-2), whereas embryonic lethality of null male (−/) start appearing in a later generation (G-3).

male offsprings at a ratio of 2 to 1. Genotype analysis revealed a significant reduction of trophinin null (–/) males in G-3. Therefore it appears that undefined factors impaired the trophinin null phenotype in early generations. Such factors might have been introduced in embryonic stem cells during harsh treatment required for transfection of the targeting vector and subsequent drug selection. Dilution of these factors, achieved by crossing with wild type mice, allowed the trophinin null phenotypes to become apparent in later generations (Nadano and Fukuda unpublished data). Further study is needed to determine if lethality of a trophinin null male embryo is the result of a failure of implantation.

References

1. Fukuda MN, Sato T, Nakayama J, Klier G, Mikami M, Aoki D, et al. Trophinin and tastin: a novel cell adhesion complex with potential involvement in embryo implantation. Genes Devel 1995;9:1199–210.
2. Izhar M, Siebert P, Oshima RG, DeWolf WC, Fukuda MN. Trophoblastic differentiation of human teratocarcinoma cell line HT-H. Devel Biol 1986;116:510–8.
3. Ishiwata I, Nozawa S, Inoue T, Okumura H. Development and characterization of established cell lines from primary and metastatic regions of human endometrial carcinomas. Cancer Res 1977;37:1777–85.
4. Suzuki N, Fukuda MN. A novel cytoplasmic protein, bystin, interacts with trophinin and tastin, the molecules with potential involvement in implantation. In: Gomel V, Leung PCK, eds. In vitro fertilization and assisted reproduction. Bologna, Italy: (Monduzzi) 1997:759–64.

12

Osteopontin in Human Endometrium: A Role in Endometrial Receptivity and Embryo Implantation?

CHRISTOS COUTIFARIS, AKINYINKA OMIGBODUN,
PIOTR ZIOLKIEWICZ, AND JOHN HOYER

It is generally accepted that extracellular matrix proteins are not only central in providing the substrate for the anchoring of cells, but, most importantly, they play either permissive or inhibitory regulatory roles in the migration of cells. It has become quite clear that these matrix proteins participate in the signaling events regulating these cellular processes by binding to integrin cell adhesion molecules expressed on the surface of cells (1). During the process of embryo implantation, the trophoblast not only is required to interact directly or indirectly with the endometrial epithelium, but in those animals (including the human) in which invasive implantation is observed, trophoblasts adhere and migrate through the stromal extracellular matrix, continuously degrading and remodeling it (2). In animals exhibiting hemochorial placentation this migratory activity of the trophoblast cells continues until invasion into the maternal vessels and replacement of the endothelial cells with trophoblasts is achieved (3).

We have recently focused our attention on the secretory matrix phosphoprotein, osteopontin (OPN), as a possible mediator of adhesive and/or signaling events relating to the regulation of human trophoblast adhesion, migration, and invasion. Osteopontin is a 45 kD phosphorylated glycoprotein that was originally found to be present in mineralized mammalian tissues such as bone (4). In fact, OPN acquired its name when it was discovered that it mediated the adhesion of osteoclasts to bone, and it was thought of as the molecular "bridge" between the cell and the bone matrix (5,6). Its widespread synthesis and secretion has since been confirmed, and it has been shown to be expressed by a variety of epithelial tissues as well as diverse populations of cells found in the mesenchyma (7,8). Although OPN's precise function as a signaling molecule is still under investigation, significant evidence points to the direction that this matrix protein may have important roles in processes involved in angiogenesis and tissue remodeling (9,10). Early work by Young et al. (11) indicated that OPN mRNA was present in extracts of secretory, but not proliferative, endometrium and that its protein was present in the decidua of pregnancy. More recently, work from our laboratory has demonstrated the regulated expression of OPN in human trophoblasts, and, specifically, the cytotrophoblasts of floating villi. These experiments have conclusively shown that the expression of this matrix protein at both the mRNA and protein levels was regulated by cyclic AMP and by progesterone (12–15). Although we have recently extended the observations of Young et al. (11) in defining more precisely the expression and regulation of OPN in human endometrial epithelium (Omigbodun et al. unpublished data), the expression of this protein in the endometrial stroma and, most importantly, the decidua of pregnancy has been less well characterized. This chapter further investigates the expression of OPN in human endometrium and specifically evaluates the regulation of the stromal expression of this protein by estrogen and progesterone.

Materials and Methods

Endometrial tissue was obtained from premenopausal women after hysterectomy performed for nonmalignant indications, such as uterine myomata. Decidua of pregnancy were obtained from gentle scraping of the placental cotyledons at the maternal fetal interface or from the surface of the fetal membranes. In addition, endometrial specimens from dilatation and curettage of patients suffering from an ectopic pregnancy were utilized. None of the procedures were performed specifically for the present investigation, and all the tissue utilized in this study was excess tissue not required for histopathologic evaluation of the specimen. Utilization of "residual" tissue for these studies has been approved by the Institutional Review Board of the University of Pennsylvania. Upon completion of the surgical procedure, the tissue specimen was quickly transported to the Pathology Laboratory, where the appropriate description and selection of tissue for histologic diagnosis was performed. Any excess endometrial/decidual tissue was placed in Dulbecco's modified eagle medium (DMEM) containing 10% heat inactivated fetal bovine serum and antibiotics. Once the tissue was transported to the research laboratory, it was liberally washed with ice cold Hank's solution, containing 1% penicillin-streptomycin and fungizone. Throughout the performance of these isolation procedures, sterility was maintained. For the cases where RNA isolation was performed, the tissue was quickly processed using the acid guanidine isothiocyanate method, and the tissue was homogenized using a polytron tissue homogenizer (16). For the separation of epithelial and stromal cells, the tissue was minced in 0.25% collagenase solution as 37°C in a shaking water bath for 90 minutes. Epithelial glands and stroma were separated using stainless steel sieves of 250 microns, 106 microns, and 38 microns in a sequential manner. Cells were isolated by back washing of the sieves. Stromal cells were obtained from the filtrate solution, because single cells passed even through the smallest (38 microns) sieve openings. Stromal cell culture was performed in medium consisting of RPMI 1640 and DMEM at 1:1 ratio supplemented with 10% FBS, 1% gentamicin, and 25 mg/ml fungizone. Cells were cultured in humidified 5% CO_2 95% air at 37°C. In some experiments, cells were exposed to estradiol (100 nM) and/or medroxyprogesterone acetate (100 nM) for 72 h prior to isolation and extraction of total RNA for Northern analysis.

For immunohistochemical staining, tissue samples were fixed in formalin and paraffin embedded, and subsequently sectioned. Staining procedures were processed in the microprobe manual immunostainer and a rat monoclonal antibody against human OPN at a concentration of 12 μg/ml was utilized (15). Characterization of this antibody has been previously described (17). Controls consisted of sections incubated with nonimmune rat serum.

Results

Indirect immunofluorescence of the human endometrial tissue confirmed previous results showing that proliferative endometrium did not express the OPN protein but secretory endometrium exhibited intense immunostaining of the epithelial cells (Fig. 12.1). With the exception of extracellular matrix

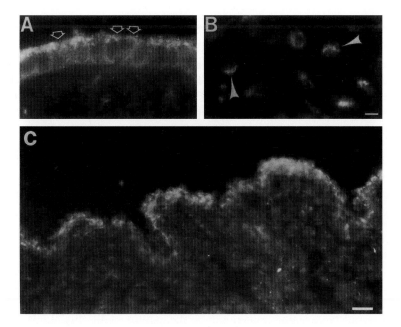

FIGURE 12.1. Indirect immunofluorescence for osteopontin (OPN) in human endometrium in the nonpregnant (A,C) and pregnant (B) state. Note the intense staining of the epithelium for OPN under both low power (C) and higher power (A). OPN appears to be localized mainly towards the apical pole of the cells (*open arrows*). During pregnancy, the majority of decidual stromal cells stain positively for OPN (D; *arrowheads*). Magnification A and B: bar = 10 microns; C: bar = 50 microns.

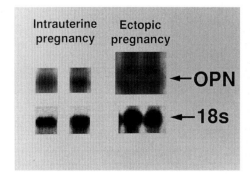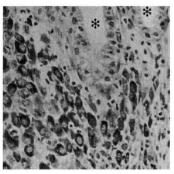

FIGURE 12.2. OPN expression and localization in human endometrium during pregnancy. Total mRNA was extracted from the decidua of two women with an intrauterine pregnancy and two women suffering from ectopic pregnancies. Note the abundant mRNA for OPN. Immunohistochemical localization (right) shows the protein to be present in the decidual cells while epithelial cells of glands (*) do not stain for OPN. Magnification ×200.

surrounding endometrial arterioles, no OPN staining was observed in endometrial stromal cells during either phase of the endometrial cycle.

Total mRNA obtained from either decidua of pregnancy or endometrial curettings from patients suffering with a tubal pregnancy exhibited high abundance of the OPN mRNA (Fig. 12.2). This finding was confirmed by immunohistochemistry, which showed strong staining of the endometrial stroma. Of particular interest was the observation that the endometrial stroma during pregnancy exhibited high levels of both OPN protein and mRNA in the stromal cells even in the absence of an intrauterine pregnancy. Thus, it appears that it is the endocrine/paracrine milieu of pregnancy rather than the juxtaposition of trophoblasts within the endometrium that regulate the expression of OPN by the endometrial decidua cells, and it can be concluded that OPN is a marker of endometrial cell decidualization.

Under basal conditions, endometrial stromal cells in culture showed very little or no OPN expression at the mRNA level. Exposure of the cells to estrogen and/or medroxyprogesterone acetate had no significant effect in stromal cells in culture isolated from secretory endometrium. Endometrial stromal cells isolated from the proliferative phase of the cycle exhibited a small induction of the OPN mRNA, which was most pronounced if the estrogen and progesterone were added sequentially to the culture media (Fig. 12.3).

Discussion

Thus, we further confirmed and extended the observations made by us and others with respect to the expression of OPN in human endometrium. Specifi-

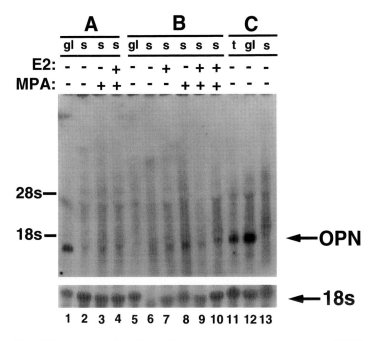

FIGURE 12.3. Effect of estradiol (E$_2$) and medroxy-progesterone acetate (MPA) on endometrial stromal cell OPN mRNA in culture. Cells were fractionated into glands (gl) and stroma (s) as described in the text from a secretory phase endometrium (A,C) and proliferative endometrium (B). Stromal cells were placed in culture and exposed for 72 h to the indicated hormone treatment. Sample C (lanes 11, 12: t, total endometrium; gl, glands; s, stroma) served as the positive and negative controls showing abundant mRNA in the epithelial cells of glands and absence of mRNA for OPN in the stroma. Note the marginal induction of OPN mRNA after treatment with estrogen and/or MPA regardless whether the two hormones were added together (lanes 4 and 9) or whether the cells were exposed to E$_2$ initially for 48 h and subsequently exposed to both E$_2$ and MPA for the subsequent 72 h (lane 10).

cally, we showed the cycle variation of OPN expression at both the mRNA and protein levels, and we further characterized the expression of OPN in the decidua of pregnancy. It is of great interest that OPN expression in the endometrium during pregnancy does not require the presence of an implanting embryo in the uterus. Even though OPN is not expressed by the stromal cells of human endometrium during the secretory phase of the menstrual cycle, the upregulation of expression during pregnancy in these cells was quite dramatic. The fact that there was marginal induction of OPN mRNA by stromal cells exposed to estrogen and/or progesterone indicates that other factors specific to pregnancy play an important role in the induction of expression of this protein. It can be concluded that although the presence of a pregnancy may be necessary for induction of the decidual expression of OPN, there is no need for the presence of an embryo within the endometrial cavity for this induction to occur. Thus, it appears that the effect is endocrine rather than paracrine and involves other factors in addition to estrogen and progesterone. Given that a modest induction of OPN by endometrial stromal cells in culture could be achieved by exposure to steroid hormones, it can also be hypothesized that the observed effect on endometrial stromal cells is a function related to the high levels of steroid hormones found during pregnancy. Nevertheless, this induction of OPN mRNA was minimal and in marked contrast to the dramatic up regulation observed with cAMP (Omigbodun et al., unpublished data). This observation suggests that, in vivo, the effect of the steroid hormones on OPN expression by stromal cells is probably mostly indirect through paracrine factors utilizing the cAMP pathway for signaling. Such mediators of steroid hormone action, as they relate to OPN expression by stromal cells during pregnancy, remain to be elucidated. It should be noted that the in vivo induction of OPN by estrogen and progesterone has been previously reported in the mouse (18).

The functional significance of our findings on the expression of OPN in human endometrium is unclear. It can be hypothesized that the epithelial expression and secretion of OPN in the secretory phase of the endometrial cycle may participate in signaling events that mediate the heptotactic migration of the trophoblast of the blastocyst and participate in the initial adhesion of this cell to the endometrial epithelium. The expression of the OPN receptors (members of the αV family of integrins) (19) by human blastocysts and trophoblasts provide the framework for possible adhesive and signaling events mediating this process (20). Further, the abundance of OPN in the decidua of pregnancy suggests the possible role for this protein in events surrounding decidualization and possibly the migration and invasion of trophoblasts during placentation. It should not be forgotten though that this is purely speculative at the present time, and the function of OPN in the decidua of pregnancy may be unrelated to the process of trophoblast adhesion and migration, but may participate in other critical events important to the decidualization process. For example, other cells found in human endometrium express members of the αV family of integrins, which may also be targets for the OPN action. Specifically, and most notably, endothelial cells are amongst the cell types expressing αV integrins, and given the possible role of OPN in angiogenesis and neovascularization, it can be hypothesized that this protein participates in the signaling events of this process, which is very active in decidualized endometrium during placentation (9,10,21). Alternatively, but not exclusively, many migratory cells of bone marrow origin are also known to express αV integrins, and it is well accepted that there is a significant migration into the endometrial stroma of such variety of cells during decidualization. These cells may be critical in the establishment of the immune tolerance of the conceptus during implantation.

In conclusion, OPN expression in human endometrium during the menstrual cycle and pregnancy appears to be regulated. At present, the functional significance of the expression of this protein in this tissue is unclear. Its spatial and temporal distribution coinciding with events associated with the process of embryo implantation make it very attractive to speculate that this matrix secretory protein plays a role in the cell biology of trophoblast attachment and migration during implantation. Nevertheless, such conclusions, even though attractive as hypotheses, are speculative at present, and further work trying to analyze further the direct effects of OPN on human trophoblast behavior needs to be completed. Although both the αV knock-out mouse can implant and the OPN knock-out female mouse is fertile, these observations do not exclude a role for this protein in human implantation. OPN expression in the mouse implantation site does not appear until after implantation has been initiated and placentation has progressed significantly, suggesting that in this experimental animal this protein may not be critical to the process (22). Alternatively, many investigators have hypothesized that the process of implantation is both complex, but also involves redundant cell adhesion molecules and their matrix proteins, thus ensuring a higher likelihood of the establishment of pregnancy. The diversity of matrix proteins present in the endometrium and the multitude of integrin heterodimers of both the αV and β1 family of integrins capable of binding the same ligands support such a general hypothesis. Certainly, both the temporal and spatial expression of OPN in human endometrium justifies further intense study into the function of this protein as it relates to either human trophoblast behavior or other processes related to the endometrium as it renders itself capable of accepting and supporting a pregnancy.

Acknowledgments. The authors wish to thank Ms. Valerie Baldwin for her help in the preparation of this manuscript. This work was supported by NIH grants HD-06274 (CC) and DK-33501(JH) and the Rockefeller Foundation (AO).

References

1. Ruoslahti E, Noble NA, Kagami S, Border WA. Integrins. Kidney Int 1994;45(Suppl 44):S17–22.
2. Aplin JD, Charlton AK, Ayad S. An immunohistochemical study of human endometrial extracellular matrix during the menstrual cycle and first trimester of pregnancy. Cell Tissue Res 1988;253:231–40.
3. Aplin JD. The cell biology of human implantation. Placenta 1996;17: 269–75.
4. Denhardt DT, Guo X. Osteopontin: a protein with diverse functions. FASEB J 1993;7:1475–82.
5. Butler WT. The nature and significance of osteopontin. Connect Tissue Res 1989;23: 123–6.
6. Reinholt FP, Hultenby K, Oldberg A, Heinegard D. Osteopontin—a possible anchor of osteoclasts to bone. Proc Natl Acad Sci USA 1990;87:4473–75.
7. Brown LF, Berse B, Van De Water L, Papadopoulos-Sergiou A, Perruzzi CA, Manseau EJ, et al. Expression and distribution of osteopontin in human tissues: widespread association with luminal epithelial surfaces. Mol Biol Cell 1992;3:1169–80.

8. Senger DR, Ledbetter SR, Claffey KP, Papadopoulos-Sergiou A, Peruzzi CA, Detmar M. Stimulation of endothelial cell migration by vascular permeability factor/ vascular endothelial growth factor through co-operative mechanisms involving the alpha v/ beta 3 integrin, osteopontin and thrombin. Am J Pathol 1996;149:293–305.

9. Giachelli CM, Liaw L, Murry CE, Schwartz SM, Almeida M. Osteopontin expression in cardiovascular diseases. Ann NY Acad Sci. 1995;760:109–26.

10. Liaw L, Skinner MP, Raines EW, Ross R, Cheresh DA, Schwartz SM, et al. The adhesive and migratory effects of osteopontin are mediated via distinct surface integrins: role of $\alpha_v\beta_3$ in smooth muscle migration to osteopontin. J Clin Invest 1995;95:713–24.

11. Young MF, Kerr JM, Termine JD, Wewer UM, Wang MG, McBride OW, et al. cDNA cloning, mRNA distribution and heterogeneity, chromosomal location, and RFLP analysis of human osteopontin (OPN). Genomics 1990;7:491–502.

12. Daiter E, Omigbodun A, Wang S, Walinsky D, Strauss JF III, Hoyer JR, et al. Osteopontin expression by human trophoblasts is regulated by cell differentiation and cyclic AMP. Endocrinology 1996;137:1785–90.

13. Omigbodun A, Daiter E, Walinsky D, Fisher L, Young M, Hoyer J, et al. Regulation of osteopontin expression in human trophoblasts. Ann NY Acad Sci 1995;760:346–9.

14. Omigbodun A, Tessler C, Ziolkiewicz P, Hoyer J, Coutifaris C. Progesterone regulates osteopontin expression in human cytotrophoblasts. Proceedings of the 51st Meeting of the American Society for Reproductive Medicine, Seattle, WA, October 1995:0–140.

15. Omigbodun A, Ziolziewicz P, Tessler C, Hoyer JR, Coutifaris C. Progesterone regulates osteopontin expression in human trophoblasts: a model of paracrine control in the placenta? Endocrinology 1997;138:4308–15.

16. Sambrook J, Fritsch EG, Maniatis T. Molecular cloning: a laboratory manual, 2d ed. Plainview, NY: Cold Spring Harbor Laboratory Press, 1989;719–25, 739–52.

17. Shiraga H, Min W, VanDusen WJ, Clayman MD, Miner D, Terrell CH, et al. Inhibition of calcium oxalate crystal growth in vitro by uropontin: another member of the aspartic acid-rich protein superfamily. Proc Natl Acad Sci USA 1992;89:426–30.

18. Craig AM, Denhardt DT. The murine gene encoding secreted phosphoprotein 1 (osteopontin): promoter structure, activity, and induction in vivo by estrogen and progesterone. Gene 1991;100:163–71.

19. Hu DD, Lin EC, Kovach NL, Hoyer JR, Smith JW. A biochemical characterization of the binding of osteopontin to integrins alpha v beta 1 and alpha v beta 5. J Biol Chem 1995;270:26232–8.

20. Campbell S, Swann HR, Seif MW, Kimber SJ, Aplin JD. Cell adhesion molecules on the oocyte and preimplantation human embryo. Hum Reprod 1995;10:1571–8.

21. Yue TL, McKenna PJ, Ohlstein EH, Farach-Carson MC, Butler WT, Johanson K, et al. Osteopontin-stimulated vascular smooth muscle cell migration is mediated by beta-3 integrin. Exp Cell Res 1994;214:459–64.

22. Waterhouse P, Parhar RS, Guo X, Lala PK, Denhardt DT. Regulated temporal and spatial expression of the calcium-binding proteins calcyclin and OPN (Osteopontin) in mouse tissues during pregnancy. Mol Reprod Devel 1992;32:315–23.

Part V

Trophoblast Factors

13

The Rabbit as a Model for Implantation: In Vivo and In Vitro Studies

LOREN H. HOFFMAN, D. RACHEL BREINAN, AND GARETH L. BLAEUER

Historically, some of the major concepts about implantation have been developed using the rabbit as the experimental animal. This includes the demonstration by Chang (1) of the requirement for synchronous development of embryos and endometrium to achieve successful implantation following blastocyst transfer to pseudopregnant hosts. An appropriate animal model generally implies that the results obtained will have relevance to many, if not all, mammals. With the focus of the research community on human health issues, an appropriate animal model may be restricted in meaning to one from which results have application to some aspect of human implantation. Other factors may influence selection of animals for a given study, particularly their availability, cost of purchase and maintenance, and length of pregnancy. Accordingly, while primates such as the rhesus monkey and baboon are regarded as good models for human reproduction, their use is impractical for many investigators. In practice the choice is often among rats, mice, and rabbits. Granted, rabbits lack a true estrous cycle, and implantation is not "interstitial" as in humans. Nevertheless, the arguably-most-critical aspects of rabbit endometrium, including its hormonal regulation, are similar to those of primates. Not only do the ostensibly negative characteristics of rabbit reproductive biology not undermine the applicability of the rabbit model to human implantation, but they also confer unique advantages—making the rabbit an excellent model for both in vivo and in vitro studies of implantation. These advantages will be discussed, along with recent progress on replicating embryo attachment using an in vitro system amenable to intervention for studying embryo-endometrial interactions.

Endometrial Preparation for Implantation

The rabbit is a reflex ovulator, and ovulation can be induced by mating or the injection of hCG/LH to induce pseudopregnancy (2). The ease of obtaining either pregnant (PG) or pseudopregnant (PSP) females and the precise timing of reproductive events constitute advantageous features of the rabbit. Both pseudopregnancy and pregnancy are characterized by a relatively constant, low level of circulating estradiol, and by progesterone concentrations which increase progressively through day 11 to 12 post ovulation (p.o.) (3). Thereafter, in PSP females luteal regression is initiated, and progesterone levels decline. In PG females implantation occurs on day 7, prior to which endometrial structural and biochemical features are comparable to those of pseudopregnancy. At prospective implantation sites, but not interimplantation regions, changes such as increased vascular permeability can be detected beginning around 6.5 days p.o. (4). Endometrial epithelial and stromal cells proliferate rapidly between days 0 to 4 p.o.; thereafter, progesterone-directed cellular differentiation and secretory activity take place (5,6). The increased number of cells is accomodated by the formation of numerous small mucosal folds, the lateral margins of which are lined by cryptal epithelium, which is structurally similar to the luminal epithelium (Fig. 13.1). This endometrial response is exquisitely progesterone-sensitive, such that the relative amplification of the endometrial surface is used as a bioassay for progestins (7). Structural and biochemical parallels between rabbit and human uteri have led to the use of PSP rabbits as a model for the luteal phase of humans (8). We proposed that the postovulatory endometrial condition in rabbits actually encompasses both proliferative (days 0–4) and secretory (after day 4) phases (5).

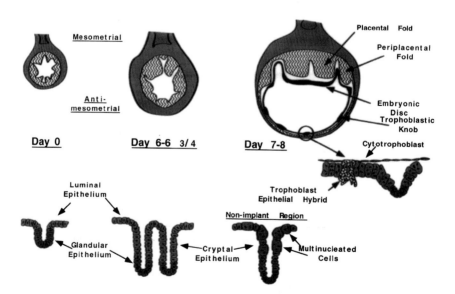

FIGURE 13.1. Features of rabbit endometrium between estrus (day 0) and implantation (day 7–8).

The distribution of progesterone receptor (PR) in rabbit endometrium between 0 and 6.75 days was examined by immunfluorescence microsopy (mouse monoclonal anti-PR, Affinity BioReagents) and is illustrated in Figure 13.2. Moderate levels of PR are present in nuclei of luminal and glandular epithelial cells, as well as in stromal cells at estrus (day 0). By day 4 of PG or PSP, the mucosal folds are well formed, and luminal, cryptal, and glandular epithelia react prominently, stromal cells moderately, with anti-PR. Just prior to implantation, day 6.75 PG, this distribution was remarkably altered. Both the luminal and cryptal epithelia over the mucosal folds were devoid of PR. Furthermore, stromal cells within the folds were likewise unstained. More

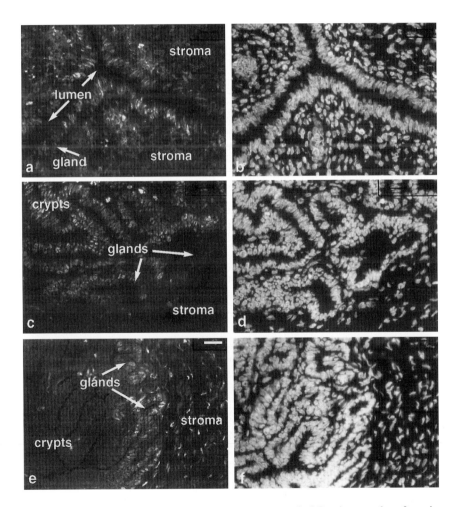

FIGURE 13.2. Fluorescence (a,c,e) and phase contrast (b,d,f) micrographs of uterine progesterone receptor distribution at estrus (a,b), day 4 PSP (c,d), and day 6.75 PG (e,f). Scale bar = 20 μm.

basally, however, the gland and deep crypt epithelial cells retained PR, as did stromal cells of the deep endometrium. Most glandular cells of the antimesometrial endometrium exhibited this pattern, while glands of the mesometrial endometrium contained few or no immunoreactive cells. These results are in agreement with a report on the distribution of PR in PSP uteri (8), but add to those findings the disparity of gland cell PR in antimesometrial versus mesometrial regions and differential staining in stromal regions on day 6.75 PG. It seems unlikely that these differences reflect our use of PG rather than PSP uteri, since the same PR distribution was seen in endometrium whether or not apposed to blastocysts.

In primates, the endometrium is stratified into four horizontal zones (9). Epithelial cells of the deep glands, zone IV, in the late secretory phase of rhesus monkey retain estrogen receptor and PR (10) and show a different pattern of steroid-related mitotic control than do cells of the more superficial zones (11). In rabbits as well, glandular epithelial cells differ structurally (5) and functionally (12,13) from those lining the lumen and crypts. This, together with the steroid receptor data above, leads us to concur with the proposal by Hegele-Hartung et al. (8) that the basal gland cells are a separate cell population from the crypt/luminal epithelium and may represent a reservoir for regenerating the epithelial surface epithelium. Accordingly, the more superficial structures, the luminal and cryptal epithelia and supporting stroma, would represent the rabbit equivalent of the zona functionalis.

Modulation of Endometrial Function by Hormones and Blastocysts

Uterine epithelial features in the rabbit which correlate with acquisition of the blastocyst-receptive state include alterations in apical membrane properties, such as decreased surface negative charge and changes in glycocalyx structure, increased affinity for certain lectins, and changes in stage-specific membrane polypeptides and in membrane-associated enzymes (14). A prominent redistribution of cell junction structures and coexpression of vimentin with cytokeratin intermediate filaments have also been documented. Denker (14) proposed that these features constitute an alteration in apical–basal polarity that prepares the epithelial cells for interaction with blastocysts at implantation. The modifications cited above, along with the appearance of specific uterine secretory products (15–17), occur during the progesterone-dominated early secretory phase. Paracrine factors important for implantation in rabbits include leukemia inhibitory factor (LIF) and platelet activating factor (PAF). For both of these the hormonal regulation of endometrial expression depends largely on progesterone, following the pattern seen in primates rather than that of rodents (18,19).

Studies recently carried out in our laboratory demonstrate the utility of rabbits as a model for analyzing implantation mechanisms, along with the regulation of endometrial products of significance to this process. These include studies on vascular endothelial growth factor (VEGF) and the epithelial transmembrane mucin Muc1. In rabbit endometrium the mRNAs for VEGF and the VEGF receptor Flk-1 are elevated just prior to implantation, 6 to 6.75 days PG (13). Furthermore, a redistribution of VEGF transcript occurs, from a uniform distribution in all uterine compartments in early preimplantation stages, to predominantly the luminal and cryptal epithelium just before implantation. This redistribution corresponds with that reported for VEGF mRNA in the secretory phase of human endometrium (20). Of additional interest was the finding that VEGF mRNA levels decreased during the implantation process, except at implantation sites. The high level maintained at implantation sites was the result, in part, to blastocyst expression of VEGF transcript, in particular to the trophoblast knobs which attach to uterine epithelium. VEGF receptor mRNA was localized to vascular elements in periimplantation stage rabbit endometrium (13). This suggests a role for trophoblast-derived VEGF in the vascular hyperpermeability associated with rabbit implantation (4) and in the subsequent expansion of the endometrial vascular bed.

Muc1 is a transmembrane mucin with antiadhesive properties that is found on the luminal surface of nonreceptive uteri in various species. In mice and pigs, Muc1 expression is up-regulated by estrogen and inhibited by progesterone, while in primates its expression is up-regulated by progesterone (21–24). In preliminary studies (Hoffman, Olson, Carson, and Chilton), it was shown that rabbit endometrial Muc1 expression is regulated as in primates, by progesterone. This would appear to have the counterproductive effect of presenting an antiadhesive epithelial surface to the blastocyst during the receptive phase. In the rabbit, Muc1 mRNA and protein expression are down-regulated locally at the site of blastocyst apposition. The evidence demonstrating this mechanism included in vitro experiments in which Muc1 immunostaining was reduced on epithelial cells apposed to trophoblast vesicles (see section on trophoblast attachment in vitro). The ability to localize and separate implantation sites from nonimplantation regions in rabbit uteri, or to obtain prospective sites (days 6.5–6.75 PG), has facilitated studies on blastocyst influences on endometrial function.

Patterns of Implantation

Rabbit blastocysts are large relative to those of most laboratory animals. They attain diameters of >5mm prior to implantation, by which time the blastocyst has expanded to fill the lumen, dilating the uterine wall (Fig. 13.3). Because the blastocyst contacts the whole uterine surface, implantation is termed "superficial" in type, a pattern shared with domestic animals, baboons, and rhesus monkeys (25). In contrast, implantation in the rat and mouse is "eccentric," and in humans it is "interstitial" (25). Rabbit blastocyst cytotrophoblast cells begin to aggregate into thickened areas, and these de-

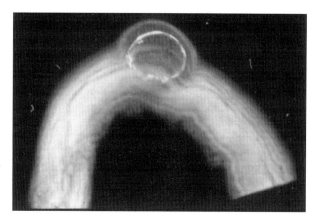

FIGURE 13.3. View of an implantation-stage rabbit blastocyst through the uterine wall (fixed and cleared specimen). Magnification ×~2.

veloping "trophoblast knobs" show evidence of cell fusion to produce syncytiotrophoblast before attachment to uterine epithelial cells begins (26,27). Blastocyst coatings break down ~7 days p.o., and trophoblast attachment to epithelial cells is initiated on the anti-mesometrial surface of the implantation chamber (26) (Fig. 13.4a). Attachment of trophoblast to the mesometrial surface is delayed until 8 days p.o. (26), and the chorioallantoic placenta develops at this location. Thus in rabbits, the trophoblast which attaches to and invades the endometrium at implantation is syncytial, as it is in primates (28). This contrasts with blastocyst attachment via cytotrophoblast, as seen in rats and mice.

Trophoblast Vesicle Attachment In Vitro

Early in vitro experiments on embryo attachment by Glenister (29) used rabbit blastocysts and organ cultures of endometrium. Unfortunately, the results did not simulate normal attachment, since nonreceptive endometrium was employed, blastocyst attachment was often to stromal tissue, and the trophoblast involved was cellular rather than syncytial. More recently, Hohn and Denker (30) improved upon this system to show that, in many respects, attachment and invasion resembled comparable processes in utero and that appropriate steroid treatment was beneficial. In those experiments, it was necessary to artificially hold blastocysts against the endometrial explants by confining them within a thin tube of dialysis material.

We have carried out a number of experiments on rabbit embryo attachment to extracellular matrix (ECM) components and to uterine epithelial cells. We have taken advantage of the large blastocyst size by subdividing them. Blastocysts are obtained by flushing uteri at 6.75 days p.o., just prior to implantation. Blastocyst coatings are removed by dissection, and trophoblastic vesicles are prepared us-

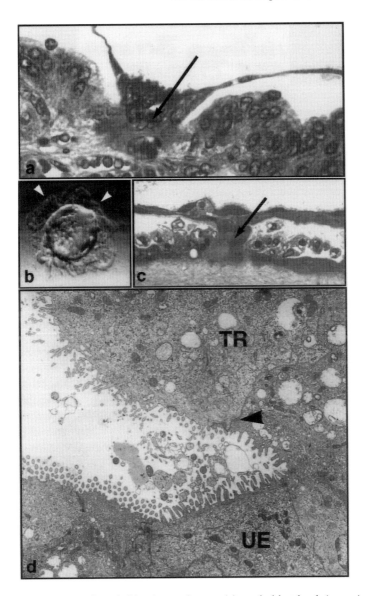

FIGURE 13.4. Features of trophoblastic attachment. (a) trophoblast knob (*arrow*) attachment to antimesometrial surface during implantation in vivo, (b) trophoblast outgrowth (*arrowheads*) from vesicle attached to ECM surface, (c) trophoblast knob (*arrow*) attaching to uterine epithelial cells and matrix in vitro, (d) electron micrograph showing the lateral margin of a trophoblast knob as seen in (c), junctions (*arrowhead*) are formed between trophoblast (TR) and uterine epithelial cells (UE).

ing microscissors to repeatedly cut blastocysts. From the 6 to 12 blastocysts obtained per female, 125 to 200 vesicles are obtained, with the apical trophoblast surface oriented externally. After vesicles recover their spherical shape during overnight incubation, they are seeded onto substrates. The smaller size and buoyancy of vesicles allow them to maintain closer apposition to the substrate during incubation than is possible with whole blastocysts. When cultured in serum-free medium, the vesicles attach to ECM-coated plastic surfaces, but not to uncoated plastic, beginning ~6 h after seeding. By 24 h significant numbers have attached. Vesicles attach well to a variety of ECM components, including collagen types III and IV, fibronectin, and laminin. Laminin seems to afford the best surface for attachment. Between 24 and 48 h, the vesicle trophoblast begins spreading to form outgrowths (Fig. 13.4b). These resemble the outgrowths from mouse blastocysts used to examine trophoblast differentiation and attachment properties (31). Similarly, rabbit trophoblast vesicles will attach to a monolayer of uterine epithelial cells. Epithelial cells are isolated from uteri of day 4 PSP females and cultured on porous filter surfaces coated with ECM as described previously (17). Attachment rate is monitored at 24 and 48 h of coculture, and attachment is typically in the 40% to 45% range. The vesicles form trophoblast knobs, as seen in vivo, and ultrastructural analysis shows that syncytial transformation at knobs has begun before attachment. Penetration of the epithelial layer and invasion of the underlying matrix is seen routinely, and where invasion takes place, trophoblast knobs are always present (Fig. 13.4c). Attachment has never been observed between cytotrophoblast and the uterine epithelial cells. Sharing of junctions between syncytiotrophoblast and uterine epithelial cells has been documented by EM analysis (Fig. 13.4d), but we have yet to see fusions between trophoblast and apical epithelial membranes as occurs in vivo (26). Steroid hormone treatment of cultures does not appear to increase the numbers or rate of vesicle attachments. Similar epithelial monolayers derived from immature rabbit uteri are reported to sustain their steroid responsiveness (32). It seems likely that the epithelial cells in our study have been suitably primed by hormone exposure in vivo prior to their isolation on day 4. These cultures produce the progesterone-dependent glycoproteins uteroglobin and haptoglobin without exogenous hormones (17). Furthermore, trophoblastic vesicle apposition to uterine monolayers induces the loss of apical Muc1 protein, as seen at implantation sites. Under modified culture conditions, the fusion of epithelial cells to form multinucleated cells has been observed, a process which occurs on day 7 PSP or PG (5,33). The influences of matrix type, hormonal treatment, and of stromal cell factors on this fusion and on vesicle attachment are still under investigation. In cocultures employing cells from estrous uteri, we have seen little vesicle attachment (~5%).

In summary, we have discussed several factors which make the rabbit an attractive animal model for studies on implantation. These include (1) the ease of obtaining precisely timed reproductive stages, (2) an analogy between endometrial regions in rabbits and the functionalis/basalis regions of primate endometrium, (3) comparable steroid hormone regulation for many endometrial functions between rabbits and primates, (4) the large blastocyst diameter, which facilitates identifying implantation sites and enables studies of blastocyst influences on the endometrium, and (5) the ability to obtain trophoblastic vesicles from preimplantation blastocysts and their development of specialized regions of syncytiotrophoblast. The vesicles interact with ECM substrates and uterine epithelial cultures in a fashion suggesting their utility for combined in vivo and in vitro studies on embryo attachment processes.

Acknowledgments. This work was supported by the National Cooperative Program on Markers of Uterine Receptivity for Blastocyst Implantation, HD29969, and by training grant HD07433 (D.R.B.).

References

1. Chang MC. Development and fate of transferred rabbit ova or blastocysts in relation to the ovulation time of recipients. J Exp Zool 1950;114:197–225.
2. Kanematsu S, Scaramuzzi RJ, Hilliard J, Sawyer CH. Patterns of ovulation-inducing LH release following coitus, electrical stimulation and exogenous LH-RH in the rabbit. Endocrinology 1974;95:247–52.
3. Browning JY, Keyes PL, Wolf RC. Comparison of serum progesterone, 20α-dihydroprogesterone, and estradiol-17β in pregnant and pseudopregnant rabbits: evidence for postimplantation recognition of pregnancy. Biol Reprod 1980;23:1014–9.
4. Hoos PC, Hoffman LH. Temporal aspects of rabbit uterine vascular and decidual responses to blastocyst stimulation. Biol Reprod 1980;23:453–9.
5. Davies J, Hoffman LH. Studies on the progestational endometrium of the rabbit. I. Light microscopy, day 0 to day 13 of gonadotrophin-induced pseudopregnancy. Amer J Anat 1973;137:423–6.
6. Murai JT, Conti CJ, Gimenez-Conti I, Orlicky D, Gerschenson LE. Temporal relationship between rabbit uterine epithelium proliferation and uteroglobin production. Biol Reprod 1981;24:649–53.
7. McPhail MK. The assay of progestin. J Physiol 1934;83:145–56.
8. Hegele-Hartung C, Chwalisz K, Beier HM. Distribution of estrogen and progesterone receptors in the uterus: an immunohistochemical study in the immature and adult pseudopregnant rabbit. Histochemistry 1992;97:39–50.
9. Bartelmez GW, Corner GW, Hartman CG. Cyclic changes in the endometrium of the rhesus monkey (*Macaca mulatta*). Contrib Embryol 1951;34:99–146.
10. Okulicz WC, Savasta AM, Hoberg LM, Longcope C. Biochemical and immunohistochemical analyses of estrogen and progesterone receptors in the rhesus monkey uterus during the proliferative and secretory phases of artificial menstrual cycles. Fertil Steril 1990;53:913–20.
11. Padykula HA, Coles LG, Okulicz WC, Rapaport SI, McCracken JA, King NW, et al. The basalis of the primate endometrium: a bifunctional germinal compartment. Biol Reprod 1989;40:681–90.
12. Olson GE, Winfrey VP, Matrisian PE, Melner MH, Hoffman LH. Specific expression of haptoglobin mRNA in implantation-stage rabbit uterine epithelium. J Endocrin 1997;152:69–80.
13. Das SK, Chakraborty I, Wang J, Dey SK, Hoffman LH. Expression of vascular endothelial growth factor (VEGF) and VEGF-receptor mRNAs in the peri-implantation rabbit uterus. Biol Reprod 1997;56:1390–9.
14. Denker HW. Trophoblast-endometrial interactions at embryo implantation: a cell biological paradox. Trophoblast Res 1990;4:3–29.

15. Anderson TL, Hoffman LH. Alterations in epithelial glycocalyx of rabbit uteri during early pseudopregnancy and pregnancy, and following ovariectomy. Amer J Anat 1984;171:321–34.
16. Beier HM. Uteroglobin and related biochemical changes in the reproductive tract during early pregnancy in the rabbit. J Reprod Fertil 1976;(Suppl)25:53–69.
17. Hoffman LH, Winfrey VP, Blaeuer GL, Olson GE. A haptoglobin-like glycoprotein is produced by implantation-stage rabbit endometrium. Biol Reprod 1996;55:176–84.
18. Yang Z, Chen D, Le S, Harper MJK. Differential hormonal regulation of leukemia inhibitory factor (LIF) in rabbit and mouse uterus. Mol Reprod Devel 1996;43:470–6.
19. Harper MJK. Platelet-activating factor: a paracrine factor in preimplantation stages of reproduction? Biol Reprod 1989;40:907–13.
20. Charnock-Jones DS, Sharkey AM, Rajput-Williams J, Burch D, Schofield JP, Fountain SA, et al. Identification and localization of alternately spliced mRNAs for vascular endothelial growth factor in human uterus and estrogen regulation in endometrial carcinoma cell lines. Biol Reprod 1993;48:1120–8.
21. Surveyor GA, Gendler SJ, Pemberton L, Das SK, Chakraborty I, Julian J, et al. Expression and steroid hormonal control of Muc-1 in the mouse uterus. Endocrinology 1995;136:3639–47.
22. Bowen JA, Bazer FW, Burghardt RC. Spatial and temporal analyses of integrin and Muc-1 expression in porcine uterine epithelium and trophectoderm in vivo. Biol Reprod 1996;55:1098–106.
23. Hey NA, Graham RA, Seif MW, Aplin JD. The polymorphic epithelial muci MUC1 in human endometrium is hormonally regulated with maximal expression in the implantation phase. J Clin Endocrinol Metab 1994;78:337–42.
24. Hild-Petito S, Fazleabas AT, Julian J, Carson DD. Mucin (Muc-1) expression is differentially regulated in uterine luminal and glandular epithelia of the baboon (Papio anubis). Biol Reprod 1996;54:939–47.
25. Wimsatt WA. Some comparative aspects of implantation. Biol Reprod 1975;12:1–40.
26. Enders AC, Schlafke S. Penetration of the uterine epithelium during implantation in the rabbit. Amer J Anat 1971;132:219–30.
27. Boving BG. Anatomical analysis of rabbit trophoblast invasion. Contrib Embryol 1962;37:33–55.
28. Enders AC. Contributions of comparative studies to understanding mechanisms of implantation. In: Glasser SR, Mulholland J, Psychoyos A, eds. Endocrinology of embryo-endometrium interactions. New York: Plenum; 1994:11–6.
29. Glenister TW. Observations on the behaviour in organ culture of rabbit trophoblast from implanting blastocysts and early placentae. J Anat 1961;95:474–85.
30. Hohn HP, Denker HW. A three-dimensional organ culture model for the study of implantation of rabbit blastocyst in vitro. Trophoblast Res 1990;4:71–95.
31. Armant DR. Cell interactions with laminin and its proteolytic fragments during outgrowth of mouse primary trophoblast cells. Biol Reprod 1991;45:664–72.
32. Mani SK, Decker GL, Glasser SR. Hormonal responsiveness by immature rabbit uterine epithelial cells polarized in vitro. Endocrinology 1991;128:1563–73.
33. Winterhager E, Busch LC, Kuhnel W. Membrane events involved in fusion of uterine epithelial cells in pseudopregnant rabbits. Cell Tissue Res 1984;235:357–63.

14

Regulation of Trophoblast Endocrine Function: The Placenta Does Its Own Thing Transcriptionally

Jerome F. Strauss III and Lee-Chuan Kao

The placenta is the most structurally diverse mammalian organ. The remarkable variation in the morphology of the placenta across species can be rationalized by the fact that the forces that drive placental evolution are different from those that impact upon the organism in postnatal life. The placenta must serve the competing needs of the mother and fetus; evolution presumably strives to increase the efficiency of this unique symbiotic relationship. Given these considerations, it is not surprising that recent advances in molecular biology have revealed that trophoblast cells employ novel mechanisms to control the expression of specific genes (1).

One of the major functions of the placenta is hormone production, a task of trophoblast lineage that is taken on prior to implantation (2). The trophectoderm secretes the signals through which the maternal organism recognizes the gestative state. The endocrine functions of the trophoblast encompass the synthesis of protein, glycoprotein, and steroid hormones. Among the protein hormones, it has long been recognized that the trophoblast forms its own versions of anterior pituitary hormones, including chorionic gonadotrophin, the placental lactogens, and variant growth hormone. Because the placental proteins are specified by unique genes, they have transcriptional regulatory mechanisms that can be distinguished from those controlling the expression of the homologous pituitary hormones.

In some species, including the human, placental progesterone production is required for the maintenance of pregnancy. Earlier investigators assumed that the rules that govern the synthesis of steroid hormones in the gonads and adrenal cortex would also apply to the placenta. This has proven to be erroneous. Indeed, the novelty of the strategies used by the trophoblast in regulating its steroidogenic activity is striking when compared to those employed by the steroidogenic cells of the gonads and the adrenal cortex. This review will focus on the unique aspects of the regulation of trophoblast steroidogenesis as a vehicle to emphasize the distinctive mechanisms exercised by the placenta to control gene expression.

Steroidogenic Factor-1 (SF-1) Is Not Expressed in the Human Placenta

The transcription of many of the genes encoding proteins involved in steroid hormone biosynthesis in the gonads and adrenal cortex is dependent on a member of the nuclear receptor family of transcription factors, steroidogenic factor 1 (SF-1), also called Ad-4-BP (3). Originally thought to be an orphan receptor, it appears that certain oxysterols may be the ligand activators of SF-1 (4). The steroidogenic cytochrome P450 enzyme gene promoters as well as the promoters of the steroidogenic acute regulatory protein (StAR) and the 3 β-hydroxysteroid dehydrogenase type II gene all contain at least one functionally important SF-1 binding element. The SF-1 binding cis elements are also important for cAMP-stimulated transcription of these genes.

While SF-1 protein and mRNA are abundant in the gonads and adrenal cortex, they are undetectable in the human placenta, suggesting that a different mechanism is used for trophoblast expression of steroidogenic enzymes (5).

Steroidogenic Acute Regulatory Protein (StAR) Is Not Expressed in the Human Placenta

The rate-limiting step in steroidogenesis is the movement of cholesterol to the inner mitochondrial membranes where the cholesterol side-chain cleavage enzyme (P450scc) resides. In the gonads and adrenal cortex this translocation is acutely increased by tropic hormones acting through the intermediacy of cAMP. The StAR protein promotes this intramitochondrial cholesterol translocation (6). The StAR gene is highly expressed in the adrenal cortex and gonads. In response to elevations in cAMP, StAR is rapidly phosphorylated by protein kinase A, increasing its steroidogenic activity (7). In addition, cAMP a increases StAR gene transcription (8). Thus, there are both short-term and long-term effects of tropic hormone action on StAR. However, StAR mRNA and protein are undetectable in the human placenta and in choriocarcinoma cells (9). The absence of StAR in the human placenta accounts for the fact that fetuses affected with loss of function mutations in the StAR gene can reach term because of the continued placental production of progesterone through StAR independent mechanisms despite deficient fetal adrenal and fetal testicular steroidogenesis (6).

The human trophoblast compensates for the absence of StAR by using two different mechanisms. A StAR homologue, MLN64, was recently shown to have StAR-like activity (10). MLN64 shares 60% amino acid sequence similarity with the C-terminus of StAR, which contains the functional domains responsible for steroidogenic activity. It is expressed in the human placenta, and its presence could account for placental pregnenolone synthesis in the absence of StAR. The other mechanism is a marked ultrastructural change in the syncytiotrophoblast mitochondria; these organelles acquire a compact configuration with tubular cristae as the cytotrophoblast cells fuse to form syncytiotrophoblast (11). The resulting change in surface to volume ratio may facilitate the delivery of cholesterol to the inner mitochondrial membranes and P450scc.

The Human Placenta Expresses Its Own Form of 3β-Hydroxysteroid Dehydrogenase

The enzyme converting pregnenolone into progesterone in the trophoblast is encoded by a different gene than the enzyme in the gonads and adrenal cortex (12). The two different 3β-hydroxysteroid dehydrogenase genes (type I and type II) differ in their coding sequences in only 12 amino acids. However, this difference produces a 10-fold difference in Km for pregnenolone, giving the placental enzyme (type I) a greater affinity for pregnenolone than the gonadal or adrenal enzymes. The fact that the placental 3 β-hydroxysteroid dehydrogenase is encoded by a different gene than the gonadal and adrenal enzyme affords another opportunity for different transcriptional regulation strategies.

Cholesterol Side-Chain Cleavage Enzyme Expression Is Controlled by Different Cis Elements in the Trophoblast

There is only one cholesterol side-chain cleavage gene in the human genome. The *cis* elements that are important for gonadal and adrenal cortical expression have been mapped and they appear to be different from those governing expression of the gene in trophoblast cells (13,14). The key *cis* element controlling trophoblast-specific expression are located between −142 to −155 in the human P450scc promoter. DNA sequences lying more 5′ (−177 to −152) contain suppresor elements.

Expression of the Aromatase Gene in the Human Trophoblast Is Driven by a Unique Promoter

The large, single aromatase gene has several different promoters. The promoter controlling placental expression of aromatase lies more than 40 kb upstream from the translational start site, whereas the promoter driving expression of aromatase in the ovary is immediately proximal to the exon containing the translation start site (15,16). This novel configuration of the aromatase promoter should caution investigators searching for placental-specific promoters in other genes. Clearly, a focus on elements close to the translational start site may miss important elements at distant sites.

Regions of the aromatase promoter that are critical for trophoblast-specific expression have been mapped and include key cis elements at -242 to -166 from the major cap site (16). This element appears to bind stimulatory as well as repressing transcription factors.

Is There a Placental Specific Cis Element and *Trans* Factor?

The notion that there is a signature cis element in genes expressed in trophoblast cells that bind a trophoblast-specific trans factor is attractive. The search for such signature sequences and trans factors has been ongoing but has yet to be fruitful with the exception of the recent discovery of a novel sequence in the α subunit gene called the junctional response element (JRE), which binds a 40 kDa trophoblast-specific nuclear factor (17). Interestingly, variations of the JRE sequence can be found in the functionally important cis elements of the human cholesterol side-chain cleavage and aromatase genes (Fig. 14.1). The JRE sequence may bind other factors in addition to the recently reported 40 kDa nuclear protein. Hum and colleagues (13) described a 55 kDa factor present in trophoblast cells, but not adrenal cortical cells, that bound to an oligonucleotide containing the human cytochrome P450scc JRE-like sequence. This factor was not trophoblast specific. Andersen et al. (18) also reported a 50 kDa protein that was present in trophoblast cells, but was not trophoblast specific, that bound to the α subunit JRE. It is possible that the DNA proteins identified in these two studies are similar. However, their relationship to the 40 kDa protein remain to be determined.

JRE-LIKE SEQUENCE	GENE	CRITICAL REGION
G**GTAATTAC**A	α subunit	-130 to -80
AG**AAATTCC**A	P450scc	-155 to -131
TA**TAATCTG**A	P450arom	-240 to -170

FIGURE 14.1. The JRE-like sequences in the human glycoprotein α subunit, P450scc, and aromatase genes. Bold nucleotides indicate conserved nucleotides. The promoter regions containing the critical *cis* elements for trophoblast-specific expression and the JRE-like sequences are identified.

The similarities in the nucleotide sequences among three genes in regions of their promoters that are critical for trophoblast-specific expression, and the suggestion that there is a trophoblast-specific nuclear factor that binds to the proposed common sequence are the first clues that a signature cis element controlling trophoblast-expressed genes exists.

Another strategy to identify trophoblast-specific trans factors is to sequence trophoblast cDNA libraries and utilize motif-based sequence analysis programs to identify novel transcription factors and their abundance. Our use of this strategy has revealed interesting features of the placental transcriptional machinery. In the term placenta there is a paucity of transcripts for homeobox and basic helix-loop-helix transcription factors, whereas a variety of transcripts for zinc finger proteins are present; many of the transcription factor mRNAs encode suppressers of transcription (e.g., ATF3, AP-2B, X2 Box repressor, the COUP-like factor ARP-1, MITF-28-related factor). SF-1 homologues have not been identified in this analysis whereas the presence of expected factors including CREB, the glucocorticoid receptor, the coactivator RIP140, IRF-2, and STAT-6, and GATA-2 and GATA-3 were confirmed. First trimester placenta has more homeobox and basic helix-loop-helix transcripts and transcriptional suppressers and dominant negative factors are prominent indicating that repression or derepression are important strategies, a finding consistent with recent studies on the transcriptional regulation of the type I 17 β-hydroxysteroid dehydrogenase gene in trophoblast cells (19) and the localization of suppressor elements near the key cis elements governing trophoblast-specific expression of P450scc (14) and P450arom (16).

Summary

The human trophoblast utilizes different transcriptional mechanisms to control expression of steroidogenic enzymes: different genes are utilized, different promoters or different cis elements. The possibility that a placental-specific cis element and cognate trans factor are critical to regulating gene expression in the placenta is supported by recent observations.

Acknowledgments. Work in the author's laboratory was supported by N.I.H. grant HD-06274.

References

1. Strauss III JF, Martinez F, Kiriakidou M. Placental steroid hormone synthesis: unique features and unanswered questions. Biol Reprod 1996;54:303–11.
2. Strauss III JF, Gafvels M, King BF. Placental hormones. Endocrinology 1995; 3:2171–206.
3. Parker K, Schimmer BP. Steroidogenic factor 1: a key determinant of endocrine development and function. Endocrin Rev 1997;18:361–77.

4. Lala DS, Syka PM, Lazarchik SB, Mangelsdorf DJ, Parker KL, Heyman RA. Activation of the orphan nuclear receptor steroidogenic factor 1 by oxysterols. Proc Natl Acad Sci USA 1997;94:4895–900.

5. Ramayya MS, Zhou J, Kino T, Segars JH, Bondy CA, Chrousos GP. Steroidogenic factor 1 messenger ribonucleic acid expression in steroidogenic and nonsteroidogenic human tissues: northern blot and in situ hybridization studies. J Clin Endocrinol Metab 1997;82:1799–806.

6. Lin D, Sugawara T, Strauss III JF, Clark BJ, Stocco DM, Saenger P, et al. Role of steroidogenic acute regulatory protein in adrenal and gonadal steroidogenesis. Science 1995;267:1828–31.

7. Arakane F, King SR, Du Y, Kallen CB, Walsh LP, Watari H, et al. Phosphorylation of steroidogenic acute regulatory protein (StAR) modulates its steroidogenic activity. J Biol Chem 1997;272:32656–62.

8. Kiriakidou M, McAllister JM, Sugawara T, Strauss III JF. Expression of steroidogenic acute regulatory protein (StAR) in the human ovary. J Clin Endocrinol Metab 1996;81:4122–8.

9. Sugawara T, Holt JA, Driscoll, Strauss III JF, Lin D, Mille, WL, et al. Human steroidogenic acute regulatory protein: functional activity in COS-1 cells, tissue-specific expression, and mapping of the structural gene to 8p11.2 and a pseudogene to chromosome 13. Proc Natl Acad Sci USA 1995;92:4778–82.

10. Watari H, Arakane F, Moog-Lutz C, Kallen CB, Tomasetto C, Gerton GL, et al. MLN64 contains a domain with homology to the steroidogenic acute regulatory protein (StAR) that stimulates steroidogenesis. Proc Natl Acad USA 1997;94:8462–7.

11. Martinez F, Kiriakidou M, Strauss III JF. Structural and functional changes in mitochondria associated with trophoblast differentiation: methods to isolate enriched populations of syncytiotrophoblast mitochondria. Endocrinology 1997;138:2172–83.

12. Labrie F, Simard J, Luu-The V, Pelletier G, Belanger A, Lachance Y, et al. Structure and tissue-specific expression of 3β-hydroxysteroid dehydrogenase/5-ene-4-ene isomerase genes in human and rat classical and peripheral steroidogenic tissues. J Steroid Biochem Mol Biol 1992;41:421–35.

13. Hum DW, Aza-Blanc P, Miller WL. Characterization of placental transcriptional activation of the human gene for P450scc. DNA Cell Biol 1995;14:451–63.

14. Moore CCD, Hum DW, Miller WL. Identification of positive and negative placenta-specific basal elements and a cyclic adenosine 3′,5′-monophosphate response element in the human gene for P450scc. Mol Endocrinol 1992;6:2045–58.

15. Simpson ER, Mahendroo MS, Means GD, Kilgore MW, Hinshelwood MM, Graham-Lorence S, et al. Aromatase cytochrome P450, the enzyme responsible for estrogen biosynthesis. Endocrin Rev 1994;15:342–55.

16. Toda K, Nomoto S, Shizuta Y. Identification and characterization of transcriptional regulatory elements of the human aromatase cytochrome P450 gene (CYP19). J Steroid Biochem Molec Biol 1996;56:151–9.

17. Budworth PR, Quinn, PG, Nilsson, JH. Multiple characteristics of a pentameric regulatory array endow the human a-subunit glycoprotein hormone promoter with trophoblast specificity and maximal activity. Mol Endocrinol 1997;11:1669–80.

18. Andersen B, Kennedy GC, Nilson JH. A cis-acting element located between the cAMP response elements and the CCAAT box augments cell-specific expression of the glycoprotein hormone α subunit gene. J Biol Chem 1990;265:21874–80.

19. Piao Y-S, Peltoketo H, Vihko P, Vihko R. The proximal promoter region of the gene encoding human 17β-hydroxysteroid dehydrogenase type I contains GATA, AP-2, and Sp1 response elements: analysis of promoter function in choriocarcinoma cells. Endocrinology 1997;138:3417–25.

15

Transcription Factors Regulating the Differentiation of the Trophoblast Cell Lineage

Ian C. Scott and James C. Cross

The trophoblast cell lineage is the first to be specified during mammalian embryogenesis. Although trophoblast derivatives do not contribute to the embryo proper, they are essential from a very early stage for several complex processes. They mediate the attachment to and implantation into the uterus of the conceptus, secrete factors that regulate the fetal and maternal environments, modulate the maternal immune response to "foreign" embryonic tissue, invade the decidual circulation, and provide an interface where the fetal/maternal exchange of nutrients and waste products can occur (1,2). Proper development of this cell type is therefore crucial for embryonic survival and growth, and defects in these early events are likely causes of a significant proportion of failures in the successful maintenance of pregnancy. For this reason, there has been considerable interest in determining the factors that regulate normal trophoblast differentiation. Development of cell lineages ultimately involves changes in programs of gene expression, which are in turn regulated by transcription factors. A large number of transcription factors that are expressed in trophoblast have now been identified (Table 15.1). This catalogue has increased recently because of the sequencing of expressed sequence tags (EST) found in placental and purified trophoblast cDNA libraries.

To determine the function of trophoblast transcription factors, one line of investigation has focused on describing the trans-acting factors that account for cell type-restricted transcription of genes encoding trophoblast-specific products, such as placental hormones. In theory, at least, this reverse line of investigation should eventually identify factors that account for trophoblast cell identity and specificity of gene expression. A second approach has been to use genetic techniques, such as the production of mutant mice by gene targeting, to test the requirements of genes for normal embryonic development. This has resulted in the identification of several genes that affect placental development (2,3). This review summarizes our current understanding of the transcription factors

TABLE 15.1. Summary of transcription factors expressed in trophoblast cells.

Family	Gene	Species	Cell type or tissue source	Reference*
bHLH	Hxt	Mouse	TGC, int. troph.	11
	Mash-2	Mouse	extr. ect., int. troph.	13
	E2A	Mouse	extr. ect.	13
	ALF1	Mouse	extr. ect., int. troph.	13
	ME2	Mouse	extr. ect., int. troph.	13
	Id-1	Mouse	extr. ect.	21
	Id-2	Mouse	extr. ect.	21
	HES-1	Mouse	extr. ect.	23
	HES-2	Mouse	extr. ect., int. troph., TGC	23
	HES-3	Mouse	extr. ect., int. troph., TGC	23
	Twist	Mouse	extr. ect.	25
	Lyl-1	Mouse	placenta	Acc. #AA016353
Zinc finger	GATA-2	Mouse	TGC	30
	GATA-3	Mouse	TGC	30
	ERR-a	Mouse	int. troph.	35
	ERR-b	Mouse	extr. ect.	36
	mSna	Mouse	int. troph.	37
	mLIMK	Mouse	TGC	56
	RIT-18	Mouse	placenta	Acc. #AA023056
	SCNA	Mouse	placenta	Acc. #AA024185
Homeobox	Cdx2	Mouse	extr. ect.	41
	Pem	Mouse	int. troph.	57
	Esx1	Mouse	extr. ect.	58
	HoxB6	Human	1st trimester placenta	59
	HoxC5	Human	1st trimester trophoblast	60
	HoxC6	Human	1st trimester trophoblast	60
	Hox3E	Human	1st trimester trophoblast	60
	HB24	Human	3rd trimester placenta	61

	GAX	Human	3rd trimester placenta	61
	MSX2	Human	3rd trimester placenta	61
	DLX4	Human	3rd trimester placenta	61
Groucho	TLE2	Mouse	int. troph., TGC	23
	TLE3	Mouse	extr. ect., int. troph., TGC	23
Pou Domain	Pit-1	Rat	rat placenta	62
	Pit-1	Human	syncytiotrophoblast	63
Others	AP-2α	Mouse	mouse placenta	64
	AP-2β	Mouse	mouse placenta	64
	TEF-1	Human	1st and 3rd trimester placenta	65
	TEF-5	Human	placenta, JEG-3 cells	66
	c-Ets1	Human	1st trimester cytotrophoblast	67

Abbreviations used: extr. ect., extraembryonic ectoderm; int. troph., intermediate trophoblast of ectoplacental cone and/or spongiotrophoblast; TGCs, trophoblast giant cells.
*Gen Bank accession numbers provided for expressed sequence tags (ESTs)

that are thought to regulate trophoblast differentiation and function based on genetic studies in mice, and discusses what these two experimental approaches have indicated about the complexities of trophoblast differentiation and gene regulation.

Trophoblast Development in Mice

Up to the formation of the blastocyst, embryogenesis proceeds similarly in different species. At the blastocyst stage, the outer epithelial cell layer, the trophectoderm, is the precursor population for subsequent trophoblast cell derivatives. It is clear that cell–cell interactions are critical for inducing trophectoderm formation and for segregating the developmental potential of these trophoblast cells from the inner cell mass (1,4). However, it remains an unanswered question as to whether there are transcription factors essential for driving these processes, as no mouse mutants in transcription factors have been described to date in which trophoblast cell lineage formation is affected. After the blastocyst stage, distinct trophoblast cell populations arise that contribute to different parts of the placenta and have different functions (Fig. 15.1). In rodents, trophoblast cells overlying the inner cell mass, polar trophectoderm, continue to proliferate and give rise to the extraembryonic ectoderm. These cells are thought to have trophoblast stem cell-like function in that they self-renew and are capable of differentiating into both terminally differentiated trophoblast cell types: labyrinthine trophoblast and trophoblast giant cells (TGCs) (4). Ectoplacental cone and spongiotrophoblast cells will differentiate into TGCs in culture suggesting that they are an intermediate population. In contrast to polar trophectoderm, the mural trophectodermal cells of blastocysts, which are not in contact with the inner cell mass, differentiate immediately into TGCs, suggesting that the inner cell mass is an initial source of mitogenic stimulation.

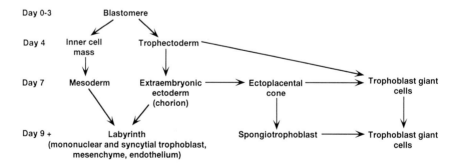

FIGURE 15.1. Diagram depicting the differentiation of the trophoblast cell lineage in mice and the names used to describe the different cell populations at different times during gestation.

The later overall anatomy of the placenta differs markedly among eutherian mammals. This fact has certainly stifled progress towards a universal understanding of placental function and development. One reason may be that attention has tended to focus on the gross anatomy and the regulation of specific placental hormones which represent physiological specializations in species, rather than on fundamental cellular processes which are clearly more widely conserved. For example, trophoblast cells in rodents and primates populate three similar groups: (1) trophoblast stem cells (primate villous cytotrophoblast and rodent extraembryonic ectoderm); (2) fused trophoblast cells (primate syncytiotrophoblast and rodent labyrinthine trophoblast); and (3) invasive cells (primate extravillous cytotrophoblast and rodent TGCs). Future work is required to determine if these cellular similarities correlate with molecular homologies in terms of the expression patterns of putative regulatory transcription factors.

Transcription Factors Expressed in Rodent Trophoblast

Specific classes of transcription factors that have been conserved throughout the evolution of multicellular organisms, in both plants vertebrate animals, function to regulate developmental processes during embryogenesis. This conservation of structure and function has become a powerful argument for using gene homologies to identify new factors with suspected regulatory functions. Members of all of these major classes of transcription factors are also expressed in the placenta.

Helix-Loop-Helix Factors

Basic-helix-loop-helix (bHLH) factors regulate cell lineage establishment and differentiation in several developmental systems including skeletal (5,6) and cardiac (7) myogenesis, neurogenesis (8) and, more recently, trophoblast development in mice (9, Cross, unpublished data).

Mash-2

Mash-2, a homologue of the *Drosophila achaete-scute* proneural genes (10), is first expressed during preimplantation development and later in the extraembryonic ectoderm of the chorion and ectoplacental cone in the early postimplantation conceptus (Fig. 15.2). *Mash-2* mRNA levels decrease coincident with trophoblast differentiation into TGCs. In addition, *Mash-2* becomes restricted to fewer and fewer cells of the midgestation placenta. Gene targeting experiments in the mouse have revealed an essential role for *Mash-2* in trophoblast development, as conceptuses lacking a functional copy of *Mash-2* die by embryonic day 10.5 because of placental failure associated with a poorly organized labyrinthine trophoblast layer, an absent spongiotrophoblast layer, and an increased number of TGCs (9). The precise function of *Mash-2* is unknown, although it may be required for maintaining the proliferative potential of trophoblast cells, since its overexpression in Rcho-1 trophoblast cells inhibits their terminal differentiation into the TGC (nonproliferative) fate (11). This activity likely depends on other factors as well. The MASH-2 protein appears to function as a classical cell-specific bHLH factor in that it homodimerizes poorly, but forms heterodimers with one of the more widely expressed bHLH E-factors with high affinity. Only these heterodimers are able to bind and activate transcription from so-called E-box DNA sequences (12,13). MASH-2/E-factor heterodimers therefore likely act in vivo as positive regulators of genes required for promoting trophoblast proliferation and/or blocking TGC differentiation.

Hxt

Hxt is strongly expressed in TGCs at all stages of development, as well as in the ectoplacental cone of early postimplantation conceptuses (11,14,15) where the expression patterns of *Hxt* and *Mash-2* significantly overlap (Fig. 15.2). *Hxt* appears to have an activity opposite to that of *Mash-2* in that *Hxt* is

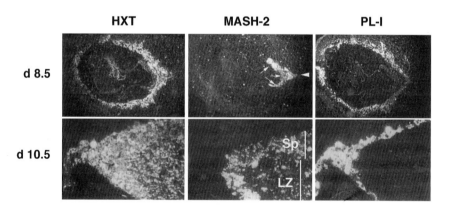

FIGURE 15.2. Expression patterns of *Hxt, Mash-2,* and *PL-I* mRNAs in mouse placentas at days 8.5 and 10.5 of gestation. In situ hybridization was performed using ^{33}P-rUTP-labeled antisense riboprobes on serial sections from day 8.5 and 10.5 conceptuses. *PL-I* expression delineates the TGC layer that surrounds the conceptuses. Note that at both day 8.5 and 10.5 *Mash-2* expression is not detectable in trophoblast giant cells. At day 8.5, it is strongly expressed throughout the extraembryonic ectoderm of the chorion and the ectoplacental cone at day 8.5; *Hxt* expression overlaps only in the ectoplacental cone. At day 10.5, *Hxt* and *Mash-2* expression overlap in the spongiotrophoblast and labyrinthine layers, but note that *Mash-2* expression is becoming localized to focal areas. Arrows, extraembryonic ectoderm; arrowhead, ectoplacental cone; Sp, spongiotrophoblast; LZ, labyrinthine layer.

sufficient to promote TGC formation (11). Recently, gene targeting of the mouse *Hxt* gene has demonstrated an essential role for *Hxt* in trophoblast development (Riley, Anson-Cartwright, Cross, unpublished ms). Mutant conceptuses arrest by day 7.5 of gestation and have smaller ectoplacental cones, decreased numbers of primary TGCs, and an absence of secondary TGCs. Trophoblast cells that are normally fated to form secondary TGCs continue to express ectoplacental cone markers indicating a molecular defect in terminal differentiation. Like *Mash-2*, genes that are downstream of *Hxt* are unknown at present, although the regulation of the HXT protein may be complex. The *Hxt* cDNA was cloned by multiple groups based on its ability to heterodimerize with E-factors (11–15). In vitro, HXT avidly forms heterodimers with E-factors, suggesting that HXT could compete for E-factor partners with MASH-2. In addition, HXT is able to homodimerize in vitro (Scott, Cross, unpublished data). Most bHLH proteins bind to so-called consensus E- or N-box elements, either as a homodimer or heterodimer with one of the E-factors. However, such activity has not been found for HXT (13,15). While it is clear that HXT/E-factor heterodimers do not bind E-box sequences, binding to a noncanonical sequence has been demonstrated in vitro (15).

bHLH Modifiers of *Hxt* and *Mash-2* Activity: E-factors and Ids

Due to the opposing activities, yet overlapping expression patterns, of *Hxt* and *Mash-2*, we have recently investigated the expression patterns of their likely dimerization partners, the E-factors, during trophoblast development. Mammalian E-factors are encoded by three genes (16–18). Interestingly, these three genes share distinct yet overlapping expression patterns in the extraembryonic ectoderm and intermediate-type trophoblast of the ectoplacental cone and spongiotrophoblast, with no detectable expression in TGCs (13). The lack of detectable E-factor expression in TGCs indicates that bHLH factors are presented with differing dimerization partners in various trophoblast populations. The Id factors are HLH proteins that lack functional basic domains and, as such, are unable to bind to DNA. Therefore, they can inhibit bHLH activity by forming inactive heterodimers with E-factors (19). In addition, they may play a more direct role in promoting cell proliferation (20). Limited information is available concerning Id factor expression in the placenta. However, at early postimplantation stages, transcripts of *Id-1* and *Id-2* are detectable in the extraembryonic ectoderm of the chorion but not in the ectoplacental cone and TGCs (21). Forced expression of Id-1 in Rcho-1 trophoblast cells inhibits their differentiation into TGCs (11). These factors may therefore act in extraembryonic ectoderm to prevent both E-factor activity and terminal differentiation. The overlapping expression patterns of *Hxt, Mash-2, Id,* and E-factor genes suggests that a range of bHLH protein interactions may occur during trophoblast development. Therefore, the activity of a given factor depends not only on its expression but also on what other factors are coexpressed in the same cell.

Regulators of *Mash-2* Expression

Little is known about mechanisms that regulate *Mash-2* from initial expression in all blastomeres of the morula to restricted expression in a subset of the tropho-blast lineage. Superficially, this appears similar to the regulation of the *achaete-scute* genes of *Drosophila*, whose expression is refined from an initially broad pattern. This is produced by the action of the *Notch/hairy(E(spl))/Groucho* sig-naling pathway (22). Recently, all elements of this pathway have been identified in trophoblast (23). *Notch-2* is expressed in the outer spongiotrophoblast and the TGC layers, and its potential downstream effectors of the bHLH (*HES-2 and -3*) and Groucho (*TLE2* and *TLE3*) protein families coincide in their expression in TGC at midgestation when *Mash-2* mRNA expression becomes restricted. As all components are expressed in the proper cell types, it is tempting to speculate that signaling via the Notch receptor pathway may be responsible for the down-regulation of *Mash-2* in TGCs.

Other Cell-Specific bHLH Factors in Trophoblast

The bHLH family presently encompasses over 250 transcription factors (24), with new members being discovered at a rapid pace. It therefore seems likely that other bHLH factors will also be found to regulate trophoblast develop-ment. Of particular interest is *Twist* and *LYL-1*. *Twist* is transiently expressed in extraembryonic ectoderm of early postimplantation mouse conceptuses (25). The details of *LYL-1* expression are not clear at present, although an EST representing *LYL-1* has been detected in a mouse placental cDNA database (unpublished results). The trophoblast functions of these factors are unknown. In *Drosophila, Twist* and the zinc-finger factor *Snail* have antagonistic ac-tivities in mesoderm (26). *LYL-1* is a close relative of *Hxt* and therefore may also play an interesting role in trophoblast.

Zinc Finger Proteins

Members of the zinc-finger transcription factor family play roles in diverse developmental systems including hematopoiesis and cardiogenesis (GATA factors), and skeletal muscle (LIM proteins) and mesoderm differentiation (Snail family members) (26–29). A number of these factors are also expressed in trophoblast and affect its development (Table 15.1).

GATA Factors

GATA-2 and *-3* are both expressed in murine trophoblast giant cells (30). Mutation of GATA factor binding sites reduces the promoter activity of a number of trophoblast-specific genes including adenosine deaminase (31), human chorionic gonadotropin (hCG)-α and -β (32,33) and placental lacto-gen-I (PL-I) (30). Loss-of-function mutations in *GATA-2* and *-3* result in a marked decrease in the expression of the TGC-specific markers PL-I and proliferin, with an associated decrease in the angiogenic activity secreted by the placenta (34). These effects are more severe with mutations in *GATA-2*, where neovascularization of the surrounding decidua is markedly reduced. These factors therefore seem to play important roles in the regulation of giant-cell specific genes required for fetal-maternal signaling.

Estrogen-Related Receptor (ERR)-α and -β

The ERRs are members of the nuclear receptor superfamily. They are expressed in distinct regions of the murine placenta; *ERR*-α in the spongio-trophoblast layer (35) and *ERR*-β in extraembryonic ectoderm cells of the chorion (36). Mutation of the *ERR*-β gene results in lethality by day 10 of gestation, with a noted absence of chorionic ectoderm, a decrease in the number of spongiotrophoblast cells, and an increase in TGC number (36). As *ERR*-β expression is limited to the extraembryonic ectoderm, it seems likely that it is responsible for mediating a chorion-derived signal that promotes proliferation of diploid trophoblast at the expense of giant cell differentiation. Determining the nature and source of the ligands for the ERR receptors will provide further insight into signaling pathways that maintain trophoblast proliferation in vivo.

Murine Snail (mSna)

mSna, a homologue of the *Drosophila Snail* and *Escargot* genes, is expressed in the ectoplacental cone (37,38) and later spongiotrophoblast, with a marked loss of expression coincident with TGC differentiation (Scott, Nakayama, Cross unpublished data). Members of the *Snail/Escargot* family bind to E-box sequences (39,40), the same sequences that are bound by many bHLH factors such as Twist, MASH-2, and possibly HXT. Therefore, the transition to TGC differentiation could be regulated via competition between transcription factors of different classes for the same target sites. Genes regulated in this manner may play central roles in trophoblast proliferation and differentiation.

Homeobox Genes

Transcription factors containing the 60 amino acid homeodomain define a large family whose members play roles in processes as diverse as patterning of the body axes, specifying positional information, and organogenesis. Homeobox-containing genes are expressed also in the developing placenta (Table 15.1), including several *Hox* genes. However, at present little is known regarding the spatial and temporal expression patterns of these factors, and only *Cdx2*, a homologue of the *Drosophila Caudal* gene, has been shown to play a role in trophoblast development to date.

Cdx2

Early in embryogenesis *Cdx2* expression is specific to trophoblast: it is detectable in extraembryonic ectoderm of the chorion at day 7 (41). Mutation of the *Cdx2* gene results in early embryonic lethality; although not well defined, mutant embryos fail at the periimplantation period between day 3.5 and 5.5 (42). The cause of the phenotype is not known, though it clearly occurs as the trophoblast lineage is specified. Because *Cdx2* expression is restricted to the trophectoderm at this stage, it is likely, but not yet proven, that lethality is because of defects in the trophoblast lineage.

Regulation of Trophoblast-Specific Target Genes

Although the transcription factors described above have been shown through genetic analysis to be essential for different aspects of trophoblast development, the direct target genes that they regulate remain largely unknown. Looking for alterations of gene expression patterns in mutant mouse placentas will give important clues in the future. Several groups have taken the reverse approach to the study of trophoblast development by studying the regulatory regions that control the expression of known trophoblast-specific genes. This has been done largely in transfected trophoblast cell lines such as Rcho-1 and JEG-3 (30,32,43) and to a lesser extent in transgenic mice (31,44,45). One pitfall with this reverse approach has been the difficulty in reconciling data from the cell culture and transgenic models. *PL-II* elements found to direct expression in trophoblast cell lines are also able to confer correct TGC-specific expression in transgenic mice (44). However, *hCG-α* elements that are sufficient to drive "trophoblast-specific" expression in JEG-3 cells are not functional in transgenic mice (46). Likewise, a *4311* enhancer element sufficient for spongiotrophoblast-specific expression in transgenic mice has no activity in JEG-3 or Rcho-1 cells (45). These data suggest that different insights may be gained by using in vitro and in vivo experimental models.

A central hypothesis that appears to have driven much of the promoter analysis to date is that trophoblast-specific genes should be regulated by trophoblast-specific transcription factors. This may be true at some level, although the concept of specificity should perhaps be blurred. Even factors like *Hxt, Mash-2,* and *Cdx2,* that have critical functions in trophoblast, are expressed elsewhere at various times during development (e.g., *Hxt* and *Mash-2* in gonads). The study of trophoblast-specific promoter and enhancer regions have likewise not yielded factors that either are expressed exclusively in trophoblast or play essential roles in trophoblast development per se. For example, AP-2, which binds to the so-called "trophoblast-specific element" found in a number of genes including adenosine deaminase, *4311, hCG-α* and -β (31,45,47), is expressed not only in trophoblast, but also in a number of other cell types in which roles have been shown by gene targeting experiments (48,49). GATA-2 and -3, for which binding sites exist in the *PL-I, hCG,* and adenosine deaminase genes (30,31,33) also serve critical hematopoietic functions (50,51).

Trophoblast development may not, therefore, be regulated by trophoblast-specific transcription factors, but by the coexpression of multiple factors whose expression patterns are not individually trophoblast specific. Interactions among members of the three transcription factor families reviewed in this chapter have been shown to be required during the development of other cell lineages (52,53). For example, erythropoeisis requires interactions between the bHLH factor SCL and the zinc finger proteins GATA-1 and Rbtn1/2 (27,54). Combinatorial interactions between transcription factors may similarly be required to produce complexes with trophoblast-specific activity. As the trophoblast lineage has arisen relatively late in evolutionary terms, it would perhaps not be surprising that development is regulated not by a host of novel factors, but by a novel combination of previously existing factors.

Conclusions

We are presently left with relatively short lists of factors independently shown either to be essential for different aspects of trophoblast development or to regulate trophoblast-specific target genes, as well as a much larger number of factors known only to be expressed in this cell type. What is now required is an elaboration of this information into a model of trophoblast development based on how these factors interact in vivo. As a first step the placental expression patterns of these genes must be determined with attention to the multiple trophoblast cell types. In addition, it is clear that these populations are not static during gestation as demonstrated, for example, by the sequential activation of the prolactin/growth hormone family genes that occurs in TGCs (55). Therefore in situ expression in trophoblast should be studied over a range of developmental periods. Finally, comparisons of expression in different species will help demonstrate what factors play conserved, and hence likely important, roles. While studying expression alone will be useful, ultimately functional studies will be required. The ability to both modify and overexpress genes in mice will be required to definitively assess the role that transcription factors play in trophoblast development. "Knock-out" technology alone will not be sufficient, as this only highlights essential roles for a specific factor, and cannot account for potential redundancy of the mammalian genome. Complementary overexpression, tissue-specific modification, dominant-negative, and loss-of-function approaches will therefore be required to properly address these questions.

References

1. Rossant J. Development of extraembryonic cell lineages in the mouse embryo. In: Rossant J, Pedersen R, eds. Experimental approaches to mammalian embryonic development. Cambridge: Cambridge University Press, 1986:97–120.

2. Cross JC, Werb Z, Fisher SJ. Implantation and the placenta: key pieces of the development puzzle. Science 1994;266:1508–18.

3. Rinkenberger J, Cross JC, Werb Z. Molecular genetics of implantation in the mouse. Devel Genetics 1997;21:6–20.

4. Rossant J. Development of the extraembryonic lineages. Semin Devel Biol 1995;6:237–47.

5. Nabeshima Y, et al. Myogenin gene disruption results in perinatal lethality because of severe muscle defect. Nature 1993;364:532–5.

6. Rawls A, et al. Myogenin's functions do not overlap with those of MyoD or Myf-5 during mouse embryogenesis. Devel Biol 1995;172:37–50.

7. Srivastava D et al. Regulation of cardiac mesodermal and neural crest development by the bHLH transcription factor, dHAND. Nat Genet 1997;16:154–60.

8. Lee JE, et al. Conversion of Xenopus ectoderm into neurons by NeuroD, a basic helix-loop-helix protein. Science 1995;268:836–44.

9. Guillemot F, Nagy A, Auerbach A, Rossant J, Joyner AL. Essential role of Mash-2 in extraembryonic development. Nature 1994;371:333 6.

10. Johnson JE, Birren SJ, Anderson DJ. Two rat homologues of Drosophila achaete-scute specifically expressed in neuronal precursors. Nature 1990;346:858–61.

11. Cross JC, et al. Hxt encodes a basic helix-loop-helix transcription factor that regulates trophoblast cell development. Development 1995;121:2513–23.

12. Johnson JE, Birren SJ, Saito T, Anderson DJ. DNA binding and transcriptional regulatory activity of mammalian achaete-scute homologous (MASH) proteins revealed by interaction with a muscle-specific enhancer. Proc Natl Acad Sci USA 1992;89:3596–600.

13. Scott IC, Cross JC. Basic helix-loop-helix factors HXT and MASH-2 have distinct expression patterns and partner preferences during murine trophoblast development. Biol Reprod 1996;54(Suppl)1:176.

14. Cserjesi P, Brown D, Lyons GE, Olson EN. Expression of the novel basic helix-loop-helix gene *eHAND* in neural crest derivatives and extraembryonic membranes during mouse development. Devel Biol 1995;170:664–78.

15. Hollenberg SM, Sternglanz R, Cheng PF, Weintraub H. Identification of a new family of tissue-specific basic helix-loop-helix proteins with a two-hybrid system. Mol Cell Biol 1995;15:3813–22.

16. Hu JS, Olson EN, Kingston RE. HEB, a helix-loop-helix protein related to E2A and ITF2 that can modulate the DNA-binding ability of myogenic regulatory factors. Mol Cell Biol 1992;12:1031–42.

17. Aronheim A, Shiran R, Rosen A, Walker MD. Cell-specific expression of helix-loop-helix transcription factors encoded by the E2A gene. Nucl Acids Res 1993;21:1601–6.

18. Soosaar A, Chiaramello A, Zuber MX, Neuman T. Expression of basic-helix-loop-helix transcription factor ME2 during brain development and in the regions of neuronal plasticity in the adult brain. Brain Res Mol Brain Res 1994;25:176–80.

19. Benezra R, Davis RL, Lockshon D, Turner DL, Weintraub H. The protein Id: a negative regulator of helix-loop-helix DNA binding proteins. Cell 1990;61:49–59.

20. Barone MV, Pepperkok R, Peverali FA, Philipson L. Id proteins control growth induction in mammalian cells. Proc Natl Acad Sci USA 1994;91:4985–8.

21. Jen Y, Manova K, Benezra R. Each member of the Id gene family exhibits a unique expression pattern in mouse gastrulation and neurogenesis. Devel Dyn 1997;208:92–106.

22. Artavanis-Tsakonas S, Matsuno K, Fortini ME. Notch signaling. Science 1995;268:225–32.

23. Nakayama H, Liu Y, Stifani S, Cross JC. Developmental restriction of *Mash-2* expression in trophoblast correlates with potential activation of the NOTCH-2 pathway. Devel Genetics 1997;21:21–30.

24. Atchley WR, Fitch WM. A natural classification of the basic helix-loop-helix class of transcription factors. Proc Natl Acad Sci USA 1997;94:5172–6.

25. Stoetzel C, Weber B, Bourgeois P, Bolcato-Bellemin AL, Perrin-Schmitt F. Dorso-ventral and rostro-caudal sequential expression of *M-twist* in the postimplantation murine embryo. Mech Devel 1995;51:251–63.

26. Leptin M. Twist and snail as positive and negative regulators during Drosophila meso-derm development. Genes Devel 1991;5:1568–76.

27. Larson RC, et al. Protein dimerization between Lmo2 (Rbtn2) and Tal1 alters thy-mocyte development and potentiates T cell tumorigenesis in transgenic mice. EMBO J 1996;15:1021–27.

28. Kuo CT, et al. GATA4 transcription factor is required for ventral morphogenesis and heart tube formation. Genes Devel 1997;11:1048–60.

29. Kong Y, Flick MJ, Kudla AJ, Konieczny SF. Muscle LIM protein promotes myogenesis by enhancing the activity of MyoD. Mol Cell Biol 1997;17:4750-60.

30. Ng YK, George KM, Engel JD, Linzer DI. GATA factor activity is required for the trophoblast-specific transcriptional regulation of the mouse placental lactogen I gene. Development 1994;120:3257–66.

31. Shi D, et al. Diverse genetic regulatory motifs required for murine adenosine deami-nase gene expression in the placenta. J Biol Chem 1997;272:2334–41.

32. Steger DJ, Buscher M, Hecht JH, Mellon PL. Coordinate control of the alpha- and beta-subunit genes of human chorionic gonadotropin by trophoblast-specific element-binding protein. Mol Endocrinol 1993;7:1579–88.

33. Steger DJ, Hecht JH, Mellon PL. GATA-binding proteins regulate the human gonado-tropin alpha-subunit gene in the placenta and pituitary gland. Mol Cell Biol 1994;14:5592–602.

34. Ma GT, et al. GATA-2 and GATA-3 regulate trophoblast-specific gene expression in vivo. Development 1997;124:907–14.

35. Sladek R, Bader JA, Giguere V. The orphan nuclear receptor estrogen-related receptor alpha is a transcriptional regulator of the human medium-chain acyl coenzyme A dehy-drogenase gene. Mol Cell Biol 1997;17:5400–9.

36. Luo J, et al. Placental abnormalities in mouse embryos lacking the orphan nuclear receptor ERR-β. Nature 1997;388:778–82.

37. Nieto MA, Bennett MF, Sargent MG, Wilkinson DG. Cloning and developmental expression of *Sna*, a murine homologue of the *Drosophila snail* gene. Development 1992;116:227–37.

38. Smith DE, Del Amo FF, Gridley T. Isolation of *Sna*, a mouse gene homologous to the *Drosophila* genes *snail* and *escargot*: its expression pattern suggests multiple roles during postimplantation development. Development 1992;116:1033–9.

39. Mauhin V, Lutz Y, Dennefeld C, Alberga A. Definition of the DNA-binding site repertoire for the *Drosophila* transcription factor SNAIL. Nucl Acids Res 1993;21:3951–7.

40. Fuse N, Hirose S, Hayashi S. Diploidy of Drosophila imaginal cells is maintained by a transcriptional repressor encoded by escargot. Genes Devel 1994;8:2270–81.

41. Beck F, Erler T, Russell A, James R. Expression of *Cdx-2* in the mouse embryo and placenta: possible role in patterning of the extra-embryonic membranes. Devel Dyn 1995;204:219–27.
42. Chawengsaksophak K, James R, Hammond VE, Kontgen F, Beck F. Homeosis and intestinal tumours in Cdx2 mutant mice. Nature 1997;386:84–7.
43. Moore CC, Hum DW, Miller WL. Identification of positive and negative placenta-specific basal elements and a cyclic adenosine 3',5'-monophosphate response element in the human gene for P450scc. Mol Endocrinol 1992;6:2045–8.
44. Shida MM, Jackson-Grusby LL, Ross SR, Linzer DI. Placental-specific expression from the mouse placental lactogen II gene promoter. Proc Natl Acad Sci USA 1992;89:3864–8.
45. Calzonetti T, Stevenson L, Rossant J. A novel regulatory region is required for trophoblast-specific transcription in transgenic mice. Devel Biol 1995;171:615–26.
46. Hamernik DL, Werth LA, Sundermann D, Zanella EL. The proximal 350 bp of 5'-flanking sequence of the human α-subunit glycoprotein hormone gene functions in the pituitary gland, but not the placenta, in transgenic mice. Endocrine 1996;5:257–63.
47. Johnson W, et al. Regulation of the human chorionic gonadotropin alpha- and beta-subunit promoters by AP-2. J Biol Chem 1997;272:15405–12.
48. Mosser M, et al. Enhanced apoptotic cell death of renal epithelial cells in mice lacking transcription factor AP-2beta. Genes Devel 1997;11:1938–48.
49. Schorle H, Meier P, Buchert M, Jaenisch R, Mitchell PJ. Transcription factor AP-2 essential for cranial closure and craniofacial development. Nature 1996;381:235–8.
50. Tsai FY, Orkin SH. Transcription factor GATA-2 is required for proliferation/survival of early hematopoietic cells and mast cell formation, but not for erythroid and myeloid terminal differentiation. Blood 1997;89:3636–43.
51. Ting CN, Olson MC, Barton KP, Leiden JM. Transcription factor GATA-3 is required for development of the T-cell lineage. Nature 1996;384:474–8.
52. Black BL, Ligon KL, Zhang Y, Olson EN. Cooperative transcriptional activation by the neurogenic basic helix-loop-helix protein MASH1 and members of the myocyte enhancer factor-2 (MEF2) family. J Biol Chem 1996;271:26659–63.
53. Molkentin JD, Black BL, Martin JF, Olson EN. Cooperative activation of muscle gene expression by MEF2 and myogenic bHLH proteins. Cell 1995;83:1125–36.
54. Osada H, Grutz G, Axelson H, Forster A, Rabbitts TH. Association of erythroid transcription factors: complexes involving the LIM protein RBTN2 and the zinc-finger protein GATA1. Proc Natl Acad Sci USA 1995;92:9585–9.
55. Hamlin GP, Lu XJ, Roby KF, Soares MJ. Recapitulation of the pathway for trophoblast giant cell differentiation in vitro: stage-specific expression of members of the prolactin gene family. Endocrinology 1994;134:2390–6.
56. Cheng AK, Robertson EJ. The murine LIM-kinase gene (*limk*) encodes a novel serine threonine kinase expressed predominantly in trophoblast giant cells and the developing nervous system. Mech Devel 1995;52:187–97.
57. Lin TP, et al. The Pem homeobox gene is X-linked and exclusively expressed in extraembryonic tissues during early murine development. Devel Biol 1994;166:170–9.
58. Li Y, Lemaire P, Behringer RR. *Esx1*, a novel X chromosome-linked homeobox

gene expressed in mouse extraembryonic tissues and male germ cells. Devel Biol 1997;188:85–95.

59. Su BC, Strand D, McDonough PG, McDonald JF. Temporal and constitutive expression of homeobox-2 gene (*Hu-2*), human heat shock gene (*hsp-70*), and oncogenes *C-sis* and *N-myc* in early human trophoblast. Am J Obstet Gynecol 1988;159:1195–9.

60. Oudejans CBM, Pannese M, Simeone A, Meijer CJM, Boncinelli E. The three most downstream genes of the Hox-3 cluster are expressed in human extraembryonic tissues including trophoblast of androgenetic origin. Development 1990;108:471–7.

61. Quinn LM, Johnson BV, Nicholl J, Sutherland GR, Kalionis B. Isolation and identification of homeobox genes from the human placenta including a novel member of the Distal-less family, *DLX4*. Gene 1997;187:55–61.

62. Lee BJ, et al. Local expression of a POU family transcription factor, Pit-1, in the rat placenta. Mol Cell Endocrinol 1996;118:9–14.

63. Bamberger AM, et al. Expression of pit-1 messenger ribonucleic acid and protein in the human placenta. J Clin Endocrinol Metab 1995;80:2021–6.

64. Mitchell PJ, Timmons PM, Hebert JM, Rigby PWJ, Tjian R. Transcription factor AP-2 is expressed in neural crest cell lineages during mouse embryogenesis. Genes Devel 1991;5:105–19.

65. Quinn G, et al. The human placenta expresses transcription enhancer factor-1 but there is no correlation with the expression of placental lactogen. J Mol Endocrinol 1996;16:205–10.

66. Jacquemin P, Martial JA, Davidson I. Human TEF-5 is preferentially expressed in placenta and binds to multiple functional elements of the human chorionic somatommatropin-β gene enhancer. J Biol Chem 1997;272:12928–37.

67. Luton D, et al. The c-ets1 protooncogene is expressed in human trophoblast during the first trimester of pregnancy. Early Hum Devel 1997;47:147–56.

Part VI

Primate Models and Human Studies

16

Hormonal Regulation of Endometrial Gene Expression in the Rhesus Monkey

WILLIAM C. OKULICZ, CHRISTOPHER I. ACE,
JANET TAST, AND CHRISTOPHER LONGCOPE

The changing pattern of estradiol (E) and progesterone (P) secretion during the primate menstrual cycle governs the hormonal regulation of endometrial growth, differentiation, shedding, and reconstruction that is an essential component of continued reproductive competence (1,2). Our laboratory has been most interested in P-dependent regulation of endometrial response in the rhesus monkey, an appropriate model for human endometrial function. P action, mediated through its cognate receptor, causes a shift from a proliferative to a secretory (differentiated) state in the endometrium that is accompanied by massive metabolic changes and structural remodeling (3–5). These features of P action on the endometrium most likely involve a cascade of signal transduction pathways that invoke the regulation of ligands, receptors, cytokines, and growth factors. One important mechanism that regulates such factors is the activation or repression of their respective gene products at the transcriptional level; a fate ultimately determined by specific promoter-binding transcription factors. This chapter describes our recent work on P-dependent regulation of endometrial gene expression and its potential relevance to implantation in the primate.

Animal Model: Rhesus Monkey

Artificial Menstrual Cycles

The development and use of artificial menstrual cycles in the rhesus monkey was first described by Hodgen (6). These studies showed that simulation of the menstrual cycle by the timed insertion and removal of silastic implants of E or P was sufficient to allow the endometrium to support implantation and eventual delivery (IVF and surrogate transfer). Both short and inadequate luteal phases similar to those found in women have been described in the rhesus monkey (7). These latter studies also provide support for the usefulness of the rhesus monkey as a model for luteal phase defects in women (8) wherein low secretory P levels lead to retarded endometrial maturation.

Our previously published studies (9–12) describe in detail the protocols for creation of adequate and inadequate cycles. These studies showed that the hormone levels produced by these protocols are coincident with those observed in the natural menstrual cycle (9). The profiles of serum E and P observed using the above protocols are shown in Figure 16.1A and B for adequate and inadequate secretory phases respectively.

Preparation of Endometrial cDNA Populations

Endometrial mRNA enriched for polyA+ mRNA was prepared and converted to cDNA by reverse transcription at three distinct hormonal periods in the cycles shown in Figure 16.1: day 13 (peak E), EcDNA; days 21 to 23 of adequate secretory phases, PcDNA; and days 21 to 23 of inadequate secretory phases, IcDNA (13,14). Fragments ranging in size from approximately 200bp to 6kb were excised from a gel (Fig. 16.2A), eluted and end-ligated with sequence specific adaptors for subsequent amplification. The adaptors also contained an EcoRI site for cloning when desired (13). The addition of sequence specific adaptors is an important approach that allows us to amplify indefinitely hormonally regulated endometrial cDNA populations from an expensive and therefore limited animal model, the rhesus monkey. We analyzed these cDNA populations to determine whether they contained genes and/or gene fragments of expected representation (housekeeping genes) using gene-specific primers for PCR analysis. Both glyceraldehyde-3-phosphate dehydrogenase (G3PDH) and actin showed a similar level of expression in all three cDNA populations (EcDNA, PcDNA, IcDNA) as shown in Figure 16.2B. These data provide supporting evidence that legitimate differences among these cDNA populations can be determined by semiquantitative PCR analysis.

Hormonal Regulation of Known Genes

E-Dominant Versus P-Dominant Endometria

PCR is an invaluable technique for the analysis of gene expression, and it is particularly useful when analyzing low abundance mRNA or when limiting amounts of tissue are available. Although absolute amounts of template are not measured, in many situations it is sufficient and simpler to compare rela-

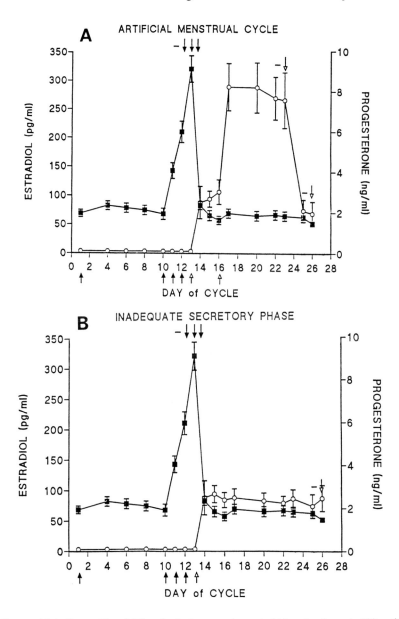

FIGURE 16.1. Serum E and P levels during an adequate (A) or inadequate (B) artificial menstrual cycle in ovariectomized rhesus monkeys. Closed squares and closed arrowheads represent the mean ± sem (*n* = 4–8) of serum E levels and implant insertion and removal respectively. Open circles and open arrowheads represent the mean ± sem (*n* = 4–8) of serum P levels and implant insertion and removal respectively. Reprinted with permission from (14).

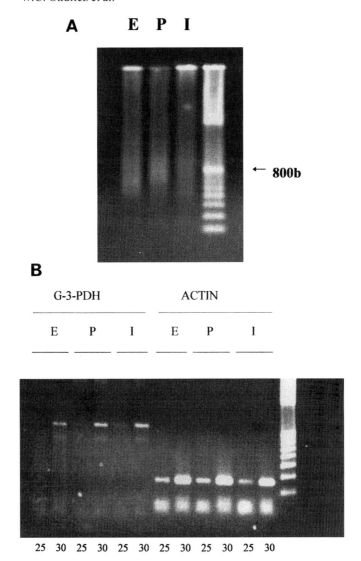

FIGURE 16.2. Ethidium bromide-stained agarose gel of E-, P-, and I-cDNA endometrial populations (A) and expression of the housekeeping genes G-3PDH and actin in EcDNA, PcDNA, and IcDNA endometrial populations (B). cDNA populations are identified by E, P, or I above the corresponding lane. Lane to the far right is a DNA molecular size ladder. In order to verify that EcDNA, PcDNA, and IcDNA populations reflect comparable levels of mRNA abundance upon which semi-quantitative PCR analysis can be based, the three populations were analyzed by PCR with gene-specific primers for G-3PDH and actin. Cycle lengths of 25 and 30 are shown from left to right for each cDNA population. Representative of three different experiments (see Table 16.1 and 16.2). Reprinted with permission from (14).

tive amounts of a particular target sequence in different samples. The essence of the approach is to sample product from the PCR at multiple points throughout the amplification process, to ensure that analysis of expected product occurs before a plateau is reached. Using this method, 2- to 10-fold differences in the level of starting mRNA are accurately detectable. The use of primers to a control transcript, such as glyceraldehyde-3-phosphate dehydrogenase (G-3-PDH), provides supporting evidence that each sample undergoes equivalent reverse transcription to cDNA and equivalent amplification in the PCR. Extensive structural remodeling occurs in the endometrium during the primate secretory phase. Because of this remodeling, P is expected to regulate a wide variety of genes that include growth factors and their receptors, extracellular matrix proteins, and enzymes involved in cellular metabolism (3,5,15–17). Our initial efforts focused on differences in EcDNA and PcDNA of genes known to be regulated by E or P or are major regulators of cellular growth and response. Table 16.1 summarizes the semiquantitative PCR analysis of the genes that we have studied and serves as a basis for the following discussion.

TABLE 16.1. Differential regulation of genes in endometrial EcDNA and PcDNA.

	-fold difference		Linear kinetic range (cyc. no.)
	Mean[a]	sd(+/–)	
Equivalent in E and P:			
G-3-PDH	1.1	0.1	30
ACTIN	1.3	0.1	25
ER	1.2	0.1	25
PR	1.2	0.2	25
EGFR	0.8	0.2	35
IGF-1	1.0	0.1	30
Down-regulated in P:			
HC3	>10[b]	nd	45
EGF	>10[b]	nd	45
RB	2.0	0.9	30
Up-regulated in P:			
PP14	>10[b]	nd	30
LIF	5.6	1.2	30
IGF-1-R	1.6	1.0	30
TGFB-2	1.9	0.8	30
TGFB-2-R	1.6	0.3	30
17-B-HSD	2.2	0.5	45

[a]The mean of three experiments, comparing E- and P-cDNA, is presented.
[b]Values >10 are estimates because PCR product was detected exclusively in only one cDNA population, and therefore the standard deviation (sd) is not presented.
Reprinted from Ace and Okulicz: Mol Cell Endocrinology 1995;115:95–103, with kind permission from Elsevier Science Ireland Ltd, Bay 15K, Shannon Industrial Estate, Co. Clare, Ireland.

Our previous studies in the rhesus monkey endometrium have documented the striking zonal changes in cell proliferation that occur during the changeover from an E- to a P-dominant endometrium (18,19). Proliferation in zones I, II, and III during peak E levels was dramatically suppressed during the midsecretory phase whereas proliferation in zone IV of the basalis increased. The results from the above studies suggest that P plays a role either directly or indirectly in the proliferation observed in the basalis during the midsecretory phase. These data prompted us to study known regulators of cellular proliferation.

Both EGF and IGF-1 have been shown to be potent mitogens in many tissues including the uterus (20,21). EGF has been described as an important growth factor that can simulate the effects of E (22). The elevated expression of EGF in EcDNA compared to PcDNA coincides with maximum endometrial proliferation at this time of the menstrual cycle (18,19,23). Although no detectable difference in EGFR was observed between EcDNA and PcDNA, a dramatic decrease in EGF gene expression (10-fold) occurred concomitant with P-inhibition of endometrial proliferation in the secretory phase. These data suggest that down-regulation of EGF expression may play a role in the decreased proliferation observed during this phase of the menstrual cycle. Similar to our results, earlier work in the human showed little or no difference in EGFR immunostaining during the menstrual cycle (24,25). Although a previous immunohistochemical study in the human did not detect differences in EGF during the menstrual cycle (25), our results suggest that P action strongly suppresses EGF gene expression in the rhesus endometrium.

IGF-1 mRNA has been shown to be present in human uterine tissue with the highest levels occurring during the proliferative phase of the menstrual cycle (26). Although we observed expression of IGF-1 during the proliferative phase in the rhesus endometrium, there was little or no difference compared to secretory phase endometrium. Previous studies on the immunohistochemical intensity and mRNA levels of uterine IGF-1-R have shown that both are maximally elevated during the late proliferative and early secretory phase in the human (27). Our results also show that IGF-1-R gene expression is up-regulated (3-fold) in secretory phase endometria. It should be noted that using RT-PCR we do not consider differences less than 1.5-fold significant.

The increased expression of TGFB-2 (3-fold) in the secretory phase is consistent with a potential physiological role because this factor has been shown to have anti-proliferative properties. These data are compatible with the decreased cellular proliferation observed during this phase of the menstrual cycle (see above). Previous studies in the human endometrium have shown similar increases in TGFB-2 protein and mRNA expression during the early and midsecretory phase (28). No significant difference was observed for TGFB-2-R between E- or P-dominant endometria.

An increased conversion of uterine estradiol to the less active estrogen, estrone, occurs during the secretory phase in the rhesus monkey (9). In addition, the protein and mRNA for the enzyme responsible for this conversion,

17-beta-hydroxysteroid dehydrogenase (17-B-HSD) was shown to be elevated during the secretory phase in the human endometrium (29,30). We also observed an increased expression of endometrial 17-B-HSD (2.9-fold) in PcDNA. The elevation of 17-B-HSD may serve as an additional mechanism whereby P-action necessary for proper maturation of the endometrium is ensured (i.e., blunting E-action).

The cell growth inhibitory mechanism of the retinoblastoma gene (RB), although not yet fully understood (31), makes it a potential regulator of the decreased endometrial proliferation (upper zones) in the secretory phase. Our data show, however, that it is down-regulated (3.2-fold) by P in the primate endometrium. Its down-regulation in PcDNA could potentially play a role in the increased proliferation in zone IV of the basalis observed during P-dominance (11).

Leukemia inhibitory factor (LIF), a secreted glycoprotein, possesses a broad range of biological activities (32). The mRNA for LIF has been shown to be present in the endometrial glands of the mouse (33) and human (34). Of particular importance for understanding endometrial function, LIF has been shown to be required for blastocyst implantation in the mouse (33). Our results show that LIF is a P-dependent factor (4.4-fold increase versus EcDNA) expressed in the rhesus endometrium during the secretory phase.

PcDNA Versus IcDNA Populations

We chose several of the above genes as well as others for further characterization in our IcDNA population, and these data are summarized in Table 16.2. To our knowledge, this was the first study to analyze the relative levels of gene expression in adequate versus inadequate endometria in a well-controlled nonhuman primate model.

It might be expected that genes that require high sustained levels of P for appropriate expression during adequate secretory phases would exhibit considerably lower levels of expression in inadequate endometria. The majority of genes tested bear out this possibility (Table 16.2). For example, PP14, a known P-dependent gene (35), was clearly underrepresented (15-fold) in our IcDNA population.

LIF, as noted above, possesses a broad range of biological activities, including an important role in implantation in the mouse and was highly up-regulated in PcDNA (see above). Our results show that LIF expression is clearly underrepresented (8.3-fold) in IcDNA compared to PcDNA. Although the precise role(s) for LIF in the endometrium is presently unknown, it may potentially serve as an important marker for appropriate endometrial maturation necessary for implantation.

As noted, the enzyme 17-B-HSD metabolizes E to the less potent, estrogen, estrone (36), and potentially helps to redirect the transition from an E-dominant to a P-dominant endometrium. The expression of this enzyme during an inadequate secretory phase was considerably lower (2.9-fold) than that in an

TABLE 16.2. Differential regulation of genes in endometrial PcDNA and IcDNA.

	-fold difference		Linear kinetic range (cyc. no.)
	Mean[a]	sd(+/−)	
Similar in P and I:			
G-3-PDH	1.1	0.1	30
ACTIN	1.3	0.1	25
HC3	no detectable bands at 50		
EGF	"	"	"
EGFR	0.8	0.2	35
Underrepresented in I:			
PP14	15	3.9	25
LIF	8.3	0.9	30
17-B-HSD	9.5	2.0	35
IGF-1	1.8	0.8	30
IGF-1-R	18	2.7	30
TGFB-2	10	2.8	30
TGFB-2-R	8.0	2.3	30
c-fos	2.7	0.9	30
c-jun	9.8	3.3	30
RB	20	7.1	35–40
Up-regulated in I:			
KGF	3.0	0.7	25

[a]The mean of three experiments comparing P- versus I-cDNA is presented.
Reprinted with permission from (14).

adequate secretory phase. These data may suggest that an inadequate endometrium is exposed to a more estrogenic milieu that may on balance result in a lower progestational state.

IGF-1 and its receptor were both found to be underrepresented (1.8 and 18-fold respectively) during an inadequate secretory phase. These results suggest that the regulation of the IGF-1-R gene requires higher sustained levels of P (normal secretory phase) for appropriate expression. The lower expression of IGF-1 in IcDNA versus PcDNA was somewhat unexpected because of its potent mitogenic action and the inhibition of endometrial proliferation observed during an adequate secretory phase. It remains unclear how this result plays a role in proper maturation of the endometrium.

Table 16.2 also shows that endometrial TGFB-2 and its receptor are underrepresented (10- and 8-fold respectively) during an inadequate secretory phase. Because proliferation generally ceases as differentiation begins, the decreased expression of TGFB-2 and its receptor could potentially play a role in retarded endometrial differentiation.

The transcription factors c-fos and c-jun (AP-1 proteins) bind DNA as homodimers or heterodimers and are considered to mediate the action of signal transduction pathways by growth factors, hormones, and cytokines (37).

In this manner, these factors serve as global mediators of transcriptional activity and might be expected to play important roles in the proper maturation of the endometrium. RB, as noted above, is an important cell-cycle/proliferation regulator (38). During an inadequate secretory phase the endometrial expression of c-fos, c-jun, and RB genes was strikingly repressed. These factors have been implicated in the regulation of many genes and gene networks, and these data indicate that a plethora of endometrial genes may be altered during an inadequate secretory phase. P inhibition of E-dependent genes represents another level of regulation that might be expected to be compromised during an inadequate secretory phase. In contrast to underrepresented genes described above, HC3 and EGF showed no differences in expression between adequate and inadequate secretory phases. As shown above, these two E-dependent genes were down-regulated in PcDNA compared to EcDNA by over 10-fold (Table 16.1). These results suggest that the inhibition of these two particular genes is very sensitive to P (i.e., low levels of P are sufficient for inhibition).

KGF is a member of the FGF gene family, and it has been shown to stimulate proliferation in epithelial cells (39). KGF is produced by mesenchymal cells. It is P-dependent and present in endometrial stromal cells in the rhesus monkey (40). We have previously shown that P up-regulates KGF expression in the rhesus endometrium by primer specific PCR analysis (EcDNA versus PcDNA) (14). Our findings in IcDNA suggest, however, that regulation of KGF differs from the other P-dependent genes that we have studied. In contrast to an underrepresentation of a gene in IcDNA, endometrial expression of KGF is substantially higher (3-fold) in IcDNA than PcDNA (Table 16.2). These data support the notion that KGF, although its expression is clearly P-dependent, is autologously down-regulated by high sustained levels of P.

Enrichment for P-Dependent Genes: Subtractive Hybridization

Subtractive hybridization utilizes two gene populations to enable isolation of uniquely expressed species in one population by subtraction of sequences common to both. We used EcDNA ("driver") to subtract complementary sequences from PcDNA ("target"), thus isolating P-specific cDNAs (for methodological details see (13)). Southern blot analysis of subtracted PcDNA (Psub.cDNA) using radiolabelled EcDNA as probe determined that four successive subtractive hybridizations were necessary for efficient removal (>95%) of driver-complementary sequences from PcDNA (data not shown). Restriction enzyme sites (EcoRI) in the adaptors (13) allow target cDNA that has been subtracted of common sequences to be cloned into compatible vectors yielding a subtracted library that contains predominantly differentially regulated cDNAs. Screening a subtracted library for hormone-dependent genes is simplified since the majority of nonspecific cDNAs have been removed.

Size and sequence of any particular cDNA fragment (independent of differential abundance) will influence the extent to which it is enriched during coupled PCR amplification and subtractive hybridization. However, because the same adaptor is used to amplify all fragments in both cDNA populations, it is assumed that; fragments from any individual gene are amplified randomly by PCR with respect to those from another gene, and that the same cDNA fragment is amplified identically in the two different cDNA populations (13). Therefore, primarily up-regulated (P-dependent) target cDNAs will be relentlessly enriched during subsequent subtraction and amplification steps as a result of differential abundance of starting mRNA level. Based on the above considerations, semiquantitative comparisons of mRNA representation between the original cDNAs are considered legitimate.

To determine efficiency of subtraction, we compared the presence of housekeeping genes in the starting PcDNA and subtracted PcDNA populations (Figure 16.3A and B, respectively). The subtraction of common genes was highly efficient because laminin and fibronectin fragments were undetectable by PCR amplification (at the cycle lengths shown). Reduction of actin was also substantial whereas levels of the P-dependent gene, PP14, remained constant. From these data we estimate that PP14 and other P-dependent cDNAs have been enriched at least 100-fold.

Of the three clones selected for sequencing and further study (H1, H3, H5) (13), H1 is novel and without homology to entries in current databases. All three fragments (H1, H3, H5) were shown to be underrepresented in IcDNA compared to PcDNA by PCR analysis (unpublished data). H5 shows extensive homology to an uncharacterized human gene KIAA0279 that is similar to the cadherin-related tumor suppressor hFAT (drosophila fat larva) (unpublished data). Certain tumor suppressor genes such as hFAT are likely to be activated by P because proliferation is inhibited in many cell-types during the secretory phase (12,41). In fact, we have shown (see above) that the tumor suppressor TGFB-2 and its receptor mRNA are increased by P in normal secretory endometria. Because cadherins are considered fundamental for establishing and maintaining multicellular structures (42), their expression in the endometrium is perhaps not surprising. Indeed, cadherin-11 has been implicated in trophoblast-endometrium interactions due to its localization and temporal expression in trophoblast and decidualizing endometrial cells during the late secretory phase in women (43).

H3 encodes the C-terminus of a new mucin-related gene (unpublished data) that shares homology to cysteine-rich repeat domains known to bind ligands and receptors in a large number of other glycoproteins. The sequence of H3 is most similar to a bovine mucin gene, gallbladder bovine mucin (GBM) (44). The 98-aa repeat-like sequence found in H3 displays considerable sequence similarity to C-terminal cysteine-rich repeats in GBM and a number of other receptor and ligand-binding proteins that contain scavenger receptor cysteine-rich repeat (SRCR) regions (45). The conserved cysteine residues in this domain are potential N-glycosylation sites and may be capable of form-

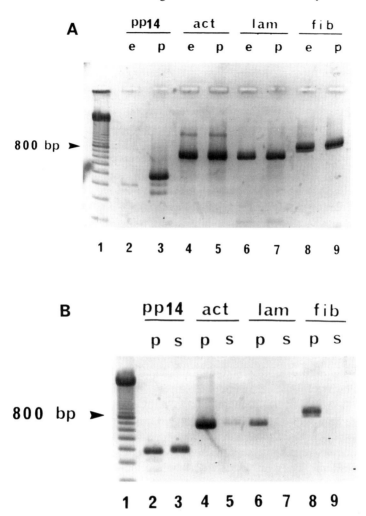

FIGURE 16.3. Verification of the efficiency of subtractive hybridization. (A) EcDNA (e) and PcDNA (p) were screened for PP14, actin, laminin, and fibronectin by sequence-specific PCR. Products for PP14 (lanes 2 and 3), actin (lanes 4 and 5), laminin (lanes 6 and 7), and fibronectin (lanes 8 and 9) were 390, 620, 630, and 720 bp respectively. (B) Starting PcDNA (p) and subtracted Psub.cDNA (s) were screened for PP14 (lanes 2 and 3), actin (lanes 4 and 5), laminin (lanes 6 and 7), and fibronectin (lanes 8 and 9). Reprinted with permission from Ace et al. (13).

ing disulfide bonds between monomers; a feature thought to be required for mucin gel formation (46). Polymorphic MUC1 mRNA and protein are maximally expressed in human endometrium (glandular and luminal epithelial cells) during the midsecretory phase of the menstrual cycle (47). The rise in MUC1 mRNA level is consistent with transcriptional activation by P and analysis of the MUC1 promotor suggests the existence of a potential P response element (48). The functional significance of elevated MUC1 expression in midsecretory endometrium remains to be determined, although the timing suggests a correlation with the periimplantation period. As noted, our novel H3 mucin-related gene was shown to be greatly underrepresented in inadequate endometrium and as such its elevated expression is associated with an adequate endometrium. The above studies implicate mucin- and cadherin-like molecules as P-dependent secretory phase proteins with potential roles in endometrial maturation and/or receptivity.

Identification of Different Levels of Endometrial Regulation by DDRT-PCR

Differential display RT-PCR (DDRT-PCR) is a recent approach for the identification of mRNAs that show differences in expression level between two or more mRNA populations. Diffferences may be discerned among cell types, tissues, developmental stages, or hormonal treatments (49). The method uses the ability of randomly chosen cDNAs to be amplified by a pair of short arbitrary (10-mer) PCR primers. The sequence of the primers dictates which panel of cDNA fragments of the total will be amplified; only those gene fragments containing sequences complementary to the primers will be amplified. The use of different primer sets results in different patterns (gene fragments) that are amplified, and we have utilized this method to broaden the scope of genes to be analyzed. Because the fragments are small (50–400 bp), they can be quickly sequenced and compared by homology to GenBank database entries. Our results support the levels of regulation identified by analysis of known genes in our E-, I-, and PcDNA populations described above.

When E-, I-, and PcDNA were compared by DDRT-PCR, we were able to identify at least four levels of mRNA regulation, as illustrated by the pattern of cDNA fragments in Figure 16.4. First, we detected fragments up-regulated by a high level of P during an adequate secretory phase similar to that shown above (Table 16.1) for PP14 and LIF (indicated by fragment 1 in Fig. 16.3). Second, there were fragments up-regulated by a low level of P in inadequate secretory phases but apparently down-regulated by an adequate level of P as shown above for KGF (e.g. fragment 2). Third, some fragments (e.g. fragment 3) were underrepresented in inadequate versus adequate secretory phases as noted above for the majority of known genes studied (see Table 16.2). Last, fragment 4 in Figure 16.3 appears to be down-regulated by P in both adequate and inadequate secretory phases compared to the proliferative phase. This result is similar to that shown above for HC3 and EGF (Tables 16.1 and 16.2). It should be noted that Figure 16.4 is a small, convenient part of one gel showing an example of each level of regulation. An examination of several DDRT-PCR gels comparing EcDNA, PcDNA, and IcDNA showed that many genes/gene fragments exhibited the four levels of regulation described above.

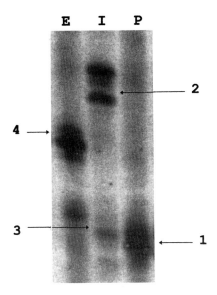

FIGURE 16.4. DDRT-PCR of primate endometial EcDNA, IcDNA, and PcDNA. (1) Indicates a gene fragment up-regulated in PcDNA compared to EcDNA and underrepresented in IcDNA; (2) Represents a fragment that is up-regulated by P (inadequate) but apparently autologously down-regulated by and adequate level of P (unpublished observation). (3) Indicates a gene fragment that is up-regulated by both an inadequate and adequate level of P; (4) Indicates a E-dependent gene fragment that is down-regulated by both a low (inadequate) and a normal (adequate) level of P. (4). Represents a fragment that is up-regulated by P (inadequate) but apparently autologously down-regulated by and adequate level of P (unpublished observation).

Summary

The most prominent functions of P in mammals are decidualization of the uterus, preparation of the endometrium for embryo implantation, and maintenance of pregnancy (1,2). The data described above focus on P regulation of endometrial gene expression in a nonhuman primate model, the rhesus monkey. Our ability to create artificial menstrual cycles in this primate animal model provides the experimental means to more precisely analyze endometrial response to P. Our data provide evidence that at least four different levels of P-dependent regulation of endometrial gene regulation can be identified in the rhesus monkey. Based on these observations it is likely that P-dependent regulation of endometrial genes involves waves of gene expression that are temporally controlled. This latter feature of P action may in part explain the restricted "window of implantation" observed in both women and nonhuman primates during the secretory phase; a temporally dependent maturation of the endometrium is required for implantation.

The above data are a first step toward a more thorough understanding of P-dependent regulation of endometrial genes and gene networks during adequate and inadequate secretory phases in the rhesus monkey. It is, however, clear from our studies (12,23,41) and those of other laboratories (50–53) that an important aspect of primate endometrial response resides in the cell-type and zonal regulation of these genes and their gene products. Future studies involving in situ hybridization and immunohistochemistry will help to resolve these important questions of endometrial physiology and their relationship to implantation.

Note Added in Proof

Additional sequence data obtained for the H3 gene and a follow-up Genbank search indicated a highly significant homology (92% identical) (Ace and Okulicz. A progesterone-induced endometrial homology of a new candidate tumor suppressor DMBT1. J Clin Endocrinol Metab 1998; in press) with the recently identified putative tumor-suppressor gene, DMBT1 (Mollenhauer J, Wiemann S, Scheurlen W et al. DMBT1, a new member of the SRCR super-family, on chromosome 10q25.3-26.1 is deleted in malignant brain tumors. Nature Gene 1997;17:32-39). Together, these studies potentially provide a molecular link to the protective effect of progesterone action on unopposed estrogen exposure in reproductive tract cancers in women.

Acknowledgment. This work was supported in part by a grant from the NICHD (HD31620).

References

1. Wynn RM, Jollie WP, eds. Biology of the uterus. 2d ed. New York: Plenum, 1989: 289–331.
2. Maslar IA. The progestational endometrium. Sem Reprod Endocrinol 1988;6: 115–28.
3. Bartelmez GW, Corner GW, Hartman CG. Cyclic changes in the endometrium of the rhesus monkey (Macaca mulatta). Contrib Embryol 1951;34:99–144.
4. Bartelmez GW. The phases of the menstrual cycle and their interpretation in terms of the pregnancy cycle. Am J Obstet Gynecol 1957;74:931.
5. Ferenczy A, Bergeron C. Histology of the human endometrium: from birth to senescence. Ann NY Acad Sci 1991;622:6–27.
6. Hodgen GD. Surrogate embryo transfer combined with estrogen-progesterone therapy in monkeys. Implantation, gestation, and delivery without ovaries. JAMA 1983;250:2167–71.

7. Wilks JW, Hodgen GD, Ross GT. Luteal phase defects in the rhesus monkey: the significance of serum FSH:LH ratios. J Clin Endocrinol Metab 1976;43:1261–7.
8. Jones GS. The luteal phase defect. Fert Steril 1976;27:351–6.
9. Longcope C, Bourget C, Meciak PA, Okulicz WC, McCracken JA, Hoberg LM, et al. Estrogen dynamics in the female rhesus monkey. Biol Reprod 1988;39:561–5.
10. Okulicz WC, Savasta AM, Hoberg LM, Longcope C. Biochemical and immunohistochemical analyses of estrogen and progesterone receptors in the rhesus monkey uterus during the proliferative and secretory phases of artificial menstrual cycles. Fertil Steril 1990;53:913–20.
11. Okulicz WC, Balsamo M, Tast J. Progesterone regulation of endometrial estrogen receptor and proliferation during the late proliferative and secretory phase in artificial menstrual cycles in the rhesus monkey. Biol Reprod 1993;49:24–32.
12. Okulicz WC, Balsamo M. A double immunofluorescent method for the simultaneous analysis of progesterone-dependent changes in proliferation (Ki-67) and the estrogen receptor in the rhesus endometrium. J Reprod Fertil 1993;99:545–9.
13. Ace CI, Balsamo M, Le LT, Okulicz WC. Isolation of progesterone-dependent complementary deoxyribonucleic acid fragments from rhesus monkey endometrium by sequential subtractive hybridization and polymerase chain reaction amplification. Endocrinology 1994;134:1305–9.
14. Okulicz WC, Ace CI, Longcope C, Tast J. Analysis of differential gene regulation in adequate *versus* inadequate secretory-phase endometrial complementary deoxyribonucleic acid populations from the rhesus monkey. Endocrinology 1996;137:(11)4844–50.
15. Gurpide E, Tseng L. Induction of human endometrial oestradiol dehydrogenase by progestins. Endocrinology 1975;97:825–33.
16. Clarke CL, Sutherland RL. Progestin regulation of cellular proliferation. Endocrinol Rev 1990;11:266–301.
17. Fay TN, Grudzinskas JG. Human endometrial peptides: A review of their potential role in implantation and placentation. Hum Reprod 1991;6:1311–26.
18. Padykula HA, Coles LG, McCracken JA, King NW, Longcope C, Kaiserman-Abramof IR. A zonal pattern of cell proliferation and differentiation in the rhesus endometrium during the estrogen surge. Biol Reprod 1984;31:1103–18.
19. Padykula HA, Coles LG, Okulicz WC, Rapaport SI, McCracken JA, King NW, Jr., et al. The basalis of the primate endometrium: a bifunctional germinal compartment. Biol Reprod 1989;40:681–90.
20. Fisher DA, Lakshmanan J. Metabolism and effects of epidermal growth factor and related growth factors in mammals. Endocrinol Rev 1990;11:418–42.
21. Murphy LJ, Ghahary A. Uterine insulin-like growth factor-1: regulation of expression and its role in estrogen-induced uterine proliferation. Endocrinol Rev 1990;11:443–53.
22. Ignar-Trowbridge DM, Teng CT, Ross KA, Parker MG, Korach KS, McLachlan JA. Peptide growth factors elicit estrogen receptor-dependent transcriptional activation of an estrogen-responsive element. Mol Endocrinol 1993;7:992–8.
23. Okulicz WC, Balsamo M, Tast J. Progesterone regulation of endometrial estrogen receptor and cell proliferation during the late proliferative and secretory phase in artificial menstrual cycles in the rhesus monkey. Biol Reprod 1993;49:24–32.
24. Berchuck A, Soisson AP, Olt GJ, Soper JT, Clarke-Pearson DL, Bast RC, Jr., et al. Epidermal growth factor receptor expression in normal and malignant endometrium. Am J Obstet Gynecol 1989;161:1247–52.

25. Chegini N, Rossi MJ, Masterson BJ. Platelet-derived growth factor (PDGF), epidermal growth factor (EGF), and EGF and PDGF β-receptors in human endometrial tissue: localization and *in vitro* action. Endocrinology 1992;130:2373–85.

26. Boehm KD, Daimon M, Gorodeski IG, Sheean LA, Utian WH, Ilan J. Expression of the insulin-like and platelet-derived growth factor genes in human uterine tissues. Mol Reprod Devel 1990;27:93–101.

27. Tang X-M, Rossi MJ, Masterson BJ, Chegini N. Insulin-like growth factor I (IGF-I), IGF-I receptors, and IGF binding proteins 1–4 in human uterine tissue: tissue localization and IGF-I action in endometrial stromal and myometrial smooth muscle cells in vitro. Biol Reprod 1994;50:1113–25.

28. Chegini N, Zhao Y, Williams RS, Flanders KC. Human uterine tissue throughout the menstrual cycle expresses transforming growth factor-b1 (TGFb1), TGFb2, TGFb3, and TGFb type II receptor messenger ribonucleic acid and protein and contains [125I]TGFb1-binding sites. Endocrinology 1994;135:439–49.

29. Maentausta O, Sormunen R, Isomaa V, Lehto VP, Jouppila P, Vihko R. Immunohistochemical localization of 17-β-hydroxysteroid dehydrogenase in the human endometrium during the menstrual cycle. Lab Invest 1991;65:582–7.

30. Casey ML, MacDonald PC, Andersson S. 17β-hydroxysteroid dehydrogenase type 2: Chromosomal assignment and progestin regulation of gene expression in human endometrium. J Clin Invest 1994;94:2135–41.

31. Goodrich DW, Lee WH. Abrogation by c-myc of G1 phase arrest induced by RB protein but not by p53. Nature 1992;360:177–9.

32. Hilton DJ, Gough NM. Leukemia inhibitory factor: a biological perspective. J Cell Biochem 1991;46:21–6.

33. Stewart CL, Kaspar P, Brunet LJ, Bhatt H, Gadi I, Kontgen F, et al. Blastocyst implantation depends on maternal expression of leukaemia inhibitory factor. Nature 1994;359:76–9.

34. Kojima K, Kanzaki H, Iwai M, Hatayama H, Fujimoto M, Inoue T, et al. Expression of leukemia inhibitory factor in human endometrium and placenta. Biol Reprod 1994;50:882–7.

35. Joshi SG. A progestagen associated protein of the human endometrium. Basic studies and potential clinical applications. J Steroid Biochem 1983;19:751–7.

36. Longcope C, Bourget C, Meciak PA, Okulicz WC, McCracken JA, Hoberg LM, et al. Estrogen dynamics in the female rhesus monkey. Biol Reprod 1988;39:561–5.

37. Curran T. Cohen P, Foulkes JG, eds.The hormonal control regulation of gene transcription. Amsterdam: Elsevier, 1991:295–308.

38. Cordon-Cardo C, Richon VM. Expression of the retinoblastoma protein is regulated in normal human tissues. Am J Pathol 1994;144:500–10.

39. Finch PW, Rubin JS, Miki T, Ron D, Aaronson SA. Human KGF is FGF-related with properties of a paracrine effector of epithelial cell growth. Science 1989;245:752–5.

40. Koji T, Chedid M, Rubin JS, Slayden OD, Csaky KG, Aaronson SA, et al. Progesterone-dependent expression of keratinocyte growth factor mRNA in stromal cells of the primate endometrium: keratinocyte growth factor as a progestomedin. J Cell Biol 1994;125:393–401.

41. Okulicz WC, Ace CI, Scarrell R. Zonal changes in proliferation in the rhesus endometrium during the late secretory phase and menses. Proc Soc Exp Biol Med 1997;214:(2)132–8.

42. Takeichi M. Cadherins: a molecular family important in selective cell-cell adhesion. Ann Rev Biochem 1991;59:237–52.

43. MacCalman CD, Furth EE, Omigbodun A, Bronner M, Coutifaris C, Strauss JF. Regulated expression of cadherin-11 in human epithelial cells: a role for cadherin-11 in trophoblast-endometrial interactions? Devel Dyn 1996;206:201–11.

44. Nunes DP, Keates AC, Afdhal NH, Offner GD. Bovine gall-bladder mucin contains two distinct tandem repeating sequences: evidence for scavenger receptor cysteine-rich repeats. Biochem J 1995;310:41–8.

45. Kanan J, Nayeem N, Binns RM, Chain BM. Mechanisms for variability in a member of the scavenger-receptor cysteine-rich superfamily. Immunogenetics 1997;46:276–82.

46. Gum JR. Mucin genes and the proteins they encode: structure diversity and regulation. Am J Respir Cell Mol Biol 1992;7:557–64.

47. Aplin JD, Hey NA. MUCl, endometrium and embryo implantation. Biochem Soc Trans 1995;23:(4)826–31.

48. Hey NA, Graham RA, Seif MW, Aplin JD. The polymorphic epithelial mucin MUC1 in human endometrium is regulated with maximal expression in the implantation phase. J Clin Endocrinol Metab 1994;78:337–42.

49. Liang P, Pardee A. Differential display of eukaryotic messenger RNA by means of polymerase chain reaction. Science 1992;257:967–71.

50. Horwitz KB, Wei LL, Sedlacek SM, d'Arville CN. Progestin action and progesterone receptor structure in human breast cancer: a review. Recent Prog Horm Res 1985;41:249.

51. McClellan MC, West NB, Brenner RM. Immunocytochemical localization of estrogen receptors in the macaque endometrium during the luteal-follicular transition. Endocrinology 1986;119:1467–75.

52. Lessey BA, Metzger DA, Haney AF, McCarty KS, Jr. Immunohistochemical analysis of estrogen and progesterone receptors in endometriosis: comparison with normal endometrium during the menstrual cycle and the effect of medical therapy. Fertil Steril 1989;51:409–15.

53. Hild-Petito S, Verhage HG, Fazleabas AT. Immunocytochemical localization of estrogen and progestin receptors in the baboon (*Papio anubis*) uterus during implantation and pregnancy. Endocrinology 1992;130:2343–3.

17

Embryo–Maternal Dialogue in the Baboon (*Papio Anubis*)

Asgerally T. Fazleabas, Ji-Yong Julie Kim,
Kathleen M. Donnelly, and Harold G. Verhage

"Endometrial receptivity" has been defined as the period during the menstrual or estrous cycle that is most favorable for blastocyst implantation. However, in the absence of a blastocyst or a blastocyst "signal," the true definition of a receptive uterus is difficult to ascertain. This is especially true for studies pertaining to the human endometrium. Towards this end, we have developed the baboon as a nonhuman primate model and attempted to identify changes in the receptive uterine endometrium both for the presence or absence of a conceptus. The window of receptivity in the baboon is between 8 and 11 days postovulation. For the purposes of our studies we have divided the receptive window into three phases. Phase I is characterized by the changes induced by estrogen and progesterone during the luteal phase of the normal menstrual cycle. Phase II is defined as modulation of the Phase I receptive endometrium by blastocyst signals. In the primate, chorionic gonadotrophin (CG) is the primary luteotrophic hormone and presumably the major embryonic "signal." Phase III of the implantation window is induced by the blastocyst interacting with the receptive endometrium. This phase is characterized by rapid trophoblast migration and the onset of decidualization of stromal fibroblasts.

This review summarizes our current in vivo studies on the three phases of uterine receptivity in the baboon and discusses the potential functional significance of these changes as they relate to blastocyst implantation.

Phase I of Uterine Receptivity

Conceptually, the phase of the menstrual or estrous cycle when the endometrium is most receptive to blastocyst implantation is thought to be associated with specific biological changes that are induced by estrogen and progesterone. In addition ovarian steroids are also thought to modulate morphological and biological changes that lead up to (prereceptive) and close (refractory) this receptive window. Figure 17.1 summarizes the qualitative changes in protein expression in the epithelial cells of the baboon endometrium during these three stages of the luteal phase.

The prereceptive phase (day 5–8 post ovulation) is characterized by the presence of both the polymorphic mucin (Muc-1) and the progesterone receptor (PR) on the luminal epithelial cells [1,2]. Estrogen influences alone do not appear to be sufficient to drive Muc-1 expression in the baboon uterus in surface or glandular epithelia of the functionalis. In contrast, combined estrogen and progesterone influences Muc-1 expression in all uterine epithelial cell types, particularly the surface epithelium. These results suggest that progesterone actions are required to support Muc-1 expression in the baboon, a suggestion previously made by Hey et al. [3] in the human. The effects of combined estrogen and progesterone actions are complex, however, because prolonged exposure to steroids (days 10–12 postovulation or in ovariectomized, estrogen-primed animals given 14 days of combined estrogen and progesterone treatment) results in the loss of Muc-1 from the surface epithelium. This loss of Muc-1 from the surface epithelium correlates with loss of progestin receptors from these cells during the postovulatory period [1,2]. Loss of Muc-1 from the surface epithelium during the receptive phase (days 8–10 postovulation) is consistent with proposed roles for mucins as antiadhesive or protectant molecules [4,5]. In this sense, high-level mucin expression at early times after ovulation (days 5–8) may aid in uterine resistance to microbial challenge during copulation. Reduction of mucin expression in surface epithelium during the receptive phase (days 8–10 postovulation) would then be necessary to permit access to appropriate receptors for embryos on the apical uterine epithelial cell surface.

In various primate species, the uterus enters the receptive phase approximately 8–10 days postovulation in a hormonal milieu rich in both estrogen and progesterone influences [4,5]. It has also been shown that these conditions result in a marked decrease in immunologically detectable estrogen and

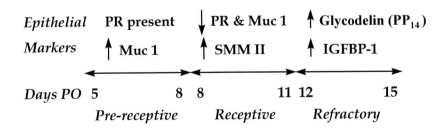

FIGURE 17.1. Graphical representation of changes in uterine epithelial marker proteins during the luteal phase in the baboon.

progesterone receptors in epithelia of both the lumen (surface) and functionalis regions; however, estrogen as well as progesterone immunoreactivity persists in the glandular epithelia of the basalis (1,6,7). Consequently, it appears that direct actions of steroid hormones on the epithelium are more likely to occur in the basalis than in any other region during the mid- to late-luteal phase. Interestingly, the downregulation of PR in the luminal epithelium and the glands closest to the uterine lumen appears to be the only consistent bio-chemical feature of uterine receptivity in the majority of mammalian species (8). Although a number of other morphological and molecular changes have been reported to be associated with the receptive phase in several mammalian species, a definite common marker other than PR has yet to be identified (9,10). For example, the $\alpha_v\beta_3$ integrin, a vitronectin receptor, appears in the epithelium of normal fertile women around the time of implantation (11), whereas in the baboon it appears well after the initial stage of embryo attach-ment (12). This observation may reflect differences between the type of im-plantation (interstitial versus superficial) in these two species. In contrast, smooth muscle myosin II expression in the luminal and glandular epithelium appears to be correlated with the receptive phase in the baboon (13).

In nonpregnant baboons and humans, the refractory phase is characterized by the synthesis of insulin-like growth factor binding protein-1 (IGFBP-1) and glycodelin PP_{14} (14–16). If pregnancy is established, the synthesis and secretion of these two proteins increases markedly. These two proteins consti-tute the major secretory products of the baboon and human endometrium during pregnancy and have been postulated to play a role in immunosuppres-sion and regulation of trophoblast migration (see (17) for review).

Phase II of Uterine Receptivity

In ruminants and pigs, the primary role of the embryonic signals is to prevent luteolysis (8,18). In contrast, chorionic gonadotrophin secreted by the pri-mate blastocyst has direct luteotrophic effects and maintains progesterone secretion by the corpus luteum during the initial stages of gestation.

Endometrial receptivity is linked with successful implantation. It is evident from studies in ruminants and pigs that the hormonally receptive primed en-dometrium is further modulated by an embryonic stimulus (8,18). These data imply that the embryo or its secretions induces functional receptivity. To test this hypothesis, we developed a simulated pregnant baboon model to determine both short-term (19) and long-term (20) effects of chorionic gonadotrophin treatment on the endometrial response. The short-term treatment mimicked blastocyst se-cretion of chorionic gonadotrophin by infusing human recombinant chorionic gonadotrophin via osmotic minipumps between days 6 and 10 postovulation. Analysis of tissues following 4 days of chorionic gonadotrophin infusion (day10 postovulation) resulted in the downregulation of smooth muscle myosin II in the luminal epithelium (see Fig. 17.1) and the induction of cellular endoreplication in this epithelial cell layer. This endoreplication is charac-terized morphologically by the appearance of epithelial plaques. Glycodelin (PP_{14}) secretion by the glandular epithelium also increases markedly in re-sponse to chorionic gonadotrophin infusion. The stromal fibroblasts below the epithelial plaque also begin to differentiate, and this process is associated with α smooth muscle actin (αSMA) expression in these cells. The exact function of these specific changes induced by chorionic gonadotrophin in the three major cell types in the endometrium have not been elucidated. We postulate that the plaque reaction in the luminal epithelium may serve to increase the surface for blastocyst/endometrial interactions.

The induction of αSMA in the stromal fibroblasts may be associated with the initial phase of decidual transformation. Cytoskeletal proteins are impor-tant in mitosis, cell growth, changes in cell shape, and also for the regulation of protein secretion (21). Alpha SMA is an important filamentous protein associated with the cytoskeleton. It is also becoming increasingly evident that integrin mediated signal transduction requires the coordination of the actin cytoskeleton with growth factor responses (22).

Decidualization in the baboon (12) and human (11) is associated with changes in integrin expression and extracellular matrix protein (ECM) syn-thesis. The expression of integrins α_1, α_3, α_5, β_1, and $\alpha_v\beta_3$ increases during decidualization, and this is accompanied by increases in fibronectin, laminin, and collagen IV at the implantation site (12). The peripheral localization of ECM proteins around decidualizing stromal cells in both baboon (12) and human (23) demonstrates that new ECM protein deposition is associated with a new cellular phenotype. The ECM may induce specific changes in integrin expression and may also participate in signal transduction (24). The interac-tion between integrins and the ECM induces changes in the actin cytoskel-eton that are thought to be critical for signal transduction (25,26). Baboon stromal cells undergoing decidualization express αSMA (13). Thus, it is conceivable that the increased expression of specific integrins and the ac-companying changes in the ECM and αSMA expression during simulated pregnancy and pregnancy may be essential for stromal cell proliferation and differentiation.

The generalized effects of long-term chorionic gonadotrophin treatment on the morphology, secretory activity, and steroid receptor localization of the nonpregnant baboon endometrium was comparable to those observed in pregnancy (20). However, the cell-specific changes in IGFBP-1 expression at the implantation site appear to require additional conceptus signals. Similar differences in expression at the implantation site compared to the nonimplantation site have been reported for basic fibroblast-growth factor in the rat uterus (27) and leukemia inhibitory factor in the rabbit uterus (28). Furthermore, differences in uterine epidermal growth factor gene expression between pregnant and ovariectomized steroid-treated mice also suggested that the blastocyst influences cell-specific gene expression in the uterus (29–31). However, as we have noted in our studies in the baboon (32,33) and as with previous studies in the mouse (34), not all of the uterine proteins were directly influenced by the conceptus. Interestingly, the genes whose expression appeared to be influenced by pregnancy in the primate (20,35) and rodent were either growth factors, their receptors, or binding proteins (29–31,35).

In summary, using a simulated-pregnant baboon model we have demonstrated that the combination of chorionic gonadotrophin and steroid hormones induces morphological changes in the endometrium that are comparable to pregnancy. In addition chorionic gonadotrophin can act directly on the endometrium to enhance the synthesis of glycodelin and IGFBP-1 by the glandular epithelium. However, additional conceptus factors appear to be necessary to initiate complete stromal cell differentiation (i.e., decidualization) and induce the changes in cell-specific expression of IGFBP-1 and IGF-I receptor that occur at the implantation site during pregnancy (20).

Phase III of Uterine Receptivity

Decidualization, or uterine stromal cell differentiation, is an essential feature of pregnancy in rodents and primates. Decidualization of stromal fibroblasts is associated with cellular proliferation followed by differentiation. Our in vivo studies (34,36) suggested that the baboon conceptus plays an obligatory role in inducing decidualization. Following implantation, the stromal fibroblasts undergo extensive modifications to form decidual cells in baboon (37), and their transformation in the baboon is associated with the sequential expression of αSMA, IGF-I receptor, and IGFBP-1 (13,34,35,37). The induction of IGFBP-1 synthesis in decidual cells at the placental–endometrial interface is a possible mechanism by which IGFs can be locally concentrated. IGF-I receptors are present in the plasma membrane of cytotrophoblast cells as early as day 18 of pregnancy in the developing placenta (37) coincident with IGFBP-1 expression in the luminal glandular epithelial cells. These two correlated events may initially enhance trophoblast proliferation and migration. The subsequent induction of IGFBP-1 in decidualized stromal cells at the maternal/fetal interface (35) may inhibit further trophoblast invasion. Thus, although the precise mechanisms by which trophoblast invasion is regulated in both the human and the baboon remain to be determined, IGFBP-1 could potentially regulate this phenomenon. IGFBP-1 binds to the $\alpha_5\beta_1$ integrin via its Arg-Gly-Asp (RGD) sequence (38). Recent in vitro studies suggest that IGFBP-1 inhibits cytotrophoblast invasion into decidualized stromal endometrium by binding to $\alpha_5\beta_1$ on cytotrophoblasts (39). We postulate that IGFBP-1, may mediate its action by binding to cell membrane receptors (40–42). The presence of the RGD tripeptide on IGFBP-1 may also enhance its interactions with the decidual cells surface and/or become a part of the decidual extracellular matrix (12). Thus, once the invading trophoblast have migrated into the spiral arteries, the trophoblasts at the cytotrophoblastic shell could induce IGFBP-1 in the underlying decidua and prevent further invasion. This type of regulation of trophoblast invasion has been demonstrated in co-cultures of human decidual and cytotrophoblast cells (39).

Summary

Using the baboon as a nonhuman primate model, we have been able to clearly demonstrate that the receptive endometrium can be further modulated by exogenous or endogenous chorionic gonadotrophin and the implanting embryo. These in vivo studies will now enable us to focus in on cellular and molecular studies in vitro and delineate the specific signaling pathways activated by chorionic gonadotrophin and the invading trophoblasts during implantation.

Acknowledgments. These studies were done as part of the National Cooperative Program for Markers of Uterine Receptivity for Blastocyst Implantation and were supported by Cooperative Agreement NIH-HD 29964.

References

1. Hild-Petito S, Verhage HG, Fazleabas, AT. Immunocytochemical localization of estrogen and progestin receptors in the baboon (*Papio anubis*) uterus during implantation and early pregnancy. Endocrinology 1992;130:2343–53.
2. Hild-Petito S, Fazleabas AT, Julian J, Carson D. Mucin (Muc-1) expression is differentially regulated in uterine lumenal and glandular epithelia of the baboon (*Papio anubis*). Biol Reprod 1996;54:939–47.
3. Hey NA, Graham RA, Seif MW, Aplin JD. The polymorphic epithelial mucin MUC1 in human endometrium is regulated with maximal expression in the implantation phase. J Clin Endocrinol Metab 1994;78:337–42.
4. Enders AC. Overview of the morphology of implantation in primates. In: Wolf R, Stouffer RL, Brenner RM, eds. In vitro fertilization and embryo transfer in primates. New York: Springer-Verlag, 1993:145–57.
5. Brenner RM, Slayden OD. Cyclic changes in the primate oviduct and endometrium. In: Knobil E, Neill JD, eds. The physiology of reproduction, 2nd ed. New York: Raven, 1994:541–69.
6. Lessey BA, Kilam AP, Metzger DA, Haney AF, Greene GL, McCarty KS. Immunocytochemical analysis of human estrogen and progesterone receptors throughout the menstrual cycle. J Clin Endocrinol Metab 1988;67:334–60.
7. Brenner RM, McClellan MC, West NB. Immunocytochemistry of estrogen and progestin receptors in the primate reproductive tract. In: Moudgal VK, eds. Steroid receptors in health and disease. New York: Plenum, 1988:47–70.
8. Bazer FW. Mediators of maternal recognition of pregnancy in mammals. Proc Soc Exp Biol Med 1992;199:373–84.
9. Tabibzadeh S, Babaknia A. The signals and molecular pathways involved in implantation: a symbiotic interaction between the blastocyst and endometrium involving adhesion and tissue invasion. Hum Reprod 1995;10:1579–602.

10. Lopata A. Blastocyst-endometrial interaction: an appraisal of some old and new ideas. Mol Human Reprod 1996;2:519–25.

11. Lessey BA, Damjanovich L, Coutifaris C, Castelbaum A, Albelda SM, Birch CA. Integrin adhesion molecules in human endometrium. Correlation with normal and abnormal menstrual cycle. J Clin Invest 1992;90:188–95.

12. Fazleabas AT, Bell SC, Fleming S, Sun J, Lessey BA. Distribution of integrins and the extracellular matrix proteins in the baboon endometrium during the menstrual cycle and early pregnancy. Biol Reprod 1997;56:348–56.

13. Christensen S, Verhage HG, Nowak, G, de Lanerolle P, Fleming S, Bell SC, et al. Smooth muscle myosin II and α smooth muscle actin expression in the baboon (*Papio anubis*) uterus is associated with glandular secretory activity and stromal cell transformation. Biol Reprod 1995;53:596–606.

14. Bell SC, Drife JO. Secretory proteins of the human uterine endometrium and decidua during menstrual cycle and pregnancy: characterization of pregnancy-associated endometrial α_1- and α_2-globulins (α_1- and α_2-PEG). In: Hau J, ed. Pregnancy proteins in animals. Berlin: Walter de Gruyter, 1986:143–64.

15. Fazleabas AT, Hild-Petito S, Verhage HG. The primate endometrium: morphological and secretory changes during early pregnancy. Sem Reprod Endocrinol 1995;13:120–32.

16. Hausermann HM, Donnelly KM, Bell SC, Verhage HG, Fazleabas AT. Regulation of the glycosylated β-lactoglobulin homologue, glycodelin [placental protein 14 (PP_{14})] in the baboon (*Papio anubis*) uterus. J Clin Endocrinol Metab 1998;83: 1226–33.

17. Fazleabas AT, Donnelly KM, Hild-Petito S, Hausermann HM, Verhage HG. (1997). Secretory proteins of the baboon (*Papio anubis*) endometrium: regulation during the menstrual cycle and early pregnancy. In: Khan FS, ed. Proceedings of a symposium on the female baboon as a model for research in reproduction. Human Reproduction Update, 1997;3:553–9.

18. Spencer TE, Ott TL, Bazer FW. Face-interferon: pregnancy recognition signal in ruminants. Proc Soc Exp Biol Med 1996;213:215–29.

19. Fazleabas AT, Donnelly KM, Fortman JD, Miller JB. Modulation of the baboon (*Papio anubis*) endometrium by chorionic gonadotrophin (CG) during the period of uterine receptivity. (Abstract #374). Biol Reprod 1997;56(Supp 1):176.

20. Hild-Petito S, Donnelly KM, Miller JB, Verhage HG, and Fazleabas AT. A baboon (*Papio anubis*) simulated-pregnant model: cell specific expression of insulin-like growth factor binding protein-1 (IGFBP-1), type I IGF receptor (IGF-I R) and retinol binding protein (RBP) in the uterus. Endocrinology 1995;3:639–51.

21. Rao KMK, Cohen HJ. Actin cytoskeletal network in aging and cancer. Mutation Res 1991;256:139–48.

22. Dedhar S, Hannigan GE. Integrin cytoplasmic interactions and bidirectional transmembrane signaling. Cur Opinions Cell Biol 1996;8:657–69.

23. Aplin JD, Charlton AK, Ayad, S. An immunohistochemical study of human endometrial extracellular matrix during the menstrual cycle and first trimester of pregnancy. Cell Tissue Res 1988;253:231–40.

24. Juliano RL, Haskill S. Signal transduction from extracellular matrix. J Cell Biol 1993;120:577–85.

25. Clark EA, Brugge JS. Integrins and signal transduction pathways: the road taken. Science 1995;268:233–9.

26. Dedhar S. Integrin-mediated signal transduction in oncogenesis: an overview. Cancer Metastasis Rev 1995;14:165–72.

27. Carlone DI, Rider V. Embryonic modulation of basic fibroblast growth factor in the rat uterus. Biol Reprod 1993;49:653–65.

28. Yang ZM, Le SP, Chen DB, Yasukawa K, Harper MJK. Expression patterns of leukemia inhibitory factor receptor (LIFR) and the gp 130 receptor component in rabbit uterus during early pregnancy. J Reprod Fertil 1995;103:249–55.

29. Das SK, Tsukamura H, Paria BC, Andrews GK, Dey SK. Differential expression of epidermal growth factor receptor (EGF-R) gene and regulation of EGF-R bioactivity by progesterone and estrogen in the adult mouse uterus. Endocrinology 1994; 134:971–81.

30. Das SK, Wang X-N, Paria BC, Damm D, Abraham JA, Klagsbrun M, et al. Heparin-binding EGF-like growth factor gene is induced in the mouse uterus temporally by the blastocyst solely at the site of its apposition: a possible ligand for interaction with blastocyst EGF-receptor in implantation. Development 1994;120:1071–83.

31. Das SK, Chakraborty I, Paria BC, Wang X-N, Plowman G, Dey SK. Amphiregulin is an implantation specific and progesterone-regulated gene in the mouse uterus. Mol Endocrinol 1995;9:691–705.

32. Fazleabas AT, Bell SC, Verhage HG. Insulin-like growth factor binding proteins: a paradigm for conceptus—maternal interactions in the primate. In: Strauss JF III, Lyttle CR, eds. Uterine and embryonic factors in early pregnancy. New York: Plenum, 1991:157–65.

33. Fazleabas AT, Hild-Petito S, Donnelly KM, Mavrogianis PA, Verhage HG. Interactions between the embryo and uterine endometrium during implantation and early pregnancy in the baboon (Papio anubis). In: Brenner RM, Wolf DR, Stouffer RL, eds. In vitro fertilization and embryo transfer in primates. New York: Springer-Verlag, 1993:169–81.

34. Dey SK, Paria BC, Das SK, Andrews GK. Trophoblast-uterine interactions in implantation: role of transforming growth factor-α/epidermal growth factor receptor signalling. In: Soares MJ, Handwerger S, Talamantes F, eds. Trophoblast cells: pathways for maternal-embryonic communication. New York: Springer-Verlag, 1993:71–91.

35. Tarantino S, Verhage HG, Fazleabas AT. Regulation of insulin-like growth factor binding proteins (IGFBPs) in the baboon (Papio anubis) uterus during early pregnancy. Endocrinology 1992;130:2354–62.

36. Enders AC, Schlafke S. Implantation in non-human primates and in the human. In: Comparative Biology, Reproduction and Development, Vol 3. New York: A.R. Liss, 1986:291–310.

37. Hild-Petito S, Verhage HG, Fazleabas AT. Characterization, localization and regulation of receptors for insulin-like growth factor (IGF)-I in the baboon uterus during the cycle and early pregnancy. Biol Reprod 1994;50:791–801.

38. Jones JI, Gockerman A, Busby WH, Wright G, Clemmons DR. Insulin-like growth factor binding protein 1 stimulates cell migration and binds to the alpha-5-beta-1 integrin by means of its Arg-Gly-Asp sequence. Proc Natl Acad Sci USA 1993;90:10553–7.

39. Irwin JC, Giudice LC. IGB binding protein-1 binds to cytotrophoblast a5b1 integrin and inhibits cytotrophoblast invasion into decidualized human endometrial stromal cell multilayers. Growth Reg 1997 (in press).

40. Lee PDK, Conover CA, Powell DR. Regulation and function of insulin-like growth factor binding protein-1. Proc Soc Exp Biol Med 1993;204:4–29.

41. Rosenfeld RG, Lamson G, Pham H, et al. Insulin-like growth factor binding proteins. Recent Prog Horm Res 1991;46:99–159.

42. Sara VR, Hall K. Insulin-like growth factors and their binding proteins. Physiol Rev 1990;70:591–614.

18

Integrins and Uterine Receptivity

Bruce A. Lessey

It is increasingly clear that successful implantation involves a complex dialogue that occurs between the endometrium and the embryo. The integrins have proven to be versatile cell surface receptors that appear to be involved at multiple functional levels, orchestrating many of the cell–cell interactions during implantation. The integrins have been shown to mediate many important physiologic duties of the cell during embryogenesis and development and are involved in cell attachment and migration as well as programmed cell death (apoptosis). The interest in integrins has gained momentum as the view of implantation has shifted to a "receptor-mediated" event (1). Cell adhesion molecules (CAMs) are actively being studied in the context of cancer cell invasion and metastasis. Given the many similarities that exist between the invasion of the embryo and the spread of cancer, it may not be surprising that the cellular interactions and migration that occurs during implantation may depend on the expression of similar specific cell adhesion receptors, their extracellular matrix (ECM) ligands, and enzymes.

Specifically, the integrin family of cell adhesion molecules are a major class of receptors for the ECM and have been shown to participate in cell–cell and cell–substratum interaction (2). These receptors are present on the plasma membrane as heterodimeric α and β glycoprotein subunits, and their numbers have increased to include at least 22 different integrins, based on subunit pairing. The integrins are increasingly being studied in the context of reproduction (for review see (3,4)). During implantation, integrins appear to have roles in signal transduction (5), maintenance of cellular polarity (6,7), and the developmental progression of placental cytotrophoblast to an invasive phenotype (8). Our studies also suggest a role in the establishment of uterine receptivity (9,10).

Endometrial Integrins

There have been many molecular markers proposed to identify the period of uterine receptivity referred to as the window of implantation. Some of these candidate factors or indices include trophinin and tastin (11), leukemia inhibitory factor (12,13), heparan sulfate proteoglycans (14), mucins such as

MUC-1 (15) or MAG (16), pinopods (17), and others. In 1992, we (9) and others (18) first described the temporal and spatial pattern of integrin expression in the endometrium of women. Since that time, numerous studies have described the changes in endometrial integrins in vivo (19–26) and in vitro (27–32) as well as in certain animal models (33–35).

The justification for the intense focus on integrins in the endometrium has been their potential involvement in adhesion molecules in embryo-endometrial interaction at the time of implantation. The window of maximal uterine receptivity is now generally thought to occur 6 to 10 days after ovulation (cycle day 20 to 24), based in part on early work by Hertig and colleagues (36) and more recently on data from Navot and coworkers, using the donor-oocyte recipient model (37,38). While many of the integrins are constitutively expressed in the endometrium involved in "housekeeping" or the maintenance of tissue architecture and cellular phenotype, we have also identified integrins with increased expression during the menstrual cycle. The coexpression of three integrins on endometrial epithelium, $\alpha 1\beta 1$, $\alpha 4\beta 1$, and $\alpha v\alpha 3$, was noted to frame the putative window of implantation (Fig. 18.1). The endometrial integrin $\alpha v\beta 3$ appears on the surface of the endometrial epithelium coincident with the opening of this window (cycle day 19 to 20) and is present first on the apical pole of the glandular and luminal epithelium at the time of initial attachment and later on the decidua of pregnancy (Fig. 18.2). This pattern of $\alpha v\beta 3$ immunostaining has subsequently been also reported by Mardon and coworkers (39) and the spatial distribution on the apical pole also confirmed by Aplin and colleagues (40). This integrin, like several others, recognizes the three amino acid sequence arg-gly-asp (RDG) in its target ligands; this amino acid sequence has been implicated in trophoblast attachment and outgrowth (41,42). Absence of $\alpha v\beta 3$ expression during the window of implantation has been reported with luteal phase deficiency (LPD) (9), and in some women with endometriosis (43), unexplained infertility (44), and hydrosalpinges (45). The selective loss of normal integrin expression is thought to reflect an altered or dysfunctional endocrine or paracrine milieu leading to implantation deficiency. These data suggest utility as both a marker of uterine receptivity as well as a potential probe to study the molecular mechanisms of implantation.

Other integrins have been evaluated in the endometrium of humans and in animal models. Although not all studies agree, a general pattern of integrin expression on different cell types is presented in Table 18.1. Any discrepancies in the literature are likely the result of the variety of antibodies that have been used to study integrins that may detect variable epitopes or alternatively spliced variant products. Occasionally, the differences in integrin expression between species have been informative. The $\alpha v\beta 3$ integrin was found in the mouse uterus at the time of implantation, but is induced by estrogen in this species (unpublished observations). In humans, this integrin is thought to be suppressed by the sex steroids in humans (see below) (31). In the baboon endometrium, $\alpha v\beta 3$ integrin expression is delayed for about two weeks com-

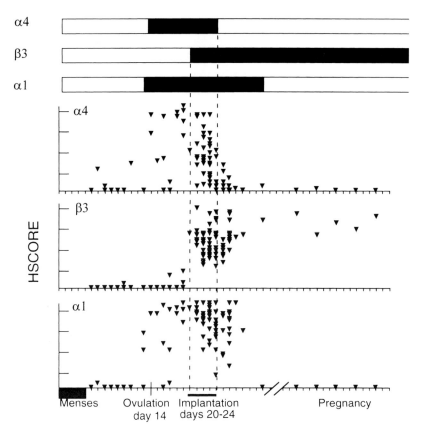

FIGURE 18.1. The pattern of cycle specific endometrial integrin expression during the menstrual cycle and early pregnancy. Note the coexpression of all three integrins ($\alpha 1\beta 1$, $\alpha 4\beta 1$, and $\alpha v\beta 3$) during the putative window of implantation. Reproduced from Lessey et al. (10) with permission from the American Society of Reproductive Medicine.

pared to the human appearing after initial attachment of the embryo has occurred (35). Acquisition of the invasive phenotype occurs about two weeks later in this species, leading to the hypothesis that endometrial $\alpha v\beta 3$ may be involved in the establishment of placental invasion in both species. Other integrins are also proving to be interesting as well and appear to have complex roles during implantation. The integrin $\alpha v\beta 5$, similar to $\alpha v\beta 3$, is present on both the endometrial and embryonic epithelium at the time of implantation (40,46). These two integrins may serve different functions, as suggested by a recent abstract at the Society for Gynecologic Investigation (47), which showed that $\alpha v\beta 5$ but not $\alpha v\beta 3$ was involved in trophoblast attachment to RL95 endometrial cells. Using these cells, Thie et al., has expanded their work on the role of apical integrins and shown that this adhesion of trophoblast is dependent on the polarization of the epithelium and an intact cytoskeleton (7). In bone, the $\alpha v\beta 5$ may provide a back up function for $\alpha v\beta 3$ which can be

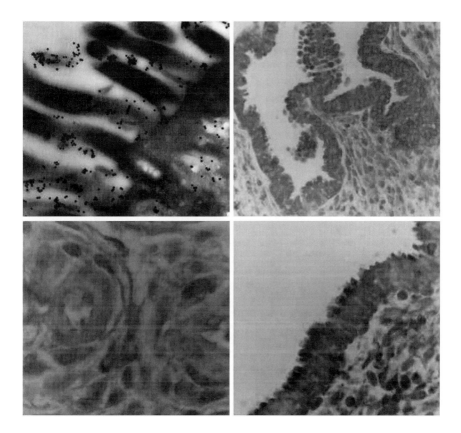

FIGURE 18.2. Distribution of the αvβ3 integrin in human endometrium. Electron microscopy (top left) demonstrates apical localization of the β3 subunit using gold particles
bound to antibodies which recognize the αvβ3 integrin. Immunostaining on glandular
(top right) and luminal epithelium (bottom left) is usually positive on cycle day 20 and
later. In the late secretory phase and in pregnancy, αvβ3 immunostaining increases on
the decidualizing stroma (bottom left).

inactivated by genetic mutation (Glanzmann's tromboasthenia). Finally, the
α5β1 integrin, which also binds RGD peptides, has been implicated as a receptor for IGF-binding protein 1 (48). It may have defined roles in limiting
invasion of the trophoblast in human implantation (49).

Regulation of Integrin Expression in the Endometrium

The regulation of integrins subunits was recently reviewed elsewhere (50).
The increased expression of secretory phase epithelial integrins in the endometrium suggests that steroid hormones likely play a role in their appearance. It is well known that estrogen and progesterone prepare the endometrium

TABLE 18.1. Temporal and spatial distribution of integrin subunits in the endometrium throughout the menstrual cycle and in pregnancy, divided by ligand preference.

	Col/LM					FN/VN						Tenascin
	α1	α2	α3	α6	β4	α4	α5	αv	β3	β5	β6	α9
Glandular												
Proliferative	○	●	●	●¶	●¶	○	○	○	○	*	○	○
Early Secretory	●	●	●	●	●	●	○	*	○	●	○	*
Mid Secretory	●	●	●	●	●	●	○	●	●	●	○	●
Late Secretory	●	●	●	●	●	○	○	●	●	●	○	●
Pregnancy	○	*	●	*	●	○	○	●	●	?	○	?
Stromal												
Proliferative	○	○	○	●	○	○	●	*	*	*	○	○
Early Secretory	*	○	○	●	○	○	●	*	*	*	○	○
Mid Secretory	*	○	*	*	○	○	●	*	*	●	○	○
Late Secretory	●	○	●	*	○	○	●	●	●	●	○	○
Pregnancy	●	○	●	●	○	○	●	●	●	●	○	○
Luminal												
Proliferative	○	*	●	●	●	○	○	○	○	*	*	●
Early Secretory	○	*	●	●	●	○	○	○	○	●	*	●
Mid Secretory	○	○	●	●	●	○	○	●	●	●	*	●
Late Secretory	○	●	●	●	●	○	○	●	●	●	*	●
Pregnancy	○	*	●	*	●	○	○	●	●	?	*	?

¶ signifies basolateral distribution of staining
● corresponds to + or ++ staining
* corresponds to ± staining
○ corresponds to - staining

for implantation. With the discovery of the α1β1 collagen/laminin receptor (VLA-1) and its expression on secretory phase endometrial epithelium (9,18), it was felt that progesterone directly up-regulates this integrin in vivo. Steroid regulation of integrins was first convincingly demonstrated in endometrial explants by Tabibzadeh and Satyaswaroop (51). In this early experiment, the α1β1 integrin was found to undergo up-regulation in explant tissue after exposure to progesterone. These data are consistent with recent studies using the Ishikawa cells as a model of endometrial epithelial cells, in which the expression of the α1 subunit was shown to be increased following estrogen and progesterone treatment (Fig. 18.3) (27,32). It is likely that the α4 subunit of the α4β1 fibronectin receptor will also be shown to be positively regulated by progesterone in the endometrium consistent with it's expression on cycle day 14 (see Fig. 18.1).

The regulation of αvβ3 in human endometrium is more enigmatic. It appeared on cycle day 20, long after the time when serum levels of estrogen and progesterone are first elevated. Furthermore, this integrin and the α1β1 collagen/laminin receptor undergo dramatic increases in expression in the decidua of pregnancy (10,23) suggesting that cell-specific differences in

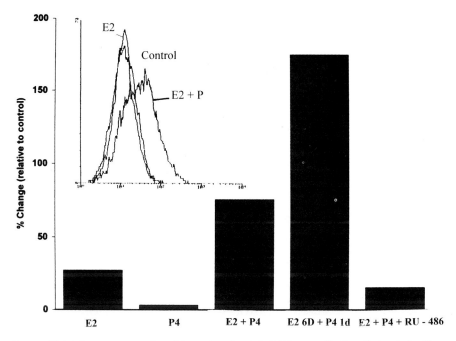

FIGURE 18.3. Flow cytometry for α1 integrin subunit in Ishikawa cells. In cells treated with estradiol (E_2; 10^{-8} M) or P alone (P_4; 10^{-6} M) there was little effect on α1 subunit expression. In contrast E_2 plus P for four days significantly increased α1 expression (lane 3 and inset). The percent change was based on the median value, as described in the Materials and Methods section. Of note, prolonged E_2 treatment with only one day of P treatment yielded maximal α1 expression. The addition of equimolar anti-progestin, RU-486, eliminated this stimulatory effect of P in E_2 primed cells (lane 5). Reproduced from Lessey et al. (10) with permission from The American Society of Reproductive Medicine.

regulation must exist. One clue came from our earlier studies on steroid receptors in the human endometrium. In 1988, we (52) and others (53,54) discovered that secretory phase endometrial epithelium selectively lost progesterone receptors (PR) while stromal cells maintained their expression of this receptor. The loss of both ER and PR is a direct effect of the rise in luteal phase serum progesterone levels and both effectively disappear by cycle day 19 to 20. We have since been able to demonstrate that the αvβ3 integrin expression at this time correlates well with the loss of epithelial PR. In women with histologic delay, such as is found with luteal phase defect, the endometrium expresses more PR than normal controls and has reduced expression of the αvβ3 integrin. Successful medical treatment that restored normal histology resulted in a return of both αvβ3 integrin expression and the normal loss of epithelial PR (55). The suggestion that the αvβ3 integrin was inversely associated with ER and PR was later shown to be the result of steroid inhibition of integrin expression (31), with decreased αvβ3 in Ishikawa cells after treatment with estrogen or estrogen plus progesterone and increased expression when the antiprogestin RU-486 was administered. Other papers have also demonstrated steroid regulation of integrin expression or activation in other model systems (56,57).

The increase in stromal integrins during decidualization reflects the change of decidual cells to an epithelial phenotype in early pregnancy. The increase in more typical epithelial integrins ($\alpha 1\beta 1$, $\alpha 3\beta 1$, $\alpha 6\beta 1$) appears to be indirectly stimulated by sex steroids. We have postulated that the increase in $\alpha 1\beta 1$ and $\alpha v\beta 3$ expression during decidualization is modulated by specific growth factors. We have used primary stromal cell cultures to demonstrate that TGF–β and EGF appear to increase $\alpha 1\beta 1$ expression in stromal cells in vitro (58). TGFα and EGF significantly enhance the expression of the $\alpha v\beta 3$ integrin in epithelial cells as well (31). Based on these and ongoing studies we now believe that the initiation of uterine receptivity depends on the local withdrawal of steroid action in the endometrial epithelium and steroid mediated paracrine effects from the stroma or from the implanting embryo. Further studies will be required to fully understand the importance of these relationships.

Integrins and the Regulation of Cellular Function In Vitro

The integrins maintain tissue architecture and cellular phenotype. Cell shape and polarity are known to be important for the maintenance of cell function (59,60). There have been several studies that demonstrate that basement membrane (Matrigel) alters cellular morphology and establishes a polarized phenotype in endometrial cells in vitro (61,62). Matrix mediated changes in gene expression have been demonstrated as well (63,64). Using the endometrial cell line, HEC 1B (65) it was demonstrated that laminin, but not collagen mediated these changes, likely through the a6β4 integrin (29).

Recent exciting data suggests that the $\alpha v\beta 3$ integrin binds and activates matrix metalloproteinases (MMP) and plasminogen activators (66,67). The position of $\alpha v\beta 3$ on the apical portion of the epithelium on the luminal surface of the endometrium (25,40) and on the outer surface of embryos (46,68) raises the possibility that this integrin serves to activate and position proteases during implantation. Proteolytic fragments that arise from MMP degradation of basement membrane serves as a signal for cell migration (69) and might stimulate trophoblast invasion. A model that reflects a role for cell adhesion molecules in initial attachment and invasion is shown in Fig. 18.4. Initial attachment may be mediated by integrins or other cell adhesion mol-

$\longrightarrow$

FIGURE 18.4. Schematic of possible involvement of cell adhesion molecules and ECM and proteases in the process of implantation in the human. As illustrated in the upper left, the embryo enters the endometrial cavity between cycle day 16 to 18 prior to implantation. Endometrial-embryonic epithelium must interact as part of the initial adhesion event (A). Models of cell–cell adhesion include integrin interaction with ECM molecules, like fibronectin or through homeotypic (integrin–integrin) or heterotypic (integrin–selectin) interactions.

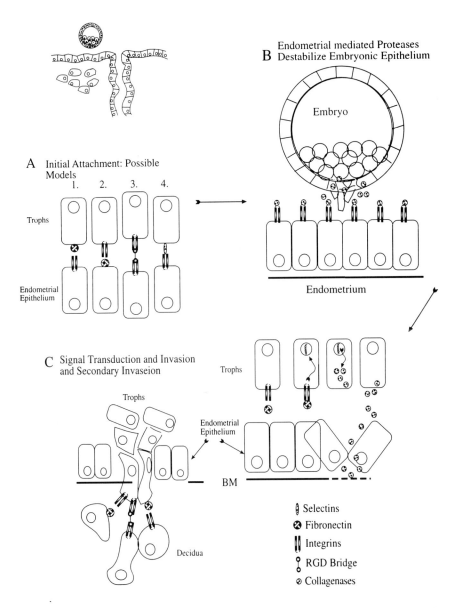

A   Initial Attachment: Possible Models

B   Endometrial mediated Proteases Destabilize Embryonic Epithelium

C   Signal Transduction and Invasion and Secondary Invaseion

Matrix metalloproteinases targeted toward the embryo by luminal integrins may degrade basement membrane and stimulate the invasive phenotype on embryonic cells (B). During the phase of invasion through the basement membrane, integrins have been shown to mediate signal transduction leading to the synthesis and secretion of matrix metalloproteinases. In the secondary invasion and attachment, intruding trophoblast cells interact with the underlying stroma and the fibrinogen rich extracellular matrix milieu (C). Multiple mechanisms of cell–cell adhesion may be postulated in this process. The up-regulation of multiple integrins in the human decidual argues for a role of these molecules in promotion and limitation on embryonic invasion.

ecules such as Trophinin (11). After proximity is established (A), the αvβ3 and MMP could destabilize the basement membrane of the embryo and pro-teolytic fragments of laminin might then stimulate cell migration (B). Upon encountering fibronectin, trophoblast α5β1 or other trophoblast integrins signal the elaboration of embryo-derived MMPs that assist in digestion and invasion into the maternal tissues (C). New integrins and CAMs are likely required to assist and to limit invasion once the decidua has been entered. In addition, biologic mimicry appears to occur as invading cytotrophoblast un-dergo transformation into the phenotype of endothelium, facilitating the in-vasion into the maternal vasculature (70).

Summary

In conclusion, the study of integrins in the endometrium has provided new insights into the timing and regulation of uterine receptivity. The develop-mental progression of the secretory endometrium is dependent on progester-one, but it appears to be the local withdrawal of progesterone support through the loss of PR that may signal the onset of uterine receptivity. A role for growth factors and cytokines is inferred by these studies. Integrins appear to interact with other endometrial proteins in ways that may stimulate or impede implantation. It is likely that the use of such markers will continue to ad-vance our understanding of implantation and lead us on a path of discovery for new treatment and diagnostic approaches to women with infertility.

Acknowledgments. Supported by NIH grants HD 30476, HD 34824. These studies were funded in part by the National Cooperative Program on Markers of Uterine Receptivity for Blastocyst Implantation.

References

1. Yoshinaga K. Receptor concept in implantation research. In Yoshinaga K, Mori T, eds. Development of preimplantation embryos and their environment. New York: A.R. Liss, 1989:379–87.
2. Albelda SM, Buck CA. Integrins and other cell adhesion molecules. FASEB J 1990;4:2868–80.
3. Bronson RA, Fusi FM. Integrins and human reproduction. Mol Hum Reprod 1996;2:153–68.
4. Sueoka K, Shiokawa S, Miyazaki T, Kuji N, Tanaka M, Yoshimura Y. Integrins and reproductive physiology: expression and modulation in fertilization, embryogensis, and implantation. Fertil Steril 1997;67:799–811.
5. Werb Z, Tremble PM, Behrendtsen O, Crowley E, Damsky CH. Signal transduc-tion through the fibronectin receptor induces collagenase and stromelysin gene expression. J Cell Biol 1989;109:877–89.

6. Thie M, Harrach-Ruprecht B, Sauer H, Fuchs P, Albers A, Denker H-W. Cell adhesion to the apical pole of epithelium: a function of cell polarity. Eur J Cell Biol 1995;66:180–91.

7. Thie M, Herter P, Pommerenke H, et al. Adhesiveness of the free surface of a human endometrial monolayer for trophoblast as related to actin cytoskeleton. Mol Hum Reprod 1997;3:275–83.

8. Damsky CH, Librach C, Lim K-H, et al. Integrin switching regulates normal trophoblast invasion. Development 1994;120:3657–66.

9. Lessey BA, Damjanovich L, Coutifaris C, Castelbaum A, Albelda SM, Buck CA. Integrin adhesion molecules in the human endometrium. Correlation with the normal and abnormal menstrual cycle. J Clin Invest 1992;90:188–95.

10. Lessey BA, Castelbaum AJ, Buck CA, Lei Y, Yowell CW, Sun J. Further characterization of endometrial integrins during the menstrual cycle and in pregnancy. Fertil Steril 1994;62:497–506.

11. Fukuda MN, Sato T, Nakayama J, et al. Trophinin and tastin, a novel cell adhesion molecule complex with potential involvement in embryo implantation. Genes Devel 1995;9:1199–210.

12. Stewart CL, Kaspar P, Brunet LJ, et al. Blastocyst implantation depends on maternal expression of leukaemia inhibitory factor. Nature 1992;359:76–9.

13. Cullinan EB, Abbondanzo SJ, Anderson PS, Pollard JW, Lessey BA, Stewart CL. Leukemia inhibitory factor (LIF) and LIF receptor expression in human endometrium suggests a potential autocrine paracrine function in regulating embryo implantation. Proc Natl Acad Sci USA 1996;93:3115–20.

14. Carson DD, Rohde LH, Surveyor G. Cell surface glycoconjugates as modulators of embryo attachment to uterine epithelial cells. Int J Biochem 1994;26:1269–77.

15. Hey NA, Li TC, Devine PL, Graham RA, Saravelos H, Aplin JD. MUC1 in secretory phase endometrium: expression in precisely dated biopsies and flushings from normal and recurrent miscarriage patients. Hum Reprod 1995;10:2655–62.

16. Kliman HJ, Feinberg RF, Schwartz LB, Feinman MA, Lavi E, Meaddough EL. A mucin-like glycoprotein identified by MAG (mouse ascites Golgi) antibodies: menstrual cycle-dependent localization in human endometrium. Am J Pathol 1995;146:166–81.

17. Nikas G, Drakakis P, Loutradis D, et al. Uterine pinopodes as markers of the "nidation window" in cycling women receiving exogenous oestradiol and progesterone. Hum Reprod 1995;10:1208–13.

18. Tabibzadeh S. Patterns of expression of integrin molecules in human endometrium throughout the menstrual cycle. Hum Reprod 1992;7:876–82.

19. Bischof P, Redard M, Gindre P, Vassilakos P, Campana A. Localization of alpha 2, alpha 5 and alpha 6 integrin subunits in human endometrium, decidua and trophoblast. Eur J Obstet Gynecol Reprod Biol 1993;51:217–26.

20. Klentzeris LD, Bulmer JN, Trejdosiewicz LK, Morrison L, Cooke ID. Beta-1 integrin cell adhesion molecules in the endometrium of fertile and infertile women. Hum Reprod 1993;8:1223–30.

21. Tawia SA, Beaton LA, Rogers PA. Immunolocalization of the cellular adhesion molecules, intercellular adhesion molecule-1 (ICAM-1) and platelet endothelial cell adhesion molecule (PECAM), in human endometrium throughout the menstrual cycle. Hum Reprod 1993;8:175–81.

22. Bridges JE, Prentice A, Roche W, Englefield P, Thomas EJ. Expression of integrin adhesion molecules in endometrium and endometriosis. Br J Obstet Gynaecol 1994;101:696–700.

23. Ruck P, Marzusch K, Kaiserling E, et al. Distribution of cell adhesion molecules in decidua of early human pregnancy: an immunohistochemical study. Lab Invest 1994;71:94–101.

24. van der Linden PJ, de Goeij AF, Dunselman GA, van der Linden EP, Ramaekers FC, Evers JL. Expression of integrins and E-cadherin in cells from menstrual effluent, endometrium, peritoneal fluid, peritoneum, and endometriosis. Fertil Steril 1994;61:85–90.

25. Lessey BA, Ilesanmi AO, Sun J, Lessey MA, Harris J, Chwalisz K. Luminal and glandular endometrial epithelium express integrins differentially throughout the menstrual cycle: implications for implantation, contraception, and infertility. Am J Reprod Immunol 1996;35:195–204.

26. Castelbaum AJ, Sawin SW, Bellardo LJ, Lessey BA. Endometrial integrin expression in women exposed to diethylstilbestrol in utero. Fertil Steril 1995;63:1217–21.

27. Lessey BA, Ilesanmi AO, Castelbaum AJ, et al. Characterization of the functional progesterone receptor in an endometrial adenocarcinoma cell line (Ishikawa): progesterone-induced expression of the $\alpha 1$ integrin. J Steroid Biochem Mol Biol 1996;59: 31–9.

28. Shiokawa S, Yoshimura Y, Nagamatsu S, et al. Expression of β_1 integrins in human endometrial stromal and decidual cells. J Clin Endocrinol Metab 1996;81:1533–40.

29. Strunck E, Vollmer G. Variants of integrin $\beta 4$ subunit in human endometrial adenocarcinoma cells: mediators of ECM-induced differentiation? Biochem Cell Biol 1996;74:867–73.

30. Sillem M, Prifti S, Schmidt M, Rabe T, Runnebaum B. Endometrial integrin expression is independent of estrogen or progestin treatment in vitro. Fertil Steril 1997;67:877–82.

31. Somkuti SG, Yuan LW, Fritz MA, Lessey BA Epidermal growth factor and sex steroids dynamically regulate a marker of endometrial receptivity in Ishikawa cells. J Clin Endocrinol Metab 1997;82:2192–7.

32. Castelbaum AJ, Ying L, Somkuti SG, Sun JG, Ilesanmi AO, Lessey BA. Characterization of integrin expression in a well differentiated endometrial adenocarcinoma cell line (Ishikawa). J Clin Endocrinol Metab 1997;82:136–42.

33. Nishida T, Murakami J, Otori T. Expression of fibronectin receptor (integrin) in the uterus of rats in relation to the estrous cycle. Histochemistry 1991;96:279–83.

34. Bruess JM, Gillett N, Lu L, Sheppard D, Pytela R. Restricted distribution of integrin $\beta 6$ mRNA in primate epithelial tissues. J Histochem Cytochem 1993;41:1521–7.

35. Fazleabas AT, Bell SC, Fleming S, Sun J, Lessey BA. Distribution of integrins and the extracellular matrix proteins in the baboon endometrium during the menstrual cycle and early pregnancy. Biol Reprod 1997;56:348–56.

36. Hertig AT, Rock J, Adams EC. A description of 34 human ova within the first 17 days of development. Am J Anat 1956;98:435–93.

37. Bergh PA, Navot D. The impact of embryonic development and endometrial maturity on the timing of implantation. Fertil Steril 1992;58:537–42.

38. Navot D, Bergh PA, Williams M, et al. An insight into early reproductive processes through the in vitro model of ovum donation. J Clin Endocrinol Metab 1991;72:408–14.

39. Rai V, Hopkisson J, Kennedy S, Bergqvist A, Barlow DH, Mardon HJ. Integrins alpha 3 and alpha 6 are differentially expressed in endometrium and endometriosis. J Pathol 1996;180:181–7.

40. Aplin JD, Spanswick C, Behzad F, Kimber SJ, Vicovac L. Integrins $\beta 5$, $\beta 3$, av are apically distributed in endometrial epithelium. Mol Hum Reprod 1996;2:527–34.

41. Armant DR, Kaplan HA, Mover H, Lennarz WJ. The effect of hexapeptides on attachment and outgrowth of mouse blastocysts cultured in vitro: evidence for the involvement of the cell recognition tripeptide Arg-Gly-Asp. Proc Natl Acad Sci USA 1986;83:6751–5.

42. Yelian FD, Yang Y, Hirata JD, Schultz JF, Armant DR. Molecular interactions between fibronectin and integrins during mouse blastocyst outgrowth. Mol Reprod Devel 1995;41:435–48.

43. Lessey BA, Castelbaum AJ, Sawin SJ, et al. Aberrant integrin expression in the endometrium of women with endometriosis. J Clin Endocrinol Metab 1994;79:643–9.

44. Lessey BA, Castelbaum AJ, Sawin SJ, Sun J. Integrins as markers of uterine receptivity in women with primary unexplained infertility. Fertil Steril 1995;63:535–42.

45. Meyer WR, Castelbaum AJ, Harris JE, et al. Hydrosalpinges adversely affect markers of uterine receptivity. Hum Reprod 1997;12:1393–8.

46. Campbell S, Swann HR, Seif MW, Kimber SJ, Aplin JD. Cell adhesion molecules on the oocyte and preimplantation human embryo. Hum Reprod 1995;10:1571–8.

47. Tran TQ, Illsley NP: Role of the $\alpha v\beta3$ and $\alpha v\beta5$ integrins in human endometrial-blastocyst attachment. Ann Meeting Soc Gynecol Invest 1997;432:187A.

48. Jones JI, Gockerman A, Busby WH, Wright G, Clemmons DR. Insulin-like growth factor binding protein 1 stimulates cell migration and binds to the alpha 5/ $\beta1$ integrin by means of its ARG-GLY-ASP sequence. Proc Natl Acad Sci USA 1993;90:10553–7.

49. Irwin JC, Giudice LC. Insulin-like growth factor binding protein-1 binds to cytotrophoblast $\alpha5\beta 1$ integrin and inhibits cytotrophoblast invasion into decidual multilayers. Soc Gynecol Invest Ann Mtg 1996;3:93A-Abst.

50. Kim LT, Yamada KM. The regulation of expression of integrin receptors. Proc Soc Exp Biol Med 1997;214:123–31.

51. Tabibzadeh SS, Satyaswaroop PG. Progestin-mediated induction of VLA-1 in glandular epithelium of human endometrium in vitro. 72nd Ann Mtg The Endocrine Society 1990;#700-Abst.

52. Lessey BA, Killam AP, Metzger DA, Haney AF, Greene GL, McCarty KS Jr. Immunohistochemical analysis of human uterine estrogen and progesterone receptors throughout the menstrual cycle. J Clin Endocrinol Metab 1988;67:334–40.

53. Garcia E, Bouchard P, De Brux J, et al. Use of immunoctyochemistry of progesterone and estrogen receptors for endometrial dating. J Clin Endocrinol Metab 1988;67:80–7.

54. Press MF, Udove JA, Greene GL. Progesterone receptor distribution in the human endometrium. Analysis using monoclonal antibodies to the human progesterone receptor. Am J Pathol 1988;131:112–24.

55. Lessey BA, Yeh IT, Castelbaum AJ, et al. Endometrial progesterone receptors and markers of uterine receptivity in the window of implantation. Fertil Steril 1996;65:477–83.

56. Li C, Ross FP, Cao X, Teitelbaum SL. Estrogen enhances $\alpha v\beta3$ integrin expression by avian osteoclast precursors via stabilization of β_3 integrin mRNA. Mol Endocrinol 1995;9:805–13.

57. Hughes PE, Renshaw MW, Pfaff M, et al. Suppression of integrin activation: a novel function of a Ras/Raf-initiated MAP kinase pathway. Cell 1997;88:521–30.

58. Grosskinsky CM, Yowell CW, Sun JH, Parise LV, Lessey BA. Modulation of integrin expression in endometrial stromal cells in vitro. J Clin Endocrinol Metab 1996;81: 2047–54.

59. Folkman J, Moscona A. Role of cell shape in growth control. Nature 1978;273: 345–9.
60. Gospodarowicz D, Greenburg G, Birdwell CR. Determination of cellular shape by the extracellular matrix and its correlation with the control of cellular growth. Cancer Res 1978;38:4155–71.
61. Bentin–Ley U, Pedersen B, Lindenberg S, Larsen JF, Hamberger L, Horn T. Isolation and culture of human endometrial cells in a three-dimensional culture system. J Reprod Fertil 1994;101:327–32.
62. Classen-Linke I, Kusche M, Knauthe R, Beier HM. Establishment of a human endometrial cell culture system and characterization of its polarized hormone responsive epithelial cells. Cell Tissue Res 1997;287:171–85.
63. Strunck E, Hopert AC, Vollmer G. Basement membrane regulates gene expression in HEC1B(L) endometrial adenocarcinoma cells. Biochem Biophys Res Commun 1996;221:346–50.
64. Hopfer H, Rinehart CA, Kaufman DG, Vollmer G. Basement membrane induced differentiation of HEC–1B(L) endometrial adenocarcinoma cells affects both morphology and gene expression. Biochem Cell Biol 1996;74:165–77.
65. Behrens P, Meissner C, Hopfer H, et al. Laminin mediates basement membrane induced differentiation of HEC 1B endometrial adenocarcinoma cells. Biochem Cell Biol 1996;74:875–86.
66. Brooks PC, Strömblad S, Sanders LC, et al. Localization of matrix metalloproteinase MMP-2 to the surface of invasive cells by interaction with integrin $\alpha v\beta 3$. Cell 1996;85:683–93.
67. Yebra M, Parry GCN, Strömblad S, et al. Requirement of receptor-bound urokinase-type plasminogen activator for integrin $\alpha v\beta 5$-directed cell migration. J Biol Chem 1996;271:29393–9.
68. Sutherland AE, Calarco PG, Damsky CH. Developmental regulation of integrin expression at the time of implantation in the mouse embryo. Development 1993;119:1175–86.
69. Giannelli G, Falk-Marziller J, Schiraldi O, Stetler-Stevenson WG, Quaranta V. Induction of cell migration by matrix metalloproteinase-2 cleavage of laminin-5. Science 1997;277:225–8.
70. Zhou Y, Fisher SJ, Janatpour M, et al. Human cytotrophoblasts adopt a vascular phenotype as they differentiate: a strategy for successful endovascular invasion? J Clin Invest 1997;99:2139–51.

19

Keratinocyte Growth Factor in the Nonhuman Primate Endometrium: Regulation and Action

Ov D. Slayden, Shin-ichi Izumi, Jeffrey S. Rubin, David L. Lacey, and Robert M. Brenner

In several reviews (1–3), we described hormonal regulation of the primate reproductive tract, including the oviduct and endometrium. Like other mucosal tissues of the tract, the endometrium is comprised of epithelial, stromal, and vascular components, each undergoing dramatic, hormonally driven changes in structure and function during the menstrual cycle. In a fertile cycle the action of these hormones ultimately prepares the endometrium for embryo implantation. Many reports now suggest that the actions of sex steroids in target tissues are mediated through locally produced growth factors in an autocrine/paracrine fashion. For example, epidermal growth factor (EGF) (4,5), insulin-like growth factor I (IGF-I) (6,7) and transforming growth factor-α (8) are regarded as possible mediators of the effects of estrogens on uterine growth. Studies from our laboratory (1,9,10) and several others (11–13) have emphasized that stromally derived factors mediate the effects of ovarian steroids on epithelial and vascular function.

Keratinocyte growth factor (KGF) is a member of the fibroblastic growth factor family (FGF-7) that fits the requirements for a mediator of stromal-epithelial interactions in the reproductive tract (14). KGF is a stromally derived, secreted peptide, which was originally purified from human embryonic lung fibroblasts (15), and acts as a mitogen for epithelial cells in culture, but not for fibroblasts, melanocytes, or endothelial cells (16,17). Recent reviews of the literature on KGF (14,18–20), support the hypothesis that KGF is a one-way paracrine regulator that can act as a stromal mediator of epithelial cell proliferation in vivo (16,21,22). However, KGF has also been noted to have effects on epithelial cell secretion and to show cytoprotective effects (23). Recently, smooth muscle cells were shown to be capable of producing KGF in cell culture (24).

KGF mRNA has been detected in a variety of reproductive tissues (16) including mouse (25), macaque (9), and human uterus (26,27), and macaque placenta (28). We found that macaque endometrial KGF was upregulated by progesterone (P) and we have proposed that KGF may mediate some actions of P in this tissue (27). KGF mRNA is also increased by P in the mouse (25) and rat (29) uterus and during the luteal phase of the menstrual cycle in human endometrium (26). However, hormonal regulation of KGF differs in different tissues. In the prostate, KGF is androgen dependent (30), in the oviduct and vagina, KGF is estrogen-dependent (31) and in the macaque placenta, KGF transcript is highest during early gestation (28), but declines in late gestation even though the steroid environment is relatively constant.

The KGF receptor (KGFR; FGFR-2b) has been isolated by expression cloning and characterized by molecular and binding studies (32–34). These studies indicate that the KGFR is a membrane-spanning tyrosine kinase that was expressed only in certain epithelial cell lines and absent from all fibroblast cell lines tested. Binding studies indicated that KGF and acidic FGF (αFGF) bind KGFR with equally high affinity. However, basic FGF (βFGF) binds KGFR with only low affinity and is effectively displaced by low concentrations of both KGF and aFGF (32). Structural analysis of mouse KGFR and human KGFR has revealed that KGFR is a splice variant of the fibroblast growth factor receptor-2 (FGFR-2)/bek gene and contains a unique 49 amino acid region near the transmembrane domain (34). Subsequent binding studies of alternate splice variants of the FGFR-2 gene have confirmed that the 49 amino acid sequence is responsible for the greater binding affinity of KGF for KGFR.

KGFR is present in the macaque endometrium, and may function as part of a KGF/KGFR paracrine system (10). To date we have found no evidence for hormonal regulation of KGFR in the endometrium. KGFR has been detected in human endometrium (26,27) and human endometrial carcinoma cells (35). In the human endometrium KGFR mRNA is reported to be increased by estrogen (26) and the relative levels of KGFR mRNA in endometrial adenocarcinoma are reported to be similar to that in cycling endometrium (35).

The effects of KGF in vivo have been studied in a variety of animal systems. For example, systemic administration of KGF stimulates rat mammary gland hyperplasia (36,37) and causes a striking increase in cell proliferation in the bladder epithelium of rats and rhesus monkeys (38). Intratracheal administration of KGF is reported to stimulate proliferation of rat type II pneumocytes and to have a cytoprotective effect on lung epithelium (14). In a preliminary report we showed that systemic administration of KGF to mice inhibited P-induced apoptosis in the uterine luminal epithelium (25).

This chapter reviews our studies of KGF regulation and localization and then describes our current progress in evaluating the effects of KGF on the macaque reproductive tract.

General Methods

Animal Treatment

Animal care throughout these studies was provided by the veterinary staff of the Oregon Regional Primate Research Center (ORPRC) in accordance with the NIH Guide for the Care and Use of Laboratory Animals. Reproductive tracts were collected by laparotomy from rhesus macaques (*Macaca mulatta*) at various time points during the menstrual cycle and from ovariectomized (spayed) animals treated sequentially with E_2 and P to induce artificial menstrual cycles (39). In adult monkeys, artificial menstrual cycles were initiated by inserting a 3 cm Silastic capsule (0.34 cm i.d.; 0.64 cm o.d.; Dow Corning, Midland, MI) packed with crystalline E_2 (Steraloids, Inc., Wilton, NH) s.c. into spayed monkeys for 14 days to produce an artificial proliferative phase. After 14 days of E_2 priming, a 6-cm Silastic capsule containing crystalline P (Steraloids Inc.) was inserted s.c. for 14 days to stimulate an artificial secretory phase. Removal of the P implant (leaving the E_2 implant in place) induced menstruation and completed a cycle. We refer to the period following P withdrawal in the artificial cycle as the luteal-follicular transition (LFT). Artificial menstrual cycles were also induced in infant rhesus macaques as above, but with smaller capsules of E_2 (1 cm) and P (2 cm). In each case serum levels of E_2 and P at the time of laparotomy were confirmed by radioimmunoassay (40). In some studies monkeys were also treated with 5-bromo-2-deoxyuridine (Br-dU) to label cells synthesizing DNA one hour before tissue collection.

Control Cell Lines

Mammalian cells including M426 human embryonic lung fibroblasts, which express KGF (15) but not KGFR (34), and MCF-7 human mammary epithelial cells, which express KGFR but not KGF, were grown to confluence and harvested for RNA extraction as previously described (9).

Probe Labeling

Probes were labeled with ^{32}P-dCTP for Northern hybridization and with Digoxigenin (Dig) dUTP for in situ hybridization by random priming of specific cDNA templates (9) with a labeling kit (Boehringer Mannheim). The human KGF cDNA (0.68 kbp) (9) coded for the 5' untranslated region and the first exon (16,41). Human KGFR cDNA (0.15 kbp) corresponding to the KGFR-specific exon (exon K) was provided courtesy of Paul Finch, Mt. Sinai Hospital, New York. Mouse glial fibrillary acidic protein (GFAP) cDNA (1.2 kbp) (42) and the 1.1 kb EcoR1/HindIII fragment of the rat ribosomal cDNA (43) were provided courtesy of Michael Melner, Department of Obstetrics and Gynecology, Vanderbilt University, Nashville, TN.

Northern Blot Analysis

Fresh tissue samples (or cells) were frozen in liquid nitrogen. The frozen samples were homogenized in 4 M guanidine thiocyanate and total RNA was isolated by cesium chloride centrifugation (44). Total RNA (20 μg) was loaded onto 1.5% agarose gels containing 0.25 M formaldehyde and 0.5 μg/ml ethidium bromide, electrophoresed at 30 V for 18 to 20 h and then transferred overnight by capillary action onto Maximum-Strength Nytran (Schleicher-Schuell, Keene, NH) or supported nitrocellulose (Gibco BRL, Gaithersburg, MD) membranes. The membranes were dried for 2 h at 80°C, prehybridized for 3 to 4 h at 42°C in hybridization medium (HM; 50% formamide, 5X SSC, 5X Denhardt's solution, 250 μg/ml salmon testis DNA, and 5% SDS). Filters were hybridized overnight at 42°C in the same solution containing ^{32}P-labeled cDNA probes, washed (final stringency: 0. 5X SSC containing 0.1% SDS at 45°C) and exposed to X-ray film (Eastman Kodak, Rochester, NY) in the presence of an intensifying screen at –80°C.

In Situ Hybridization of KGF mRNA

Expression of KGF mRNA was localized by in situ hybridization with dig-dUTP-labeled probes as previously described (9,28).

KGFR Detection by RT-PCR

Based on GenBank sequence No.M80634, two 20-mer oligonucleotide PCR primers were synthesized, which flank nucleotides 1360 to 1617 of the human KGFR cDNA. Total RNA samples (5 μg each) were reverse transcribed with SuperScriptTM RNase H - Reverse Transcriptase (Gibco BRL) and primer 1(5'-TCTTGGTCGTGTTCTTCATT-3'). Thirty-five PCR cycles were carried out in the presence of primers 1 and 2 (5'-TACCTCAAGGTTCT CAAGCA-3'), 200 mM of dNTP, and 2.5 U of Taq DNA polymerase (Promega, Madison, WI) in 100 μl buffer (50 mM KCl, 10 mM Tris-HCl [pH 9.0], 0.1% Triton X-100, 1.5 mM MgCl$_2$). Each cycle consisted of 1 min at 94°C, 2 min at 55°C, and 2 min at 72°C, except that the first denaturation step was carried out for 8 min and the last elongation reaction for 9 min. In each PCR run, H$_2$O was substituted for RNA in one sample and total RNA from M426 cells (negative control) and B5/859 cells (positive control) was also analyzed. The PCR products (5 μl) were electrophoresed on 1.5% agarose gels in parallel with a 1kbp DNA Ladder (Gibco, BRL) and then transferred to Maximum-Strength Nytran. The KGFR-specific bands were identified by Southern hybridization with random primed ^{32}P-dCTP-labeled probes prepared from exon K of the human KGFR cDNA (34). Blots were hybridized overnight at 42°C in hybridization medium, and then washed (final stringency: 0.5X SSC/0.1% SDS at 55°C). The hybridizing PCR products were isolated and subcloned, and the DNA sequence of the monkey KGFR cDNA was determined (45).

Immunohistochemistry

A chimeric KGF-HFc fusion molecule containing KGF and the hinge region-Fc portion of an IgG molecule was used as a probe to detect KGF-specific binding in tissue sections (46). This reagent was supplied courtesy of Dr. William LaRochelle, NIH. Cryostat sections of endometrium were incubated with the chimeric molecule overnight at 4°C. KGF-HFc bound to specific binding sites in sections through its KGF link was detected through reaction with an anti-IgG biotinylated second antibody. Second antibody complexes were detected with an avidin-biotin kit (Vector Laboratories, Burlingame CA).

To detect Br-dU incorporation into nuclei, frozen sections were fixed in 4% paraformaldehyde, washed, and treated with 2M HCl for 30 min. Sections were incubated with mouse anti Br-dU antibody (ICN, Costa Mesa, CA) and then reacted with an anti-IgG biotinylated second antibody. Second antibody complexes were detected with an avidin-biotin kit (Vector Laboratories). To localize cells undergoing DNA fragmentation, frozen sections were analyzed by terminal transferase labeling of DNA fragments with Dig-dUTP, with the ApoTag in situ apoptosis detection kit (ONCOR, Gaithersburg MD).

Morphological Analysis

Glycolmethacrylate (GMA) sections of monkey uterus were prepared and stained with hematoxylin as described previously (39). Low power photographs were made with an Olympus OM-system 38-mm macrolens and high-power micrographs were made with Zeiss planapochromatic lenses on Technical Pan film (Eastman Kodak, Rochester, NY). Prints were digitized with a Hewlett Packard Scanjet 4c/T. Digital images were adjusted for sharpness and contrast with Adobe Photoshop (Adobe Systems, Seattle, WA) and photomicrographs were printed with a Sony Mavigraph dye sublimation printer (Sony Corp., Japan).

Morphometrics

Abundance of endometrial apoptotic cells in GMA sections and the abundance of Br-dU-positive cells in immunohistochemical preparations were determined by a trained observer who used an ocular micrometer grid to define microscope fields and counted between 1200 and 5000 cells per animal with the aid of a mechanical tabulator. Endometrial gland areas and spiral artery areas were determined with the Optimas 3.0 (Optimas Inc, Seattle, WA) image analysis software package, on digital images captured through a MTI CCD 72 digital camera (Dage Corp., Michigan City, ID).

KGF and KGF Receptor Expression in the Endometrium

Progesterone Upregulates Endometrial KGF

Our studies indicate that KGF transcript is upregulated by P in the monkey endometrium. We also detected KGF transcript at low levels in monkey myometrium, but expression of myometrial KGF was essentially unchanged under different hormonal conditions. Figure 19.1 shows Northern blot analysis depicting endometrial KGF mRNA expression in rhesus monkeys. KGF transcript was barely detectable in endometrium of animals treated with E_2 alone, but was abundant in the endometrium after treatment with E_2 + P (Fig. 19.1A). Upregulation of KGF transcript was evident within 1 day of P treatment and KGF mRNA continued to increase many fold over the subsequent 6-week treatment period. To further show that KGF expression was P dependent, we measured KGF transcript in samples of RNA from monkey endometrium collected after P withdrawal during the LFT. Withdrawal of P during the LFT resulted in a decrease in KGF transcript (Fig. 19.1B). Endometrial KGF transcript was also higher during the luteal phase than the follicular phase of the natural menstrual cycle (Fig. 19.1C). Figure 19.1C also shows that upregulation of KGF by P was blocked by the P antagonist RU-486. Moreover, treatment with E_2 for 14 days and then for 14 days with P alone (Fig. 19.1C, lane E,P) also stimulated KGF expression, indicating that E_2 is not required for P to stimulate KGF mRNA.

We also measured KGF protein in endometrial tissue with a sensitive two-site ELISA assay (9,10). KGF protein was significantly more abundant in endometria from animals in the luteal phase, or treated with E_2 + P than in endometria from the follicular phase or from animals treated only with E_2 (data not shown). These data indicate that both KGF transcript and KGF protein are elevated by P stimulation.

---→

FIGURE 19.1. Northern blot analysis of total RNA from endometria from various hormonal treatments hybridized with ^{32}P-labeled KGF cDNA. (A) Compared to E_2 alone (14 days; lane 1) KGF mRNA (2.4 kb) was slightly upregulated by 1 day of E + P treatment (lane 2), and continued to increase substantially in E + P treated monkeys (compare lane 3, E_2 + 3 days P; Lane 4, E_2 + 7 days and lane 5, E_2 + 14 days P. Extending P treatment to 6 weeks further increased KGF transcript (lane 6). All blots showed a strong signal for KGF transcript in total RNA from M426 cells (positive control) and no signal from MCF-7 cell RNA (negative control; data not shown). The lower portion of the figure shows the signal after reprobing for 18 S RNA confirming that equivalent amounts of RNA were present in all lanes. (B) Withdrawal of P and continuation of E_2 treatment resulted in a decrease in KGF transcript on days 1 and 6 of the LFT. Hybridization with a probe for 18S RNA shows that each lane contains equivalent total RNA. (C) lane 1. E_2, then E_2 + P; lane 2. E_2, then E_2 + P + RU-486; lane 3. E_2, followed by P alone (E_2, P); lane 4. Follicular phase of the menstrual cycle; lane 5. Luteal phase of the menstrual cycle. KGF signal was elevated in P-dominated tissues whether E_2 was present or absent. The effect of P was antagonized by RU-486.

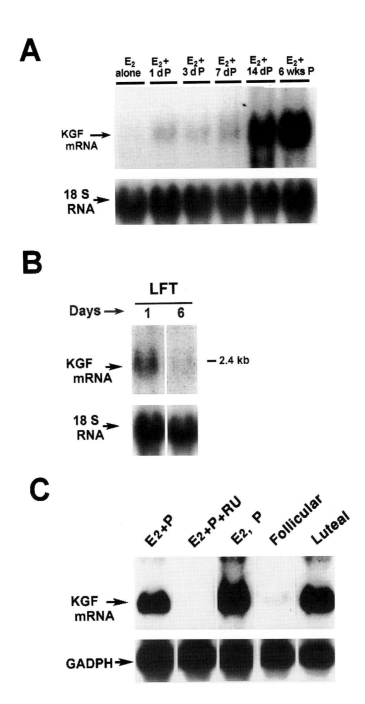

The lower portion of the figure illustrates the signal on these blots after reprobing with a cDNA probe against GAPDH to show equal loading. Reprinted with permission from Koji et al. (9).

KGF Localization in the Endometrium

We performed in situ hybridization to characterize cellular localization of KGF transcript in the uterus (9). Endometrial glandular epithelial cells were negative for KGF mRNA under all hormonal conditions. KGF mRNA was most intensely expressed in the stromal cells of the basalis region, and the perivascular stroma and musculature of spiral arteries (Fig. 19.2). In animals that were in the follicular phase, spayed, or E_2 treated, the KGF mRNA signal was nondetectable in stromal cells of all endometrial zones except for a few stromal cells closely associated with spiral arteries. In P-treated (or luteal phase) animals, only the stromal cells of the basalis zone showed a strong

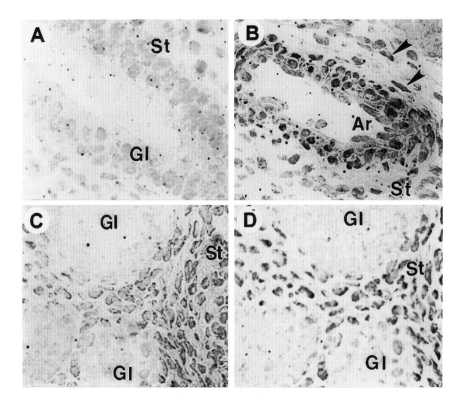

FIGURE 19.2. In situ hybridization of KGF mRNA with dig-labeled cDNA in E_2 + P-treated endometrium. All original magnifications were ×400. (A) Functionalis. The glands and the periglandular stroma are negative for KGF signal. (B) Spiral artery. The signal in the cytoplasm of the smooth muscle cells of the artery wall is present. (C) Basalis. The glands are negative, but the stroma shows a substantially increased, distinct signal for KGF mRNA. (D) Basalis. This is a phase micrograph of the identical section as in (C). The signal in the stroma is enhanced by phase microscopy, while the glands remain negative. Reprinted with permission from Koji et al. (9).

cytoplasmic signal for KGF mRNA (Figs. 19.2B,C). Under all hormonal conditions, there was a distinct, invariant cytoplasmic signal for KGF mRNA in the muscular-stromal walls of the spiral arteries. During P-domination, the stromal cells in the perivascular regions around the spiral arteries also showed a small increase in the level of hybridization signal.

Expression of KGF Receptor in the Endometrium

Expression of KGFR transcript in the endometrium was below the limits of sensitivity of Northern blot analysis. Therefore, we applied the use of RT-PCR technology to obtain information on KGFR expression in the endometrium (45). The RT-PCR technique detected KGFR mRNA in the endometrium (Fig. 19.3), and from human B/589 cells (positive control). No signal was detectable from samples prepared from total RNA from rhesus monkey brain (not shown) or from human M426 cells (negative control). Treatment with E_2 or E_2 + P, or phase of the menstrual cycle, had no detectable effect on total amount of KGFR transcript in endometrium.

However, ligand histochemistry with the KGF-HFc reagent revealed specific hormonal effects on KGF-specific binding. In estrogenized animals, binding by KGF-HFc occurred on the basolateral membrane region of the luminal and glandular epithelial cells in both the functionalis and basalis zones (Fig. 19.4A). But after E_2 + P treatment, binding disappeared from the functionalis and was only evident in the deepest regions of the basalis (Fig. 19.4B) and in

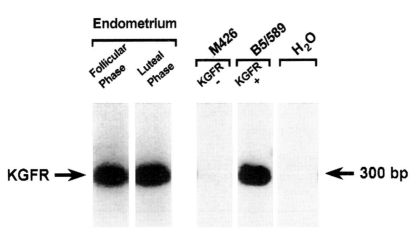

FIGURE 19.3. Southern blot analysis of RT-PCR cDNA products prepared from human and rhesus monkey total RNA. The RT-PCR technique detected KGFR mRNA in samples of total RNA from rhesus monkey endometrium from both follicular phase (lane 1) and luteal phase (lane 2) of the menstrual cycle, and in human B5/589 cells (positive control; lane 5). No signal was amplified from total RNA from human M426 cells (negative control; lane 4).

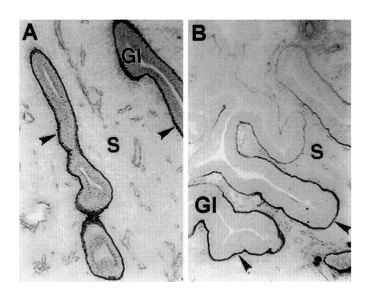

FIGURE 19.4. KGF binding activity in endometrium as indicated by ligand histochemistry with the KGF-HFc fusion molecule. (A) 14 days E_2 treatment. There is an intense signal in the basement membrane region (arrowheads) of the glands. (B) Sequential 14 days of E_2 then 14 days of E_2 + P treatment. The deepest basalis glands retained their binding capacity but there was a marked P-induced diminution in signal, marked by the large arrow, where the lower basalis blends into the functionalis. Specific staining for KGF binding was detected along the basal cell membrane of the epithelial cells. The micrographs are of the basalis region near the myometrial border. Gl = gland; S = stroma. Magnification = ×250.

the walls of the spiral arteries. When sections were incubated with a control fusion molecule that lacked the KGF ligand (HFc alone) no binding activity was detected (data not shown).

Placental KGF/KGFR Expression

We have reported that KGF and KGFR transcript were expressed in the rhesus monkey placenta (28). Northern blot analysis indicated that the KGF mRNA was most abundant in early gestation (45 days) samples and least abundant by late gestation (157 days; Fig. 19.5). However, KGFR mRNA was detectable by RT-PCR at all stages of gestation.

In situ hybridization of KGF mRNA in placenta during early gestation, revealed that KGF mRNA was strongly expressed in the placental mesenchymal cells located on the periphery of the mesenchymal cores of both anchoring and floating placental villi (28). The majority of these KGF mRNA positive stromal cells were located immediately subjacent to the cytotrophoblasts (Fig. 19.6a). In contrast, in situ hybridization detected KGFR mRNA in the cytotrophoblasts of both anchoring and floating villi (Fig. 19.6b) as well as in the intermediate

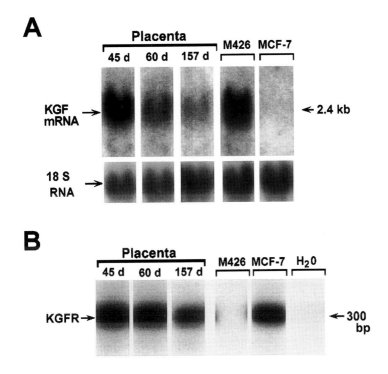

FIGURE 19.5. Detection of KGF and KGFR transcript in rhesus monkey placenta total RNA. (A) Northern blot analysis of KGF mRNA in monkey placentas collected at 45, 60, and 157 days of gestation and in control cell lines. The intensity of the KGF mRNA signal decreased with increasing placental age. 18S expression did not vary with gestational age. (B) RT-PCR analysis of KGFR mRNA in monkey placenta from various gestational ages. RNA from placenta (A) was reverse-transcribed and PCR-amplified. Southern hybridization indicated that KGFR transcripts were detectable at all gestational ages with a suggestion of lower expression in the oldest placentas. The lane designated H_2O is a negative control in which water was used in place of RNA in the RT-PCR procedure. A strong signal was detected with RNA from KGFR-positive B5/859 cells and no signal was detected with RNA from KGFR-negative M426.

cytotrophoblasts that constitute portions of the trophoblastic cell columns. This distribution of KGFR was confirmed by autoradiography of sections that had been incubated with ^{125}I-labeled KGF (data not shown).

Effects of Exogenous KGF

From the preceding results it is clear that KGF mRNA is most abundant in the progestin-treated (secretory) endometrium and localized to stromal cells in the basalis and the perivascular sheath. In such endometria, ligand binding

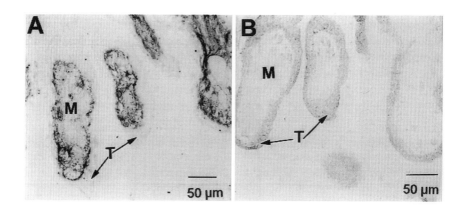

FIGURE 19.6. In situ hybridization for KGF and KGFR mRNAs in rhesus macaque placental tissue sections at 34 days gestation. All magnifications are ×400. (A) KGF mRNA. Note the strong KGF mRNA hybridization signal in stromal cells subjacent to cytotrophoblast in the anchoring villus. (B) KGFR mRNA localization in an adjacent anchoring villus section. KGFR mRNA is detectable in both layers of the trophoblastic epithelium and in the intermediate cytotrophoblasts (ICTB) of the columnar portions of the anchoring villis. Reprinted with permission from (28).

histochemistry suggested that KGF binding sites were present primarily in the glands of the endometrial basalis but also in the walls of the spiral arteries. We considered both the basalis glands and the spiral arteries as potential targets for P-stimulated KGF action.

During the LFT of the artificial menstrual cycle, P levels fall and the abundance of endometrial KGF transcript also decreases ~9-fold. The subsequent menstruation that follows is accompanied by regression of the spiral arteries, sloughing of the upper endometrial zones and regression of the basalis glands through epithelial apoptosis. Several reports indicate that KGF induces cytoprotective actions (23), and we reported that KGF could suppress apoptosis in the mouse uterine luminal epithelium (25). Therefore, we hypothesized that in macaques, the apoptotic process in the basalis and regression of the spiral arteries might be due to KGF withdrawal. To test this hypothesis we administered KGF during the LFT and examined its effects on the regressing endometrium. To minimize the amount of KGF needed, we first administered KGF systemically to juvenile (1 year old, noncycling) rhesus monkeys weighing ~1kg. In a second experiment we infused KGF directly into the reproductive tracts of ovariectomized adult monkeys.

In experiment 1, ovariectomized juvenile monkeys were treated sequentially with 1-cm long Silastic capsules of E_2 and 2 cm long Silastic capsules of P to induce artificial menstrual cycles as described earlier. During the test cycle, the juvenile monkeys were injected with recombinant human KGF (5 mg/kg) or vehicle (PBS) daily IV for 5 days, beginning 1 day before P withdrawal. At the end of treatment (LFT day 4) the juvenile monkeys were injected with Br-dU (50 mg/kg) to label cells synthesizing DNA, and the reproductive tracts were collected one hour later. Samples of endometrium were frozen and cryosectioned for immunohistochemistry or fixed and embedded in GMA for morphological analysis.

In experiment 2, spayed-artificially cycled adult monkeys were laparotomized on the day of P withdrawal and an oviductal cannula leading to a subcutaneous port was installed. The reproductive tract was flushed (via the oviduct) with either 0.5 mg/ml KGF or vehicle (Hanks Balanced Salt Solution; Gibco BRL) and the P implants were removed. KGF (0.5 mg) or vehicle (1 ml) was flushed through the tract daily for 4 days, and tracts were collected on day 4 of the LFT and processed as described above.

Results of KGF Administration

Sequential treatment of juvenile monkeys with small Silastic implants produced normal adult serum levels of E_2 (~50–100 pg/ml) and P (~4–5 ng/ml) and induced normal proliferative and secretory states in the endometrium during the artificial menstrual cycle. Withdrawal of P, as anticipated, resulted in a 2-day menstruation beginning on day 2 of the LFT.

Systemic replacement of KGF during the LFT in juvenile monkeys did not prevent menstruation. KGF treatment did stimulate a significant ($p < 0.05$) increase in endometrial gland area (see Table 19.1). KGF also significantly inhibited epithelial apoptosis in the basalis zone ($p < 0.05$; Table 19.1), confirmed by staining for DNA fragmentation with the ApoTag Kit (31). KGF also prevented atrophy of the spiral arteries, as indicated by the larger arterial area in the sections from the KGF-treated infants compared to the vehicle controls. This effect was primarily the result of significant differences in the thickness of the arterial walls (Table 19.1). However, there was no evidence that KGF enhanced cell proliferation (Br-dU incorporation; Table 19.1) in either the residual functionalis or basalis zones.

The results of KGF infused directly into the uterine lumen during the LFT were similar to the effects seen after systemic administration. Additional animals need to be added to each group for statistical validity, but the trends seem clear. KGF infusion did not inhibit menstruation, but did result in enlarged, sacculated glands with evidence of increased secretory activity, a reduction in the abundance of apoptotic cells in the basalis zone and hypertrophy of the walls of the spiral arteries, all as compared to vehicle infused monkeys (Table 19.2).

Discussion

During the natural or artificial menstrual cycle in rhesus macaques, the basalis is quiescent until the early luteal phase, when a wave of mitotic activity

TABLE 19.1. Morphometric effects of systemic administration of 5 mg/kg KGF daily i.v. on the endometrium in the juvenile monkey during the LFT.[1]

	Control $n = 4$	KGF-treated $n = 3$
Basalis Br-dU labeling (%)[2]	11.3 ± 2.31^a	7.37 ± 3.9^a
Apoptotic index (%)[2]	3.6 ± 0.6^a	1.36 ± 0.45^b
Basalis gland area (%)[3]	15.1 ± 2.8^a	24.5 ± 2.6^b
Spiral artery area (%)[3]	0.89 ± 0.48^a	5.55 ± 0.7^b
Spiral artery wall thickness (u^2)[4]	1777 ± 232^a	5893 ± 1575^b

[1] Values represent mean $\pm$ SE and statistical comparisons were made by Student's t-test. Means with differing superscripts are statistically different ($p < 0.05$).
[2] Abundance of Br-dU-positive cells in immunohistochemical preparations and the abundance of apoptotic cells in GMA sections are expressed as a percentage of total basalis epithelial cells counted.
[3] Endometrial gland areas and spiral areas are expressed as a percentage of total basalis area in sections at ×100 original magnification.
[4] Spiral artery thickness values represent the mean thickness of 24 arterial crossections per animal at ×250 original magnification.

begins. This wave of cell proliferation is the result of the action of P subsequent to estrogen-priming. With continued P administration the mitotic activity in this zone diminishes and the basalis glands hypertrophy and show indications of greatly increased secretory activity (1,47). P also stimulates both proliferation and hypertrophy of the spiral artery system during the luteal phase. When P levels decline, menstruation and sloughing of the functionalis ensue, the basalis atrophies and regresses by apoptosis, and the spiral arteries regress.

TABLE 19.2. Morphometric effects of infusing 0.5 mg KGF daily 4 days during the LFT on the endometrium of adult monkeys.[1]

	Control $n = 2$	KGF-treated $n = 2$
Apoptotic index (%)	4.8 ± 0.83	3.05 ± 0.55
Gland area (%)[2]	18.1 ± 1.4	33.5 ± 3.7
Spiral artery area (%)[2]	2.89 ± 1.48	7.15 ± 1.5
Spiral artery wall thickness[3] (u^2)	2515 ± 383	9969 ± 2003

[1] All values represent mean $\pm$ SE to indicate variance between animals ($n = 2$). Statistical comparisons were not made because of small sample size.
[2] Gland areas and spiral artery areas are expressed as a percentage of total basalis area in sections at ×100 original magnification.
[3] Spiral artery thickness values represent the mean thickness of 20 arterial cross sections per animal at ×250 original magnification.

Replacement of KGF did not block menses, so the decline of KGF is unlikely to play a key role in menses induction. Also, KGF did not increase proliferation of either the basalis or the spiral arteries above control levels. This finding suggests that either KGF is not a mitogen for these tissues, or that the basalis epithelium becomes refractory to any mitogenic actions of KGF as the cycle progresses. Normally mitotic activity in the basalis begins in the early luteal phase as KGF rises but then declines while KGF continues to increase. KGF might be a mitogen for these cells in the early luteal phase, but the cells may differentiate, increase their secretory capacity and lose their sensitivity to any mitogenic actions of KGF. Tests of KGF administered for longer periods during the follicular phase, and/or during the early luteal phase are required to dissect the mitogenic role of KGF in the endometrium.

However, our results clearly showed that exogenous KGF stimulated hypertrophy of both the basalis glands and the spiral arteries, and suppressed basalis epithelial cell death. The morphology of the basalis glands strongly suggested that KGF also led to an increase in secretory activity compared to controls. Additional information on whether specific secretory products were enhanced by KGF is needed, as such products may play important roles in implantation and pregnancy. We have previously shown that KGF inhibits P-stimulated apoptosis in the uterine luminal epithelium of mice (25) and other laboratories have shown that KGF inhibits cell death in lung epithelium. Such effects, as well as the secretory changes, fit the role of KGF as an epithelial cytoprotective factor. The molecular mechanisms underlying these cytoprotective and secretory effects are important areas for future research. These results add to the evidence suggesting that KGF is a pleiotropic growth factor with multiple actions that vary in different target tissues.

The most striking effect of KGF treatment was the large increase in the thickness of the spiral arterial walls as compared to arteries in vehicle-treated controls. Growth of the spiral arteries is extensive during P treatment and the steady increase in growth of these arteries parallels the continuous increase in KGF under P influence. The cellular makeup of spiral arteries includes fibroblasts, smooth muscle cells, and endothelial cells, and none of these cell types has been considered as a normal target of KGF action. Consequently, this effect of KGF is either an indirect one, perhaps mediated by an epithelial product, or a direct one unique to this specialized vascular system. The walls of the spiral arteries appear to have KGF-binding activity, but more definitive evidence from in situ hybridization studies is needed to confirm the presence of KGFR in these cells.

Regardless of the underlying mechanism, the spiral arteries clearly respond to KGF, a response that may be very important in the establishment of pregnancy in primates. The embryonic trophoblast invades and canalizes the spiral arteries during the early stages of implantation (48), and this invasion may require arteries fully stimulated by KGF.

The arteries themselves produce KGF, and the trophoblastic epithelium of the villi of 30-day old macaque placentas expressed KGFR mRNA and bound ^{125}I-KGF (28). Consequently, KGF produced by cells in and around the spiral arteries might not only enhance arterial hypertrophy, but facilitate the proliferation and/or migration of the embryonic trophoblast during arterial invasion.

KGF might also play a role in the proliferation of the surface epithelium that results in the temporary epithelial plaque that forms during implantation in this species (49). Because the surface epithelium lacks progesterone receptors during the luteal phase (3,50,51), it is likely that the P-dependent proliferation of these cells is mediated indirectly by the P receptor-positive stromal elements. Whether the KGF/KGFR system is involved in this or other aspects of implantation is currently unknown.

In summary, our search for hormonally regulated, stromally derived growth factors in the endometrium has been rewarding. We have identified a stromal factor, KGF, that is upregulated by P in the endometrium and has dramatic effects on the glands of the basalis and the unique spiral arteries of the primate endometrium. Moreover, the KGF/KGFR paracrine system is expressed by the villous trophoblast of the macaque placenta at very early gestational stages.

Progesterone is the key hormone essential for implantation and pregnancy in all mammalian species. All P-dependent endometrial growth factors, including KGF, should be considered as playing important roles in implantation and early gestation. Our results are the first to show effects of exogenous KGF on the primate endometrium, and they provide insight into the pleiotropic effects of this paracrine agent. Further research is needed to determine whether any of these effects facilitate primate implantation and/or early gestation.

Acknowledgments. We gratefully acknowledge the Animal Care Technicians in the Division of Laboratory Animal Medicine for care of the animals during this study, Kuni Mah for immunocytochemistry, and Angela Adler for word processing assistance. This study was supported by NIH grants HD07675 (ODS), HD19182 (RMB),and RR00163. The Morphology, Hormone Assay, Cell Culture and Molecular Biology Core laboratories provided by Population Center grant P30 HD18185 were invaluable to these studies.

References

1. Brenner RM, Slayden OD. Cyclic changes in the primate oviduct and endometrium. In: Knobil E, Neill JD, eds. The physiology of reproduction. New York: Raven Press, 1994:541–69.
2. Brenner RM, West NB, McClellan MC. Estrogen and progestin receptors in the reproductive tract of male and female primates. Biol Reprod 1990;42:11–9.
3. Brenner RM, McClellan MC, West NB, Novy MJ, Haluska GJ, Sternfeld MD. Estrogen and progestin receptors in the macaque endometrium. In: Bulletti C, Gurpide E, eds. The primate endometrium. New York Academy of Sciences, 1991:149–66.

4. Huet-Hudson YM, Chakraborty C, De SK, Suzuki Y, Andrews GK, Dey SK. Estrogen regulates the synthesis of epidermal growth factor in mouse uterine epithelial cells. Mol Endocrinol 1990;4:510–23.

5. Nelson KG, Takahashi T, Bossert NL, Walmer DK, McLachlan JA. Epidermal growth factor replaces estrogen in the stimulation of female genital-tract growth and differentiation. Proc Natl Acad Sci USA 1991;88:21–5.

6. Murphy LJ, Murphy LC, Friesen HG. Estrogen induces insulin-like growth factor-I expression in the rat uterus. Mol Endocrinol 1987;1:445–50.

7. Ghahary A, Chakrabarti S, Murphy LJ. Localization of the sites of synthesis and action of insulin-like growth factor-I in the rat uterus. Mol Endocrinol 1990;4:191–5.

8. Nelson KG, Takahashi T, Lee DC, Luetteke NC, Bossert NL, Ross K, et al. Transforming growth factor-α is a potential mediator of estrogen action in the mouse uterus. Endocrinology 1992;131:1657–64.

9. Koji T, Chedid M, Rubin JS, Slayden OD, Csaky KG, Aaronson SA, et al. Progesterone-dependent expression of keratinocyte growth factor mRNA in stromal cells of the primate endometrium: keratinocyte growth factor as a progestomedin. J Cell Biol 1994;125:393–401.

10. Brenner RM, Slayden OD, Koji T, Izumi S, Chedid M, Csaky KG, et al. Hormonal regulation of the paracrine growth factors HGF and KGF in the endometrium of the rhesus macaque. In: Beier HM, Harper MJK, Chwalisz K, eds. The endometrium as a target for contraception. New York: Springer-Verlag, 1997:22–49.

11. Cunha GR, Bigsby RM, Cooke PS, Sugimura Y. Stromal-epithelial interactions in adult organs. Cell Differ 1985;17:137–48.

12. Bigsby RM, Cunha GR. Estrogen stimulation of deoxyribonucleic acid synthesis in uterine epithelial cells which lack estrogen receptors. Endocrinology 1986;119: 390–6.

13. Cunha GR, Chung LWK, Shannon JM, Taguchi O, Fujii H. Hormone-induced morphogenesis and growth: role of mesenchymal-epithelial interactions. Recent Prog Horm Res 1983;39:559–98.

14. Rubin JS, Bottaro DP, Chedid M, Miki T, Ron D, Cheon G, et al. Keratinocyte growth factor. Cell Biol Int 1995;19:399–411.

15. Rubin JS, Osada H, Finch PW, Taylor WG, Rudikoff S, Aaronson SA. Purification and characterization of a newly identified growth factor specific for epithelial cells. Proc Natl Acad Sci USA 1989;86:802–6.

16. Finch PW, Rubin JS, Miki T, Ron D, Aaronson SA. Human KGF is FGF-related with properties of a paracrine effector of epithelial cell growth. Science 1989;245:752–5.

17. Halaban R, Funasaka Y, Lee P, Rubin J, Ron D, Birnbaum D. Fibroblast growth factors in normal and malignant melanocytes. Ann NY Acad Sci 1991;638:232–43.

18. Rubin JS, Bottaro DP, Chedid M, Miki T, Ron D, Cunha GR, et al. Keratinocyte growth factor as a cytokine that mediates mesenchymal-epithelial interaction. In: Goldberg I, Rosen E, eds. Epithelial mesenchymal interactions in cancer. Basel: Birkhauser, 1995.

19. Aaronson SA, Bottaro DP, Miki T, Ron D, Finch PW, Fleming TP, et al. Keratinocyte growth factor. A fibroblast growth factor family member with unusual target cell specificity. Ann NY Acad Sci 1991;638:62–77.

20. Chevalier S, Aprikian AG, Beauregard G, Defoy I, Nguyen LT. Action, localization and structure-function relationship of growth factors and their receptors in the prostate. Reprod Med Rev 1996;5:73–105.

21. Werner S, Peters KG, Longaker MT, Fuller-Pace F, Banda MJ, Williams LT. Large induction of keratinocyte growth factor expression in the dermis during wound healing. Proc Natl Acad Sci USA 1992;89:6896–900.

22. Staiano-Coico L, Krueger JG, Rubin JS, D'limi S, Vallat VP, Valentino L, et al. Human keratinocyte growth factor effects in a porcine model of epidermal wound healing. J Exp Med 1993;178:865–78.

23. Hines MD, Allen-Hoffmann BL. Keratinocyte growth factor inhibits cross-linked envelope formation and nucleosomal fragmentation in cultured human keratinocytes. J Biol Chem 1996;271:6245–51.

24. Winkles JA, Alberts GF, Chedid M, Taylor WG, DeMartino S, Rubin JS. Differential expession of the keratinocyte growth factor (KGF) and KGF receptor genes in human vascular smooth muscle cells and arteries. J. Cell Phys (in press).

25. Sakata H, Izumi S-I, Mah KA, Slayden OD, Rubin J, Brenner RM. Keratinocyte growth factor (KGF) inhibits progesterone-induced apoptosis in the mouse uterine luminal epithelium. In: Program and Abstracts of 29th Annual Meeting of SSR, London, Ontario, Canada, July 27–30, 1996 (Abstr).

26. Siegfried S, Pekonen F, Nyman T, Ammälä M. Expression of mRNA for keratinocyte growth factor and its receptor in human endometrium. Acta Obstet Gynecol Scand 1995;74:410–4.

27. Pekonen F, Nyman T, Rutanen E. Differential expression of keratinocyte growth factor and its receptor in the human uterus. Mol Cell Endocrinol 1993;95:43–9.

28. Izumi S, Slayden OD, Rubin JS, Brenner RM. Keratinocyte growth factor and its receptor in the rhesus macaque placenta during the course of gestation. Placenta 1996;17:123–35.

29. Cullinan K, Koos RD. Expression of basic fibroblast growth factor (bFGF), vascular endothelial growth factor (VEGF), and keratinocyte growth factor (KGF) in the rat uterus-stimulation by estrogen. Biol Reprod 1991;44 (Suppl 1): 186 (Abstr 536).

30. Yan G, Fukabori Y, Nikolaropoulos S, Wang F, McKeehan WL. Heparin-binding keratinocyte growth factor is a candidate stromal to epithelial cell andromedin. Mol Endocrinol 1992;6:2123–8.

31. Slayden OD, Rubin J, Lacey D, Brenner RM. Keratinocyte growth factor (KGF) stimulates epithelial cell proliferation in the primate oviduct and vagina. In: Program and Abstracts of 30th Annual Meeting of SSR, Portland, Oregon, August 2–5, 1997: 103 (Abstr 84).

32. Bottaro DP, Fortney E, Rubin JS, Aaronson SA. A keratinocyte growth factor receptor-derived peptide antagonist identifies part of the ligand binding site. J Biol Chem 1993;268:9180–3.

33. Miki T, Fleming TP, Bottaro DP, Rubin JS, Ron D, Aaronson SA. Expression cDNA cloning of the KGF receptor by creation of a transforming autocrine loop. Science 1991;251:72–5.

34. Miki T, Bottaro DP, Fleming TP, Smith CL, Burgess WH, Chan AM, et al. Determination of ligand-binding specificity by alternative splicing: two distinct growth factor receptors encoded by a single gene. Proc Natl Acad Sci USA 1992;89:246–50.

35. Siegfried S, Pekonen F, Nyman T, Ämmälä M, Rutanen EM. Distinct patterns of expression of keratinocyte growth factor and its receptor in endometrial carcinoma. Cancer 1997;79:1166–71.

36. Ulich TR, Yi ES, Cardiff R, Yin S, Bikhazi N, Biltz R, et al. Keratinocyte growth factor is a growth factor for mammary epithelium *in vivo*. The mammary epithelium of lactating rats is resistant to the proliferative action of keratinocyte growth factor. Am J Pathol 1994;144:862–8.

37. Yi ES, Bedoya AA, Lee H, Kim S, Housley RM, Aukerman SL, et al. Short communication. Keratinocyte growth factor causes cystic dilation of the mammary glands of mice. Am J Pathol 1994;145:1015–22.

38. Yi ES, Shabaik AS, Lacey DL, Bedoya AA, Yin S, Housley RM, et al. Keratinocyte growth factor causes proliferation of urothelium in vivo. J Urol 1995;154:1566–70.

39. Slayden OD, Hirst JJ, Brenner RM. Estrogen action in the reproductive tract of rhesus monkeys during antiprogestin treatment. Endocrinology 1993;132: 1845–56.

40. West NB, Hess DL, Brenner RM. Differential suppression of progesterone receptors by progesterone in the reproductive tract of primate macaques. J Steroid Biochem 1986;25:497–503.

41. Kelley MJ, Pech M, Seuanez HN, Rubin JS, O'Brien SJ, Aaronson SA. Emergence of the keratinocyte growth factor multigene family during the great ape radiation. Proc Natl Acad Sci USA 1992;89:9287–91.

42. Lewis SA, Balcarek JM, Krek V, Shelanski M, Cowan NJ. Sequence of a cDNA clone encoding mouse glial fibrillary acidic protein: structural conservation of intermediate filaments. Proc Natl Acad Sci USA 1984;81:2743–6.

43. Low KG, Allen RG, Melner MH. Association of proenkephalin transcripts with polyribosomes in the heart. Mol Endocrinol 1990;4:1408–15.

44. Current Protocols in Molecular Biology. New York: Greene Publishing Associates, and John Wiley, 1994.

45. Slayden OD, Izumi S, Wilson I, Vijayaraghavan S, Rubin JS, Finch P, Brenner RM. Keratinocyte growth factor (KGF) and KGF receptor (KGFR) mRNAs in the cervix, placenta, and decidua of rhesus macaques. In: Abstracts of SSR Annual Meeting. Ann Arbor, Michigan, July 24–27, 1994: 121 (Abstr 267).

46. LaRochelle WJ, Dirsch OR, Finch PW, Cheon H-G, May M, Marchese C, et al. Specific receptor detection by a functional keratinocyte growth factor-immunoglobulin chimera. J Cell Biol 1995;129:357–66.

47. Okulicz WC, Balsamo M, Tast J. Progesterone regulation of endometrial estrogen receptor and cell proliferation during the late proliferative and secretory phase in artificial menstrual cycles in the rhesus monkey. Biol Reprod 1993;49:24–32.

48. Enders AC, King BF. Early stages of trophoblastic invasion of the maternal vascular system during implantation in the macaque and baboon. Am J Anat 1991;192: 329–46.

49. Enders AC, Hendrickx AG. Implantation and early embryonic development in primates. In: Brans YW, Kuehl TJ, eds. Nonhuman primates in perinatal research. New York: John Wiley, 1988:139–60.

50. Hild-Petito S, Verhage HG, Fazleabas AT. Immunocytochemical localization of estrogen and progestin receptors in the baboon (*Papio anubis*) uterus during implantation and pregnancy. Endocrinology 1992;130:2343–53.

51. Okulicz WC, Savasta AM, Hoberg LM, Longcope C. Biochemical and immunohistochemical analyses of estrogen and progesterone receptors in the rhesus monkey uterus during the proliferative and secretory phases of artificial menstrual cycles. Fertil Steril 1990;53:913–20.

20

Molecular Lesions in Infertility

Siamak Tabibzadeh and Ardeshir Babaknia

Receptivity of Human Endometrium to Implantation

Exquisite mechanisms control the processes that drive endometrium through the characteristic phases of the menstrual cycle and prepare this tissue for the implantation (1). Implantation is a complex process that initially requires the interaction of the blastocyst and subsequently, the developing embryo and placenta, with the endometrium. In implantation, both endometrial and embryonic factors are involved. During the menstrual cycle, endometrium becomes receptive to implantation during a defined period called the "receptivity period" or "implantation window." Outside this window, endometrium remains either neutral or refractory to implantation (2–3). Therefore, the acquisition of endometrial receptivity is a regulated process. A receptive endometrium is likely to establish a dialogue with the implanting blastocyst and to actively participate in the implantation process. For example, the trophoblasts of the implantation state blastocysts can invade, quite deeply, tissues other than endometrium (4). Despite the invasive behavior in vitro, in some animals, such as the pig, the trophoblasts attach to—but do not invade—the uterine epithelium (5). When transplanted ectopically in the uterine wall, however, the same cells can invade tissues. Therefore, it is likely that endometrium is actively involved in the regulation of the blastocyst implantation.

Molecular Repertoire of Endometrial Receptivity

It is speculated that two sets of molecules may exist in endometrium. One set of molecules makes endometrium receptive whereas a second set makes endometrium resistant to implantation. Therefore, presence or absence of the "implantation window" may depend on the regulated and timed expression of these molecules in endometrium.

The identity of the molecules that participate in endowing to endometrium its receptivity or refractoriness to implantation is being revealed. Among these factors are adhesion molecules (6–7), cytokines (8–10), metalloproteases (12), heat shock proteins (13–14), and trophinin and tastin (15).

We recently identified a molecule, α crystallin B chain, of the heat shock protein family whose progressive expression during the secretory phase in human endometrium was initiated at the time of the opening of the implantation window. The α crystallin B chain mRNA was absent during the proliferative phase. On the other hand, the expression of its mRNA first appeared in the secretory phase, progressively increased during this phase, and peaked in the late secretory endometria (14). Western blot analysis confirmed that the α crystallin B chain protein expression follows the pattern of the mRNA expression. Immunoreactive α crystallin B chain protein first appeared in the surface epithelial cells of human endometrium within the "implantation window." Within the same period, there was no significant immunoreactivity in the underlying glandular cells. During the mid and late secretory phases, the intensity of staining in the epithelial cells was enhanced, and an intense immunoreactivity was developed in the glandular epithelium. α crystallin B chain was virtually an epithelial product and no immunoreactivity for this protein was detectable in the stromal cells, endothelial cells, or lymphoid cells. α crystallin B chain protects cells against cytotoxic factors such as TNF-α Therefore, it seems reasonable to speculate that the function of the α crystallin B chain in human endometrium may be to protect endometrium against the cytotoxic effects of this cytokine.

Endometrium is regularly shed if implantation fails. Therefore, it is conceivable that a specific molecular repertoire prepares endometrium for the menstrual shedding. The same molecular repertoire may signal the closure of the implantation window and make endometrium refractory to implantation. Little information is available regarding the molecules that make endometrium resistant to implantation. However, it has been suggested that MUC1 may act as an antiadhesion molecule during embryo attachment in the mouse (16). We have identified TNF-α as a member of the premenstrual/menstrual molecular repertoire that may play a role in the menstrual shedding. This assumption is based on the following observations. TNF-α is expressed by the human endometrium (17–18). In situ hybridization and immunohistochemical staining showed that most of the TNF-α mRNA and immunoreactivity is confined to the endometrial glands (17–18). Northern blot analysis showed that the amount of the TNF-α mRNA progressively increases toward the menstrual phase (19). We also showed that the amount of the TNF-α released into the endometrial cavity also progressively increased towards the late secretory phase (9). In addition, TNF-α was present in the menstrual discharge in amounts far exceeding those found in the peripheral circulation (11). Furthermore, TNF-α is cytotoxic and by virtue of damaging the endothelial cells, causes edema (20) and bleeding in various organs (21). Injection of the TNF-α into a mouse causes endometrial bleeding and apoptosis in the endometrium that are reminiscent of human menstruation (12). TNF-α also causes epithelial dissociation (22), apoptosis (9), and converts the F actin to G actin in the endometrial epithelial cells (22), changes that are seen in the late secretory and menstrual phases (23–24). Taken together, these findings suggest that TNF-α may be implicated in the glandular dissociation and menstrual bleeding during the menstrual phase (12).

We have recently identified a novel gene of the TGF-β superfamily, endometrial bleeding associated factor (*ebaf* or TGF-B4) whose expression, in human endometrium, is confined to the late secretory and menstrual phases (25). The expression of this gene was not seen in endometrium in the proliferative, early, and mid-secretory phases (25). The TGF-B4 mRNA expression was confined to predecidualized stromal cells in the upper layers of endometrium underlying the surface epithelium. In the same endometria, the stroma in the basal part of the endometrium overlying the myometrium failed to exhibit evidence of mRNA expression. In these endometria, with exception of few glands located near the surface epithelium, virtually no TGF-B4 mRNA expression could be identified in the epithelial cells. The TGF-B4 mRNA was expressed in the endometria of patients with endometrial bleeding regardless whether they were in the proliferative, early, or mid-secretory phases. These findings suggest that the expression of this gene is linked to the endometrial bleeding justifying the conclusion that this gene may belong to the premenstrual molecular repertoire (25).

Molecular Lesions in Infertility

Various types of infertility may influence the regulatory mechanisms which are involved in implantation and lead to lesions in the molecular repertoire required in this process. For example, the aberrant expression of $\alpha_v\beta_3$ (6) has been described in infertility. We recently showed that a 2.1 kb TGF-B4 mRNA was aberrantly expressed in the endometria of infertile patients. Reverse transcription-polymerase chain reaction followed by Southern blot analysis showed a variety of aberrant expression of the TGF-B4 mRNA isoforms in the endometria of infertile patients. The available evidence, therefore, suggests that infertility is associated with lesions in the molecular repertoire that is expressed during the periods of receptivity and refractoriness of the endometrium to the implantation.

Acknowledgment. This work was supported by the Public Health Research Grant CA46866 (to S. Tabibzadeh).

References

1. Tabibzadeh S, Babaknia. A The signals and molecular pathways involved in implantation, a symbiotic interaction between blastocyst and endometrium involving adhesion and tissue invasion. Mol Hum Reprod 1995;10:1579–602.
2. Psychoyos A. The implantation window: basic and clinical aspects. In: Mori T, Aono T, Tominaga T, Hiroi M, eds. Perspectives on assisted reproduction. Rome, Italy: Ares-Serono Symposia, 1993;4:57–62.

3. Strauss JF III, Gurpide E. The endometrium: regulation and dysfunction. In: Yen S, Jaffe R, eds. Reproductive endocrinology, 3rd ed. Philadelphia: W.B. Saunders, 1991; 309–56.

4. Denker W-W. Implantation: a cell biological paradox. J Exp Zool 1993;266:541–58.

5. Dantzer V. Electon microscopy of the initial stages of placentation in the pig. Anat Embryol (Berl) 1985;172:281–93.

6. Tabibzadeh S. Patterns of expression of integrin molecules in human endometrium throughout the menstrual cycle. Hum Reprod 1992;7:876–82.

7. Lessey BA, Danjanovich L, Coutfaris C, Castelbaum A, Albelda SM, Buck CA. Integrin adhesion molecules in the human endometrium. Correlation with the normal and abnormal menstrual cycle. J Clin Invest 1992;90:188–95.

8. Tabibzadeh S, Kong QF, Babaknia A, May LT. Progressive rise in the expression of interleukin-6 in human endometrium during the menstrual cycle is initiated during the implantation window. Mol Hum Reprod 1995;10:2793–9.

9. Tabibzadeh S, Kong QF, Satyaswaroop PG, Zupi E, Marconi D, Romanini C, et al. Distinct regional and menstrual cycle dependent distribution of apoptosis in human endometrium. Potential regulatory role of T cells and TNF-alpha. Endocrine 1994;2: 87–95.

10. Stewart CL, Kaspar P, Brunet LJ, Bhatt H, Gadil I, Kontgen F, et al. Blastocyst implantation depends on maternal expression of leukemia inhibitory factor. Nature 1992;10:359:76–9.

11. Tabibzadeh S, Babaknia A, Liu R, Zupi E, Marconi D, Romanini C. Site and menstrual cycle-dependent expression of proteins of the TNF receptor family, and BCL-2 oncoprotein and phase specific production of TNF-α in human endometrium. Hum Reprod 1995;277–86.

12. Tabibzadeh S. The signals and molecular pathways involved in human menstruation: a unique process of tissue destruction and remodeling. Mol Hum Reprod 1996;2:77–92.

13. Tabibzadeh S, Kong QF, Satyaswaroop PG, Babaknia A. Heat shock proteins in human endometrium throughout the menstrual cycle. Hum Reprod 1996;11: 633–40.

14. Gruidl M, Buyuksal I, Babaknia A, Fazleabas AT, Sivarajah S, Satyaswaroop PG, et al. The progressive rise in the expression of α crystallin B chain in human endometrium is initiated during the implantation window; modulation of gene expression by steroid hormones. Mol Hum Reprod 1997;3:333–42.

15. Fukuda MN, Sato T, Nakayama J, Klier G, Mikami M, Aoki D, et al. Trophinin and tastin, a novel cell adhesion molecule complex with potential involvement in embryo implantation. Genes Devel 1995;9:1199–210.

16. Surveyor GA, GendlerSJ, Pemberton L, Das SK, Chakraborty I, Pimental R-A, et al. Expression and steroid hormonal control of muc-1 in the mouse uterus. Endocrinology 1995;136:3639–47.

17. Tabibzadeh S. Ubiquitous expression of TNF-alpha/Cachectin in human endometrium. Am J Rep Immunol 1991;26:1–5.

18. Hunt JS, Chen H-L, Hu X-L, Tabibzadeh S. Tumor necrosis factor-alpha mRNA and protein in human endometrium. Biol of Reprod 1992;47:141–7.

19. Phillipaeux M-M, Piguet PF. Expression of tumor necrosis factor-α and its mRNA in the endometrial mucosa during the menstrual cycle. Am J Pathol 1993;143:480–6.

20. Remick DG, Kunkel SL. Pathopysiologic alteration induced by tumor necrosis factor. Int Rev Exp Pathol 1994;34B:7–25.

21. Shalaby MR, Laegried WW, Ammann AJ, Liggitt HD. Tumor factor necrosis factor-α associated unterine endothelial injury *in vivo*. Influence of dietary fat. Lab Invest 1989;61:564–70.
22. Tabibzadeh S, Kong QF, Kapur S, Leffers H, Ridley A, Aktories K, et al. TNF-alpha induces dyscohesion of epithelial cells. Association with disassembly of actin filaments. Endocrine 1995;3:549–56.
23. Tabibzadeh S, Kong QF, Kapur S, Satyaswaroop PG, Aktories K. TNF-alpha mediated dyscohesion of epithelial cells is associated with disordered expression of cadherin/β-catenin and disassembly of actin filaments. Mol Hum Reprod 1995;10:994–1004.
24. Tabibzadeh S, Babaknia A, Kong QF, Zupi E, Marconi D, Romanini C, Satyaswaroop PG. Menstruation is associated with disordered expression of Desmoplakin I/II, cadherin/catenins and conversion of F to G actin in endometrial epithelium. Hum Reprod 1995;10:776–84.
25. Kothapalli R, Buyuksal I, Wu S-Q, Chegini N, Tabibzadeh S. Detection of *ebaf*, a novel human gene of the TGF-β superfamily; association of gene expression with endometrial bleeding. J Clin Invest 1997;99:2342–50.

Part VII

Transcriptional Regulation of Fetal–Maternal Recognition

21

The Role of *Abdominal B* (*AbdB*) *Hoxa* Genes During Implantation

LIANG MA, GAIL V. BENSON, HYUNJUNG LIM,
SUDHANSU K. DEY, AND RICHARD L. MAAS

Successful implantation in mammals depends critically on the establishment of a receptive environment in the uterus and on reciprocal and synchronized interactions between uterine and embryonic tissues (for reviews, see (1,2)). A suitable maternal environment for implantation is established and strictly regulated by the combined action of estrogen and progesterone, being initiated by a nidatory pulse of estrogen acting on a uterus already prepared by progesterone. Prior to implantation, the uterus undergoes dramatic morphologic changes in response to estrogen from ovarian follicles and progesterone from corpora lutea. The requirement for progesterone in priming the uterus is demonstrated by hormone deprivation in which the blastocysts remain in a state of diapause, a suspended state of low metabolism, and only after endometrial preparation by progesterone has been completed is estrogen effective in inducing a state of receptivity (reviewed in (1)). A second surge of estrogen secreted from the ovarian follicles just prior to implantation triggers the start of implantation. Lactation or ovariectomy eliminates this estrogen surge and prevents the attachment reaction and the blastocysts remain in a delayed implantation state (3). Although the molecular mechanisms responsible for implantation remain unclear, targeted mutagenesis in mice has implicated one subfamily of mammalian homeobox genes, the *Abdominal B* (*AbdB*) *Hox* genes, as important components of the implantation mechanism.

Mammalian *AbdB Hox* genes share substantial sequence homology to the *Drosophila Abdominal B* (*AbdB*) gene, which is the most 5' gene within the *Drosophila* homeotic complex. 16 *AbdB*-like genes, the products of gene duplication, are located on four different chromosomes at the 5' end of the *Hox* a, b, c, and d clusters (reviewed in (4)). As revealed from mice carrying targeted mutations, several *AbdB Hox* genes have important functions in reproductive tract development (5–7). Mice lacking *Hoxa-11* are infertile and display abnormal urogenital tract morphogenesis (8,9), whereas *Hoxa-13* mutant mice are embryonic lethal and exhibit developmental defects in the limb and in the posterior part of the Müllerian duct (10,11). We have recently characterized the expression and function of one of these *AbdB* genes, *Hoxa-10*, both during reproductive tract development and during pregnancy. *Hoxa-10* deficient mice exhibit developmental abnormalities in the anterior part of the uterus and also defects in implantation, vascular permeability and decidualization processes (7).

This chapter shows that in the adult mouse uterus, *Hoxa-10* is activated by progesterone and repressed by estrogen in a manner consistent with its dynamic endogenous expression pattern. This regulation is blocked by the progesterone antagonist RU-486. Examination of neighboring *Hoxa-9* and *a-11* genes show that they are both activated by progesterone, whereas estrogen represses *Hoxa-9* and activates *Hoxa-11*. Interestingly, *Hoxa-10* expression is transiently restricted to the antimesometrial pole by the combined action of estrogen and progesterone in ovariectomized mice, suggesting that *a-10* expression may provide an implantation cue. Consistent with this hypothesis, we observed a significant number of abnormal implantations in *Hoxa-10* mutant females. These data provide evidence that members of the *Hox* and hormone nuclear receptor families are functionally related during embryo implantation and that *AbdB Hoxa* genes constitute one class of the maternal genes involved in providing a suitable implantation environment.

Materials and Methods

Steroid Treatments

17β-estradiol (E2, sigma) or progesterone (P4) were dissolved in sesame oil and injected subcutaneously (0.1 ml/mouse) into ovariectomized IRS female mice (Taconic). Some mice received a combination of the same doses of E2 and P4. Control animals received oil or no injection. Mice were sacrificed at 2, 4, 6, 8, 16, and 24 h following injection, and uteri were fixed in 4% paraformaldehyde for in situ hybridization or collected for RNA extraction. For experiments involving RU-486 (gift of Roussel-Uclaf, Romainville, FR), P4 (2 mg/mouse) was injected subcutaneously for 2 days with or without E2 (100 ng/mouse) on the second day of P4 treatment. Mice were injected subcutaneously with 400 μg RU-486 with each P4 injection; control mice received vehicle alone (0.1 ml oil/ mouse). Procedures for radioactive in situ hybridizations, RNase protection assay, and information for antisense riboprobes for *Hoxa-9, -10, -11* and β-actin, are described elsewhere (Ma et al., unpublished manuscript).

Results

Expression of Hoxa-10 in the Pre- and Periimplantation Uterus

To study the role of *Hoxa-10* during periimplantation, in situ hybridization was used to examine the expression pattern of *Hoxa-10* in wild type uteri from day 0.5–7.5 of pregnancy (13). *Hoxa-10* is expressed in a dynamic pattern, consisting

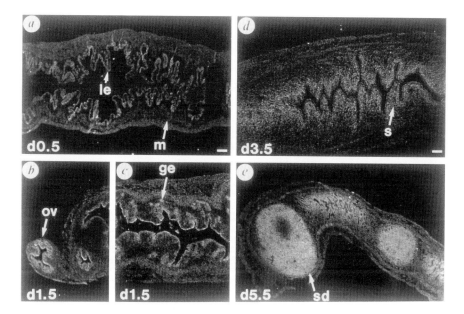

FIGURE 21.1. Analysis of *Hoxa-10* expression during early pregnancy by in situ hybridization analysis. Expression of *Hoxa-10* is detected in the luminal and glandular epithelium of the uterus at days 0.5 (a) and 1.5 p.c. (c). Expression is also present in the distal oviduct at day 1.5 p.c. (b). Endometrial expression shifts to the stroma underlying the epithelium at day 3.5 (d) and the stromal-derived decidua at day 5.5 p.c. (e). Weak expression is detected in the myometrium throughout. Abbreviations: ge, germinal epithelium; le, luminal epithelium; m, myometrium; ov, oviduct; s, stroma; sd, secondary decidua. Scale bar, 200 μm (a,e); 100 μm (b, c, d). Reproduced from Satokata et al. (12).

of sequential epithelial and stromal phases in the adult uterus. At days 0.5 and 1.5 p.c., strong expression is seen in the luminal and glandular epithelium, with a reduced level in the myometrium (Fig. 21.1a, c). Subsequently, at day 2.5 p.c., *Hoxa-10* expression begins to shift to the underlying stroma and is detected only in the stroma underlying the epithelium by day 3.5 p.c. (Fig. 21.1d). Strong *Hoxa-10* expression persists after implantation at days 4.5 to 5.5 p.c. in the developing decidua and the intervening stroma, and is later restricted to the secondary decidua, with expression decreasing on days 6.5 to 7.5 p.c. (Fig. 21.1e).

Periimplantation Failure in Hoxa-10 *Mutant Females*

Hoxa-10 mutant mice were previously prepared using standard ES cell technology by inserting a neomycin resistance gene into the *Hoxa-10* homeobox (12). Homozygotes are viable but express an anterior homeotic transformation of lumbar vertebrae (L1→T13) and severe defects in reproduction. Male homozygotes are sterile and exhibit either unilateral or bilateral cryptorchidism (12,13) in addition to an anterior transformation of the distal ductus deferens into epididymis (7). Female homozygotes are either sterile or have reduced fertility. The proximal 25% uterus is transformed to histologically resemble the more anterior oviduct structure. Altered gene expression of uterine markers, *Msx1* and *c-myc* in the transformed region confirms the histologic observation (7). These transformations occur at the anterior boundary of *Hoxa-10* gene expression consistent with the role of *Hox* genes in conferring tissue identity. To determine whether the morphologic transformation in *Hoxa-10* mutant females causes the reduced fertility phenotype, wild type blastocysts were transferred directly into the distal uterus of *Hoxa-10* mutants, bypassing the transformed region. These experiments did not rescue blastocyst survival, suggesting that the morphologic transformation alone cannot account for the reproductive phenotype in *Hoxa-10* mutant females and that *Hoxa-10* mutant uterus is defective in supporting implantation (7). Further analysis of *Hoxa-10* mutant females during the periimplantation period revealed a significant decrease in blastocyst attachment, in uterine vascular permeability, and in decidualization (7). To exclude the possibility that these defects resulted from abnormal hormone levels in *Hoxa-10* mutant females, endogenous estrogen and progesterone levels in these mutant mice were measured, and no significant differences were found compared to wild type mice (unpublished data). These periimplantation defects therefore represent an intrinsic requirement for *Hoxa-10* function in adult uterus and suggest a failure to initiate a normal hormonal response during implantation and decidualization.

Hoxa-10 *Expression Is Regulated by Both Estrogen and Progesterone*

Because embryo implantation is under strict regulation by estrogen and progesterone, we sought to understand the functional relationship between ovarian steroids and *Hoxa-10*. Using ovariectomized females, we found that 4 h following injection of 17β-estradiol (250 ng), basal *Hoxa-10* expression was sharply reduced to 50% of control levels (Fig. 21.2). In situ analysis showed that the stromal expression of *Hoxa-10* is strongly repressed whereas expression in the circular muscle layer is still detected (Fig. 21.3C). By eight hours the repression by E_2 starts to disappear and by 16 h, diffuse *Hoxa-10* expression is detected throughout the stroma.

Contrary to the repressive effects of estradiol, progesterone activates *Hoxa-10* expression after 4 h of exposure (Fig. 21.2), with maximal activation peaking at 8 h. By in situ hybridization, increased expression was first observed in the subepithelial stroma, which then expanded to deeper layers of the stroma and finally reached the circular muscle (Fig. 21.3B). Interestingly, when both estrogen and progesterone were injected ($E_2 + P_4$), they produced *Hoxa-10* expression levels comparable to control levels (Fig. 21.2),

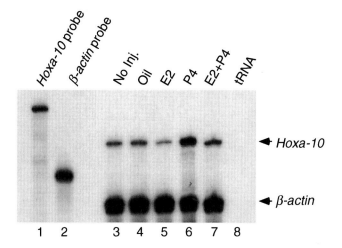

FIGURE 21.2. Hormonal regulation of *Hoxa-10* expression. Ovariectomized mice were either uninjected or injected with oil, 250 ng E2, 1 mg P4, or $E_2 + P_4$. 4 h after injection, uteri were dissected and RNA extracted. Twenty µg of RNA for each treatment were analyzed by RNase protection assay. lane 1 and lane 2 represent undigested probes for *Hoxa-10* and β-actin respectively. Protected fragments for *Hoxa-10* and β-actin are indicated.

and *Hoxa-10* expression became localized to a thin layer of sub-epithelial stroma at the antimesometrial pole of the uterus after 4 h of exposure (Fig. 21.4C, *arrow*). This restricted expression pattern is transient, and was not seen at either 2 or 8 h posttreatment.

The rapidity of regulation suggested that it might be a direct effect mediated by the estrogen and progesterone receptors. To test whether the progesterone receptor (PR) is directly involved in regulating *Hoxa-10* expression, we coadministered the progesterone antagonist RU-486 with progesterone and found that RU-486 significantly blocks the progesterone mediated activation of *Hoxa-10* expression. This result strongly implicates the progesterone receptor (PR) in the positive regulation of *Hoxa-10* expression in the adult uterus by progesterone.

Regulation of Other AbdB Hoxa Genes by Estrogen and Progesterone

AbdB Hoxa genes include *Hoxa9-13* and are all expressed in the adult mouse reproductive system (14). To test whether other *AbdB Hoxa* genes are also regulated by estrogen and progesterone, we used both in situ hybridization and RNase protection to examine the expression levels of *Hoxa-9, -11,* and *-13* in the adult uterus in response to estrogen and progesterone treatment.

Hoxa-10   Hoxa-11

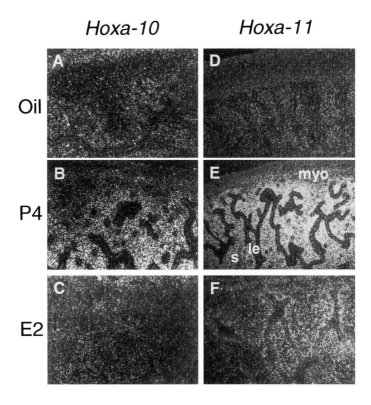

FIGURE 21.3. In situ hybridization showing the regulation of *Hoxa-10* and *Hoxa-11* gene expression by both estrogen and progesterone. Compared to oil controls (A, D), progesterone activates both *Hoxa-10* (B) and *Hoxa-11* (E) gene expression, while estrogen represses *Hoxa-10* expression (C) but activates *Hoxa-11* expression (F). s, stroma; le, luminal epithelium; m, myometrium.

RNase protection was performed by incubating antisense riboprobes of *Hoxa -9, -10, -11, -13,* and *RPL19* (internal control) with total RNAs from hormone treated uteri. This assay allows direct comparison of expression levels of different *AbdB Hoxa* genes after steroid administration. The basal expression levels of *Hoxa-10* and *Hoxa-11* are the highest, with *Hoxa-9* being weaker (50%) and *Hoxa-13* the weakest (~1/50 of *a-10)*. Quantitation of the RNase protection bands revealed that after 6 h of steroid treatment, progesterone also activates *Hoxa-9* and *a-11,* whereas estrogen represses *Hoxa-9* but activates *Hoxa-11. Hoxa-13* expression did not respond to either estrogen and progesterone. The activation by progesterone is weak for *Hoxa-9* (~1.5 fold), with progressively stronger activation for *Hoxa-10* (~2 fold) and *Hoxa-11* (~3.9 fold). Estrogen represses both *Hoxa-9* and *a-10* by 0.6 fold but activates *Hoxa-11* by 1.5 fold. In situ hybridization confirmed the above observations and showed that *Hoxa-11* expression is upregulated by both E_2 and P_4 in the stroma (Fig. 21.3E,F).

Abnormal Implantation in *Hoxa-10* Mutant Mice

The finding that *Hoxa-10* expression was transiently restricted to the antimesometrial pole after estrogen and progesterone treatment suggests that *Hoxa-10* expression may provide an important implantation cue. Although 11 of 14 asynchronous 3.5 p.c. uteri examined by in situ hybridization in transverse sections showed strong and unbiased *Hoxa-10* expression in the stroma (Fig. 21.4A), consistent with the above hypothesis, 3 of 14 uteri exhibited either localized or stronger *Hoxa-10* expression at the antimesometrial pole (Fig. 21.4B). The endogenous localization however, was extended throughout more of the stroma and was not confined to the subepithelial stroma as seen in the $E_2 + P_4$ treated uteri (Fig. 21.4C). Nevertheless, this observation suggests the possibility that transient antimesometrial *Hoxa-10* expression could provide a cue for implantation, which occurs in the rodent uterus invariantly at the antimesometrial pole. If this hypothesis is correct, one would expect that elimination of *Hoxa-10* function in mice might result in loss of implantation cues with implantation occurring elsewhere besides the antimesometrium. Interestingly, we observed a significant number of abnormally located implantation sites in *Hoxa-10* deficient mice in which some embryos were attached to epithelium at the mesometrial pole of the uterus at 4.5 p.c. and 26% of later embryos were observed to be positioned abnormally within the decidua (15).

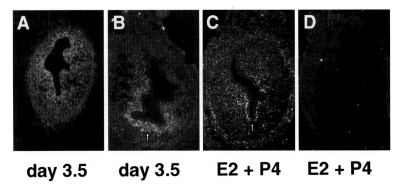

day 3.5   day 3.5   E2 + P4   E2 + P4

FIGURE 21.4. Antimesometrial expression of *Hoxa-10* during implantation. Day 3.5 p.c. uteri showing a progesterone dominated type pattern of *Hoxa-10* expression (A) and restriction of expression to the antimesometrial pole (B) similar to that seen following combined 17β-estradiol and progesterone treatment (C). Adjacent sections hybridized with a sense control riboprobe did not demonstrate any signal (D).

Discussion

Role of Hoxa-10 *During Implantation*

Hoxa-10 deficient females exhibit reduced fertility phenotypes. Although about 30% of mutant females eggs fail to be fertilized, the remaining 70% of mutant females have near normal numbers of blastocysts in the uterine lumen at the time of implantation. Although unproven, we hypothesize that the existence of oviductal malformations in *Hoxa-10* mutant females may underlie the reduction in fertilization efficiency. However, the subsequent failure of the majority of the embryos to implant into the mutant uterus undoubtedly reflects a maternal requirement for *Hoxa-10* function during the peri-implantation period.

In rodents, two asymmetrical events mark the maternal contributions to the implantation and decidualization processes. First, blastocysts always attach to epithelium at the antimesometrial pole of the uterus with subsequent implantation occurring in an invariant orientation (2). Second, after blastocyst attachment, morphological differences become apparent between the two poles of the uterus, typified by the increase in edema in the antimesometrial stroma (2). Decidualization first begins in the antimesometrial stroma immediately underneath the contacted epithelium and then extends to the deeper stromal layers of the antimesometrial pole and finally to the stroma of the mesometrial pole. The establishment of the decidual asymmetry depends in part on the local induction of genes by the blastocyst (16), but also on the regional differences preprogrammed into the uterus, because decidualization induced by an artificial stimulus undergoes the same antimesometrial to mesometrial progression (17,18). The mechanism for both asymmetrical processes is unclear. That *Hoxa-10* expression is transiently localized to the antimesometrial pole of the implanting uterus suggests the possibility that *Hoxa-10* may have a role in this recognition process. This transiently biased expression of *Hoxa-10* to the antimesometrial pole was observed in only 3 of 14 asynchronous uteri, however, suggesting that either this may be a natural variation among different individuals or may reflect a very narrow window of regulation. Consistent with the latter view, *Hoxa-10* expression was localized to the subepithelial stroma 4 h after $E_2 + P_4$ treatment, but not after either 2 or 8 h. The window for implantation is known to be narrow and highly dependent on hormonal regulation. Other genes, COX-2, HB-EGF, betacellulin and epiregulin have been previously reported to be expressed at the antimesometrial pole during implantation (16,19,20). However, their expression is present only surrounding implanting blastocysts and not detected in $E_2 + P_4$ treated uteri or in pseudopregnant females, suggesting that their expression may be specifically induced by the blastocyst. In addition, we observed a significant number (26%) of abnormal sites of implantation in *Hoxa-10* mutant females, which could also suggest that the possibility that the cues for proper implantation may have been lost.

On the other hand, because *Hoxa-10* expression is only restricted antimesometrially following combined estrogen and progesterone, it is not clear whether *Hoxa-10* plays a role in localizing embryos to the antimesometrial pole, since embryos are usually positioned in the antimesometrial crypts even in the absence of estrogen during delayed implantation (1). Therefore, it is possible that the abnormal implantation sites in *Hoxa-10* mutant females may simply result from a general failure of implantation and are unrelated to the asymmetric expression of *Hoxa-10*. The fact that the majority of embryos in *Hoxa-10* mutant females underwent correct implantation at the antimesometrial pole suggests that *Hoxa-10* cannot be the only molecule functioning in this process, if at all. Nonetheless, the results presented here could suggest a mechanism for the antimesometrial orientation of implantation, and this question remains for future investigation.

Steroidal Regulation of Hoxa-10 *Is Consistent with Its Role During Implantation*

Both increased vascular permeability and decidualization are hormone regulated events that are among the earliest responses of the sensitive maternal endometrium to deciduogenic stimuli. Nidatory estrogen secretion is required to initiate the increased vascular permeability response (reviewed in (1)), and in progesterone receptor knockout mice, decidualization in response to an artificial stimulus is abolished (21). Both responses are severely impaired in *Hoxa-10* deficient females, suggesting that *Hoxa-10* may constitute one component in the steroidal regulation of these responses during early implantation. These findings suggest that *Hoxa-10* expression could be regulated by both estrogen and progesterone in adult uterus.

At 0.5 day p.c., the uterus is exposed to the prenidatory secretion of estrogen and endogenous *Hoxa-10* is expressed in the luminal epithelium but not in the underlying stroma. This is consistent with the finding that estrogen is able to repress *Hoxa-10* expression in the stroma of ovariectomized mice after 4 h of exposure. At day 2.5 p.c. corpora lutea form and secrete progesterone, and endogenous *Hoxa-10* expression shifts from the epithelium to the underlying stroma. The upregulation of *Hoxa-10* expression by progesterone in the stroma of ovariectomized mice also agrees with the dynamic shift of *Hoxa-10* expression from epithelium to stroma. Finally, in ovariectomized mice, estrogen and progesterone together are able to restrict *Hoxa-10* expression to the antimesometrial pole of the uterus. Therefore, it is likely that the dynamic *Hoxa-10* expression pattern during periimplantation is under the regulation of both estrogen and progesterone.

Two other *AbdB Hoxa* genes, *Hoxa-9* and *-11* are also expressed in the adult uterus. Although *Hoxa-9* deficient mice exhibit no reproductive phenotype, *Hoxa-9* and *Hoxd-9* double mutants have reduced fertility, suggesting a functional redundancy between the two paralogous genes (22). Thus *Hoxa-9*, *-10*, and *-11* have all been implicated as functioning during reproduction. Because both *Hoxa-10* and *Hoxa-11* are strongly activated by progesterone, it is possible that *Hoxa-10* and *-11* are two *AbdB Hoxa* genes which have particularly important functions during embryo implantation. Further dissection of the regulatory regions spanning the *AbdB Hoxa* cluster should provide insights into the regulation of *AbdB Hox* gene function during implantation.

Although the precise cellular function for *Hox* genes is unknown, there is evidence to suggest that vertebrate *Hox* genes may provide positional information by affecting the rate of cell proliferation (reviewed in (23)). Both *Hoxd-13* knockout mice and *Hoxd-11* and *Hoxa-11* double knockout mice exhibit limb phenotypes that can be explained by a defect in cell proliferation or condensation (24,25). Consistent with this hypothesis, *Hoxa-11* deficient mice have thin, abnormally shaped uteri and no endometrial glands (8,9), whereas *Hoxa-13* knockout mice exhibit agenesis of the caudal Müllerian duct. Both phenotypes can be explained by a defect in cell proliferation. Although *Hoxa-10* mutant mice do not exhibit structural phenotypes suggestive of cell proliferation defects, the impaired decidual response in *Hoxa-10* mutant females could reflect a role for *Hoxa-10* in the hormonal control of cell proliferation.

Acknowledgments. L.M. and G.V.B contributed equally to this work. This work was supported by the Howard Hughes Medical Institute and by NICHD grant HD35580 to R.L.M, and by NICHD grants HD12304 and HD29968 to S.K.D. L.M. was supported by NIH NRSA (1F32 HD08264-01). G.V.B. was supported by an NIH training grant (T32 HD07390). H.L. is a Kansas Health Foundation Predoctoral Fellow.

References

1. Psychoyos A. Endocrine control of egg implantation. In: Greep RO, Astwood EB, Geiger SR, eds. Handbook of Physiology, Vol. 7. Washington, DC: American Physiological Society, 1973:187–215.
2. Abrahamson PA, Zorn TMT. Implantation and decidualization in rodents. J Exp Zool 1993;266:603–28.
3. McLaren A. A study of blastocysts during delay and subsequent implantation in lactating mice. J Endocrinol 1996;42:453–63.
4. Favier B, Dollé P. Developmental functions of mammalian Hox genes. Mol Hum Reprod 1997;3:115–31.
5. Dollé P, Izpisúa-Belmonte J-C, Brown JM, Tickle C, Duboule D. Hox-4 genes and the morphogenesis of mammalian genitalia. Genes Devel 1991;5:1767–76.
6. Hsieh-Li HM, Witte DP, Weinstein M, Branford W, Li H, Small K, et al. Hoxa11 structure, extensive antisense transcription, and function in male and female fertility. Development 1995;121:1373–85.

7. Benson GV, Lim H, Paria BC, Satokata I, Dey SK, Maas R. Mechanisms of female infertility in Hoxa-10 mutant mice: uterine homeosis versus loss of maternal Hoxa-10 expression. Development 1996;122:2687–96.

8. Small KM, Potter S. Homeotic transformations and limb defects in Hoxa11 mutant mice. Gene Devel 1993;7:2318–28.

9. Gendron, RL, Paradis H, Hsieh-Li HM, Lee DW, Potter SS, Markoff E. Abnormal uterine stromal and glandular function associated with maternal reproductive defects in Hoxa-11 null mice. Biol Reprod 1997;56:1097–105.

10. Fromental-Romain C, Warot X, Messaddeq N, LeMeur M, Dollé P, Chambon P. Hoxa-13 and Hoxd-13 play a crucial role in the patterning of the limb autopod. Development 1996;122:2997–3011.

11. Warot X, Fromental-Ramain C, Fraulob V, Chambon P, Dollé P. Gene dosage-dependent effects of the Hoxa-13 and Hoxd-13 mutations on morphogenesis of the terminal parts of the digestive and urogenital tracts. Development 1997;124:4781–91.

12. Satokata I, Benson GV, Maas RL. Sexually dimorphic sterility phenotypes in Hoxa10-deficient mice. Nature 1995;374:460–3.

13. Rijli FM, Matyas R, Pellegrini M, Dierich A, Gruss P, Dollé P, Chambon P. Cryptorchidism and homeotic transformations of spinal nerves and vertebrae in Hoxa-10 mutant mice. Proc Natl Acad Sci USA 1995;92:8185–9.

14. Taylor HS, Vanden Heuvel GB, Igarashi P. A conserved Hox axis in the mouse and human female reproductive system: late establishment and persistent adult expression of the Hoxa cluster genes. Biol Reprod 1997;57:1338–45.

15. Benson GV. The role of Hoxa-10 in reproductive tract morphogenesis and uterine implantation. Ph.D. thesis dissertation, 1996.

16. Chakraborty I, Das SK, Wang J, Dey SK. Developmental expression of the cyclo-oxygenase-1 and cyclo-oxygenase-2 genes in the peri-implantation mouse uterus and their differential regulation by the blastocyst and ovarian steroids. J Mol Endo 1995;15:107–22.

17. Finn C, Hinchliffe J. Reaction of the mouse uterus during implantation and deciduoma formation as demonstrated by changes in the distribution of alkaline phosphatase. J Reprod Fert 1964;8:331–8.

18. Ledford B, Rankin J, Markwald R, Bagget B. Biochemical and morphological changes following artificially stimulated decidualization in the mouse uterus. Biol Reprod 1997;15;529–35.

19. Das SK, Wang XN, Paria BC, Damm D, Abraham JA, Klagsbrun M, et al. Heparin-binding EGF-like growth factor gene is induced in the mouse uterus temporally by the blastocyst solely at the site of its opposition: a possible ligand for interaction with blastocyst EGF-receptor in implantation. Development 1994;120:1071–83.

20. Das SK, Das N, Wang J, Lim H, Schryver B, Plowman GD, et al. Expression of betacellulin and epiregulin genes in the mouse uterus temporally by the blastocyst solely at the site of its apposition is coincident with the "window" of implantation. Devel Biol 1997;190:178–90.

21. Lydon JP, DeMayo FJ, Funk CR, Mani SK, Hughes AR, Montgomery CA Jr, et al. Mice lacking progesterone receptor exhibit pleiotropic reproductive abnormalities. Genes Devel 1995;9:2266–78.

22. Fromental-Ramain C, Warot X, Lakkaraju S, Favier B, Haack H, Birling C, et al. Specific and redundant functions of the paralogous Hoxa-9 and Hoxd-9 genes in forelimb and axial skeleton patterning. Development 1996;122:461–72.

23. Duboule D. Vertebrate Hox genes and proliferation: an alternative pathway to homeosis? Curr Opin Genet Devel 1995;5:525–8.
24. Dollé P, Dierich A, LeMeur M, Schimmang T, Schuhbaur B, Chambon P, et al. Disruption of the Hoxd-13 gene induces localized heterochrony leading to mice with neotenic limbs. Cell 1993;75:431–41.
25. Davis AP, Witte DP, Hsieh-Li HM, Potter SS, et al. Absence of radius and ulna in mice lacking Hoxa-11 and Hoxd-11. Nature 1995;375:791–6.

22

Possible Role of the Transcription Factor Oct-3/4 in Control of Human Chorionic Gonadotropin Expression

Limin Liu, Douglas Leaman, and
R. Michael Roberts

During a study on the regulation of interferon-τ genes in choriocarcinoma cells, an hCGα-CAT construct was included as an internal control to check transfection efficiencies. Although Oct-3/4 coexpression had little effect on expression from an IFN-τ promoter that carried several potential Oct binding sequences, the hCGα-CAT construct was strongly silenced. This serendipitous discovery led to the data reported in this chapter and two earlier papers (1,2).

Chorionic gonadotropin (CG) is responsible for preventing the regression of the corpus luteum in higher primates (3). The timing and quantity of hCG release are considered key factors in determining whether a human pregnancy succeeds or fails (3,4). CG binds the same receptor as luteinizing hormone (LH), and there is now considerable evidence that this receptor is not confined to the ovary, but is present in numerous other organs and tissues, including endometrium, brain, blood vessels, and even placenta itself. CG may thus influence a wide variety of physiological processes during pregnancy. In particular, CG could play a direct role in implantation by inducing epithelial modifications at trophoblast contact points and initiating decidualization (6).

CG consists of an α-subunit (CGα), common to all the glycoprotein hormones, and a β-subunit (CGβ) responsible for biological specificity. Whereas there is only a single CGα gene, there are six hCGβ subunit genes (7,8). Of the latter, hCGβ5 is the one predominantly expressed in the human placenta and in choriocarcinoma cells (9). Clearly, the two subunits must be synthesized simultaneously if biologically active CG is to result, although little is known about how such coordinated synthesis is achieved.

Transcriptional Activation of hCG Production

Transcriptional regulation appears to be paramount in the control of hCG production (7). Most studies have concentrated on the transactivation of the genes, rather than on how transcription can be silenced. The hCGα-subunit gene, in particular, has received much scrutiny because it is expressed in both trophoblast and pituitary. Multiple regulatory elements (10–17) are involved in controlling trophoblast expression (Fig. 22.1A), including two random repeats of a cAMP response element (CRE), a complex, upstream regulatory element (URE) consisting of at least two subdomains that bind different sets of transcription factors, the α-activator (αACT) element, the junctional regulatory element (JRE), and the CCAAT region. The transacting factors that bind the elements have, for the most part, not been identified. Two exceptions are the CRE-binding protein (CREB) (7) and AP-2, which binds within the URE (17).

The hCGβ5 gene has been less studied. Like hCGα, expression is enhanced in response to cAMP (18), but no well-defined cis elements have been identified (7,19). The hCGβ5 gene contains at least two regions (a and b in Fig. 22.1B) that bind putative transcription factors and that contribute to cAMP responsiveness within the critical -311 to -200 promoter/enhancer segment (Fig. 22.1b). It contains no consensus CRE motifs (TGACGTCA). AP-2, which transactivates hCGβ, also binds within the a and b regions (-311 to -279 and -221 to -200) (17). Other than Oct-3/4, the subject of this chapter, AP-2 is the only transcription factor that has so far been recognized that might have a role in coordinate expression of the two subunit genes (17). Indeed, what is the most surprising feature of the promoter elements for the two subunit genes is how little they resemble each other (Fig. 22.1A and B). There are no common conserved elements that might link both to trophoblast expression. In addition, the hCGβ5 gene has no TATA element. Instead, it contains a possible initiator element (c in Fig. 22.1B) at the transcription start site.

Transcription Factor Oct-3/4

The Oct-3/4 transcription factor is a member of the POU family of transcription factors, which are characterized by possessing a conserved POU DNA-binding domain (23–27). The latter is a two-unit structure consisting of a POU-specific domain (POUs) and a POU-type homeodomain (POU$_{HD}$) (26).

Expression of Oct-3/4 is primarily restricted to totipotent/pluripotent early embryonic cells (24,27,28). Low expression of both Oct-3/4 mRNA and protein has been detected in mouse oocytes and fertilized eggs, but nuclear localization of Oct-3/4 begins in late 1-cell embryos, at the time the embryonic genome is first activated, and becomes more pronounced in 8-cell embryos, when Oct-3/4 expression is substantially increased (28). Oct-3/4 is expressed in all cells of the embryo until the late morula stage. It is rapidly down-regulated in the trophectoderm of the blastocyst. Once hatching from

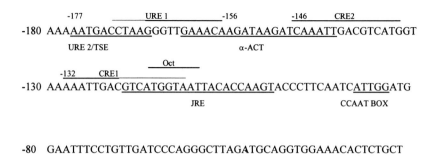

A   The hCGα Gene Promoter

```
        -177              URE 1              -156        -146      CRE2
      -180 AAAAATGACCTAAGGGGTTGAAACAAGATAAGATCAAATTGACGTCATGGT
          URE 2/TSE                              α-ACT
                                    Oct
          -132      CRE1
      -130 AAAAATTGACGTCATGGTAATTACACCAAGTACCCTTCAATCATTGGATG
                              JRE                      CCAAT BOX



                                              +1
      -30  GGTATAAAAGCAGGTGAGGACTTCATTAACTGCAGTTACTGAGAACTCAT
            TATA
```

B   The hCGβ5 Gene Promoter

```
      -330  ATGTCCTCTGAGGCTTCGGCCCCCGTGGGCAGGACACACCTCCTGCGGGCC
                                a
      -280  TATTCAATAATCAGTTAAATCACCTGAAGCACACGCATTTCCGGGGACCGCT
                  Oct
      -230  CCGGGCATCCTGGCTTGAGGGTAGAGTGGGCGGAGGTTCCTAAGGGAGAG
                b
      -180  GTGGGGCTCGGGCTGAATCCCTCGTTGGGGGGCATCTGGGTCAAGTGGCT

      -130  TCCCTGGCAGCACAGTCACGGGGAGGCCCTCTCTCATTGGGCAGAAGCTA

      -80   AGTCCGAAGCCGCGCCCCTCCTGGGAGGTTGAACTGTGGTGCAGGAAAGC
                        +1
      -30   CTCAAGTAGAGGAGGGGTTGAGGCTTCAATCCAGCACTTTGCTC
                                      c
```

FIGURE 22.1. (A) The hCGα gene promoter. Shown here are the transcription start site (+1) and various cis-elements important for expression of the gene in trophoblast cells. (B) The hCGβ gene promoter. It has no TATA element, but contains a possible initiator element (c) at the transcription start site. The two underlined regions a and b may be involved in cAMP regulation of the promoter.

the zona pellucida occurs at about day 4.5 post coitum, Oct-3/4 is expressed exclusively in the inner cell mass and not in trophectoderm. After implantation, Oct-3/4 mRNA is detectable only in the primitive ectoderm at day 5.5 p.c. and in primordial germ cells after day 8.5 p.c. (24). Data are lacking in other species, including the human.

Oct-3/4 is expressed in undifferentiated murine embryonic stem (ES) cells and embryonic carcinoma (EC) cells, but it is rapidly down-regulated when these cells differentiate (23,24,29,30). Retinoic acid (RA) treatment, which causes such differentiation, represses the Oct-3/4 gene promoter (29,30), most likely as the result of a retinoic acid-repressible enhancer located about 1 kb upstream of the transcriptional start site.

The expression pattern of Oct-3/4 and its correlative relationship with cell pluripotency suggests that Oct-3/4 is important for maintaining cells in an undifferentiated state in early embryogenesis and that silencing of its expression may be necessary for subsequent cell differentiation. For the most part, the genes to which Oct-3/4 is directed remains to be determined, and it remains unclear whether Oct-3/4 acts primarily as an activator or repressor of gene expression. In F9 cells it can act as both, depending upon the genetic context in which it is placed within reporter genes. Finally, there is evidence that some POU-containing proteins, including Oct-1, can regulate transcription through their cooperative interactions with other transcription factors (31–35) and need not bind DNA directly to exert their effects.

Oct-3/4 Inhibition of Endogenous hCG Production in JAr Cells

To study the effect of Oct-3/4 on expression of endogenous hCG genes, JAr cells were stably transfected with an Oct-3/4 gene. Total RNA was isolated from both stable Oct-3/4 clones and stable control clones, and subjected to a ribonuclease protection assay. When quantitated by densitometry and normalized to β-actin mRNA, whose concentration appeared to be identical in all clones whether or not they expressed Oct-3/4, the hCGα and hCGβ mRNA contents of the clones expressing Oct-3/4 was about 23% and 6% respectively of that in the controls (1,2).

The production of hCG protein (measured in a radioimmunoassay specific for the hCGB subunit) was dramatically reduced in the clones expressing Oct-3/4 (Fig. 22.2). For clones S1 and S4, values were 8.3% and 3.2% respectively of the production of two control lines (C1 and C2) ($p < 0.001$). These data indicated that Oct-3/4 selectively reduced the expression of hCG and its subunits in JAr cells.

Oct-3/4 Inhibition of the hCGα Promoter

A -170hCGα promoter was sufficient to provide full expression (Fig. 22.3A) and cAMP responsiveness (Fig. 22.3B) to a CAT reporter gene in JAr cells. Silencing by Oct-3/4 was directed at the shortest promoter tested (Fig. 22.3A) and occurred in a dose-dependent manner (Fig. 22.3B). The inhibitory effect of Oct-3/4 was not reversed in the presence of cAMP.

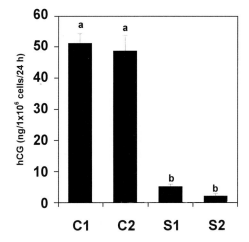

FIGURE 22.2. Reduced endogenous hCG production in JAr cells stably transfected with pcDNA3-Oct-3/4. Clones S1 and S4 had been stably transfected with pcDNA3-Oct-3/4; C1 and C2 with pcDNA3. Amounts of hCG secreted by the stable clones were measured by a radioimmunoassay that utilized monoclonal antibodies specific to the hCGβ subunit (1). The results are the means (± SEM) of four independent experiments. Values marked with different letters are statistically different ($p < 0.001$).

To define more precisely where Oct-3/4 effects in the promoter were manifested, various truncated constructs were tested in a cotransfection assay similar to those shown in Figure 22.3B, except the reporter gene in this case was human growth hormone (hGH). Whereas the -170 construct was inhibited ~70% by Oct-3/4, there was no inhibition of a -99 construct, which lacked both the URE and CREs, and of a -148 construct, which had the CREs but not the URE (see Fig. 22.1A for diagram of promoter).

To confirm that the Oct-responsive site was upstream of the CRE, selected regions of the hCGα promoter were tested for their abilities to act as enhancers to a thymidine kinase (TK) promoter driving a hGH reporter gene (1). As expected, the full URE/CRE region could increase TKGH activity (9-fold) in JAr cells, and coexpression of Oct-3/4 reduced this enhanced activity by about 70%. Again, activity from a construct lacking the URE was unaffected by Oct-3/4 coexpression. In addition, a deletion mutant, lacking the segment -160 to -155 (-160/-155, μ VIII hCGα-CAT) (36), was not inhibited by Oct-3/4 (unpublished data). These data firmly established that a site at the proximal end of the URE 1 segment of the promoter was the likely target for Oct-3/4 silencing of the hCGα gene, despite the fact that this region contained no known Oct binding sequences.

Electrophoretic mobility shift assays (EMSA) performed with Oct-3/4 synthesized by coupled in vitro transcription and translation showed that an Oct-3/4 binding site was present in the -170/-53 promoter fragment, but that it was not located in the URE where it was expected. Instead, the Oct-3/4 binding site was

A

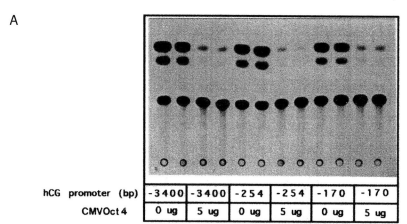

hCG promoter (bp)	-3400	-3400	-254	-254	-170	-170
CMVOct 4	0 ug	5 ug	0 ug	5 ug	0 ug	5 ug

B

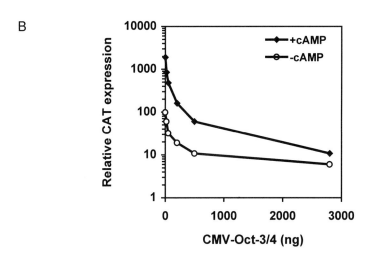

FIGURE 22.3. (A) Effect of Oct-3/4 cotransfection of hCGα-subunit promoter activity. Five μg of each expression plasmid, containing a CAT reporter gene fused to αhCG promoter fragments of the lengths indicated, were transfected into JAr cells alone, or with 5 μg of a CMV-Oct-3/4 expression plasmid. A pXGH5 plasmid (1 μg) was included in all transfections as a reference. Acetylated and non-acetylated forms of 14C-chloramphenicol were separated by thin layer chromatography (TLC). The results from duplicate plates for each treatment are presented. (B) Dosage-dependent inhibition of -170hCGα-CAT by Oct-3/4 cotransfection in JAr cells. Plasmids p-170hCGα-CAT (2μg) and pTKGH (0.3 μg) were cotransfected with 0, 25, 50, 150, 450, or 2850 ng pCMV-Oct-4 in JAr cells in either absence or presence of 8-Br-cAMP. CAT activity was normalized by hGH expression and expressed as a percentage of the activity obtained in absence of pCMV-Oct-3/4 cotransfection and absence of 8-Br-cAMP induction. Similar results were obtained in several independent experiments.

positioned between -117 and -110 (Fig. 22.1A). This site is identical at six positions to the consensus Oct motif (ATTTG/A CAT, sense; ATGC/TAAAT, antisense), and when this site was mutated by substituting A at -111 and T at -110, the -170/-53 promoter could no longer bind Oct-3/4. Importantly, however, reporter gene expression was as fully repressed by Oct-3/4 as in controls.

Oct-3/4 probably exerts its effects indirectly in the proximal region of the URE, which is believed to bind at least two, ill-defined proteins, the URE1-binding protein (16,36) and the αACT-binding protein (7). One mechanism for Oct-3/4 inhibition could be that it interacts with one or more of these transcriptional activators and influences their abilities either to bind the promoter itself or to associate with CREB (31). The latter transactivates the downstream CRE elements upon which the URE depends exclusively for its enhancing activity (12–14). Alternatively, Oct-3/4 could squelch, or repress by some other means, transcriptional coactivators necessary for proper functioning of the URE-associated factors.

Oct-3/4 Inhibition of the hCGβ Promoter

Oct-3/4 but not Oct-2 reduced CAT expression from the -305hCGβ promoter shown in Figure 22.1B by about 90% in JAr cells (1). 8-Br-cAMP, which doubles CAT expression in controls, did not reverse this repression. A series of hCGβ promoters with truncations were then used to define more precisely the site targeted by Oct-3/4. They indicated that the region responsible was within the -305/-249 region and most probably in the 30 bases between -249 and -279.

EMSA assays and methylation protection assays established that there was indeed an Oct binding site of relatively low affinity in this 30 base region. For example, a probe that had been methylated in the antisense strand at positions -276 and -269 bound Oct-3/4 less well than a nonmethylated probe. Also, a region (-275 to -268) was identical at seven nucleotides out of eight to the optimal Oct-1 POUs-binding sequence (36). Moreover, when the sequence 5′-AATC (-272 to -269) within the hCGβ promoter was mutated to 5′-ccag, Oct-3/4 could no longer repress reporter gene expression or bind the promoter (1). The putative -277/-268 Oct site (TCAATAATCA) of the hCGβ5 promoter is identical at 7 out of 10 nucleotides to a weak Oct-3/4 binding sequence found in two enhancer-promoter units of the mouse genome that are active in undifferentiated P19 embryonal carcinoma cells but inactive in differentiated P19 cells (37). The presumptive POUs motif is also placed just one base upstream from a stretch of six A/T nucleotides (Fig. 22.1B) that might be capable of interacting with the POU homeodomain of Oct-3/4.

Oct-3/4, therefore, seems to have an intrinsic ability to repress the hCGβ promoter by a mechanism that involves its direct binding to DNA. It is unclear whether, once bound, it inhibits the general transcriptional machinery directly or whether it recruits some other inhibitory factor.

All functional hCGβ genes possess TATA-less promoters (19), and it could be for this reason that the hCGβ5 gene tested was repressed by Oct-3/4 while another octamer-containing promoter, the one for thymidine kinase which possesses a conventional TATA box (38), was not affected by Oct-3/4 co-transfection. Some special transcription factor is probably required specifically for proper functioning of such TATA-less promoters (39,40) and could be the target of Oct-3/4 inhibition.

Conclusions

The genes for both the hCGα subunit and the hCGβ subunits are silenced by the embryonic transcription factor Oct-3/4, a protein that is expressed primarily in undifferentiated, potentially totipotent cells of the embryo. This inhibition by Oct-3/4 may explain why these genes are not expressed in the inner cell mass of the human embryo but expressed in trophectoderm. Surprisingly the mechanisms by which silencing of the two genes is achieved differs. With hCGα, the inhibition, while targeted to the URE, does not involve direct binding to the promoter. By contrast, a well-defined Oct element is present in the hCGβ subunit promoter and is necessary for gene silencing.

Acknowledgments. The research was supported by NIH grants HD-21896 and HD-29843.

References

1. Liu L, Roberts RM. Silencing of the gene for the β-subunit of human chorionic gonadotropin by the embryonic transcription factor Oct-3/4. J Biol Chem 1996;271: 16683–9.
2. Liu L, Leaman D, Villalta M, Roberts RM. Silencing of the gene for the α-subunit of human chorionic gonadotropin by the embryonic transcription factor Oct-3/4. Mol Endocrinol 1997;11:1651–8.
3. Ogren L, Talamantes F. The placenta as an endocrine organ: polypeptides. In: Knobil E, Neill JD, eds. The Physiology of reproduction, 2d ed. New York: Raven, 1994:875–945.
4. Hearn JP, Webley GE, Gidley-Baird AA. Chorionic gonadotropin and embryo-maternal recognition during the periimplantation period in primates. J Reprod Fertil 1991;92:497–509.
5. Rao CV, Sanfilippo JS. New understanding in the biochemistry of implantation: potential direct roles of luteinizing hormone and human chorionic gonadotropin. Endocrinology 1997;7:107–11.
6. Fazleabas AT, Donnelly KM, Fortman JD, Miller JB. Modulation of the baboon (*Papio anubis*) endometrium by chorionic gonadotropin (CG) during the period of uterine receptivity. Biol Reprod 1997;56(Suppl 1):176 (Abstr).
7. Jameson JL, Hollenberg AN. Regulation of chorionic gonadotropin gene expression. Endocrinol Rev 1993;14:203–19.

8. Boothby M, Ruddon RW, Anderson C, McWilliams D, Boime I. A single gonadotropin α-subunit gene in normal tissue and tumor-derived cell lines. J Biol Chem 1981;256:5121–7.

9. Bo M, Boime I. Identification of the transcriptionally active genes of the chorionic gonadotropin β gene cluster in vivo. J Biol Chem 1992;267:3179–84.

10. Silver BJ, Bokar JA, Virgin JB, Vallen EA, Milsted A, Nilson JH. Cyclic AMP regulation of the human glycoprotein hormone alpha-subunit gene is mediated by an 18-base pair element. Proc Nat Acad Sci USA 1987;84:2198–202.

11. Deutsch PJ, Jameson JL, Habener JF. Cyclic AMP responsiveness of human gonadotropin-α gene transcription is directed by a repeated 18-base pair enhancer. J Biol Chem 1987;262:12169–74.

12. Delegeane AM, Fedand LH, Mellon PL. Tissue-specific enhancer of the human glycoprotein hormone α-subunit gene: dependence on cyclic AMP-inducible elements. Mol Cell Biol 1987;7:3994–4002.

13. Jameson JL, Powers AC, Gallagher GD, Habener JF. Enhancer, promoter element interactions dictate cyclic adenosine monophosphate mediated, cell-specific expression of the glycoprotein hormone α-gene. Mol Endocrinol 1989;3:763–72.

14. Andersen B, Kennedy GC, Nilson JH. A cis-acting element located between the cAMP response elements and CCAAT box augments cell-specific expression of the glycoprotein hormone alpha subunit gene. J Biol Chem 1990;265:21874–80.

15. Kennedy GC, Andersen B, Nilson JH. The human α-subunit glycoprotein hormone gene utilizes a unique CCAAT binding factor. J Biol Chem 1990;265:6279–85.

16. Steger DJ, Altschmied J, Boscher M, Mellon PL. Evolution of placenta-specific gene expression: comparison of the equine and human gonadotropin α-subunit genes. Mol Endocrinol 1991;5:243–55.

17. Johnson W, Albanese C, Handwerger S, Williams T, Pestell RG, Jameson JL. Regulation of the human chorionic gonadotropin alpha- and beta-subunit promoters by AP-2. J Biol Chem 1997;272:15405–12

18. Jameson JL, Lindell CM. Isolation and characterization of the human chorionic gonadotropin β-subunit (CGβ) gene cluster: regulation of a transcriptionally active CGβ gene by cyclic AMP. Mol Cell Biol 1988;8:5100–7.

19. Otani T, Otani F, Krych M, Chaplin DD, Boime I. Identification of a promoter region in the CGβ gene cluster. J Biol Chem 1988;263:7322–9.

20. Steger DJ, Boscher M, Hect JG, Mellon PL. Coordinate control of the α- and β-subunit genes of human chorionic gonadotropin by trophoblast-specific element-binding protein. Mol Endocrinol 1993;7:1579–88.

21. Albanese C, Kay TWH, Toccoli NM, Jameson JL. Novel cyclic adenosine 3′, 5′-monophosphate response element in the human chorionic gonadotropin β-subunit gene. Mol Endocrinol 1991;5:693–702.

22. Pestell RG, Hollenberg AN, Albanese C, Jameson JL. C-Jun represses transcription of the human chorionic gonadotropin α and β genes through distinct types of CREs. J Biol Chem 1994;269:31090–6.

23. Okamoto K, Okazawa H, Okuda A, Sakai M, Muramatsu M, Hamada H. A novel octamer binding transcription factor is differentially expressed in mouse embryonic cells. Cell 1990;60:461–72.

24. Rosner MH, Vigano MA, Ozato K, Timmons PM, Poirier F, Rugby PW, et al. A POU-domain transcription factor in early stem cells and germ cells of the mammalian embryo. Nature 1990;345:686–92.

25. Scholer HR, Dressler GR, Balling R, Rohdewohld H, Gruss P. Oct-4: a germline-specific transcription factor mapping to the mouse t-complex. EMBO J 1990;9: 2185–95.

26. Verrijzer CP, Van der Vliet PC. POU domain transcription factors. Biochim Biophys Acta 1993;1173:1–21.

27. Scholer HR, Ruppert S, Suzuki N, Chowhurdy K, Gruss P. A new type of POU domain in germ line-specific protein. Nature 1990;344:435–9.

28. Palmier SL, Peter W, Hess H, Scholer HR. Oct-4 transcription factor is differentially expressed in the mouse embryo during establishment of the first two extraembryonic cell lineages involved in implantation. Devel Biol 1994;166:259–67.

29. Okazawa H, Okamoto K, Ishino F, et al. The Oct-3 gene, a gene for an embryonic transcription factor, is controlled by a retinoic acid repressible enhancer. EMBO J 1991;10:2997–3005.

30. Pikarsky E, Sharir H, Ben-Shushan E, Bergman Y. Retinoic acid represses Oct-3/4 gene expression through several retinoic acid-responsive elements located in the promoter-enhancer region. Mol Cell Biol 1994;14:1026–38.

31. Meyer TE, Habener JF. Cyclic adenosine 3′,5′-monophate response element binding protein (CREB) and related transcription-activating deoxyribonucleic acid-binding proteins. Endocr Rev 1993;14:269–90.

32. Gstaiger M, Knoepfel L, Georgiev O, Schaffner W. Hovens CM. A B-cell coactivator of octamer-binding transcription factors. Nature 1995;373:360–2.

33. Strubin M, Newell JW, Matthias P. OBF-1, a novel B-cell-specific coactivator that stimulates immunoglobulin promoter activity through association with octamer-binding proteins. Cell 1995;80:497–506.

34. Luo Y, Roeder RG. Cloning, functional characterization, and mechanism of action of the B-cell-specific transcriptional coactivator OCA-B. Mol Cell Biol 1995;15: 4115–24.

35. Verrijzer CP, Alkema MJ, Van Weperen WW, Van Leeuwen HC, Strating MJJ, van der Vilet PC. The DNA binding specificity of the bipartitie POU domain and its subdomains. EMBO J 1992;11:4993–5003.

36. Pittman RH, Clay CM, Farmerie TA, Nilson JH. Functional analysis of the placenta-specific enhancer of the human glycoprotein hormone α-subunit gene. J Biol Chem 1994;269:19360–8.

37. Bhat K, McBurney MW, Hamada H. Functional cloning of mouse chromosomal loci specifically active in embryonal carcinoma stem cells. Mol Cell Biol 1988;8: 3251–9.

38. McKnight SL, Gavis ER, Kingsbury R, Axel R. Analysis of transcriptional regulatory signals of the HSV thymidine kinase gene: identification of an upstream control region. Cell 1981;25:385–98.

39. Weis L, Reinberg D. Transcription by RNA polymerase II: initiator-directed formation of transcription-competent complexes. FASEB J 1992;6:3330–9.

40. Roy AL, Malik S, Meisterernst M, Roeder RG. An alternative pathway for transcription initiation involving TfIi-I. Nature 1993;365:355–9.

23

Molecular Mechanisms Regulating Uterine Decidualization and Implantation: Cell–Cell and Cell–Extracellular Matrix Interactions

VIRGINIA RIDER

Implantation of the mammalian embryo and development of the placenta are interactive processes that depend on two-way communication between genetically distinct individuals. Since the pioneering embryo transfer experiments of Chang (1), the importance of developmental synchrony between the uterus and embryo for successful implantation has been appreciated. Although the strictness of this relationship varies somewhat among species, some degree of maturity of both the embryo and the uterus is required for the initiation of implantation. An important correlate of uterine maturation in many species, including the human, is the proliferation and differentiation of uterine stromal cells just before implantation. This process is called decidualization. Decidualization is initiated prior to breachment of the basement membrane by the blastocyst, and decidual cells are in intimate contact with the embryo during its implantation into the uterine wall. As a normal part of placentation, some decidual cells subsequently undergo apoptosis to accommodate the growing conceptus.

The deciduate type of placenta, formed in rodents and humans, results from intimate connection of the fetal and maternal tissues, and the maternal tissue is shed with the placenta at birth (2). The extent of trophoblast invasion varies greatly among the different species that form hemochorial placentas. The invasive characteristics among these groups depends on the aggressive nature of the trophoblast and the degree of resistance offered by the decidua (3). In spite of the importance of the decidua in species that employ invasive implantation, the mechanisms that regulate its formation and regression are poorly understood (3). Moreover, the function(s) of the decidua is not known. Recent evidence suggests that the decidua can exert control over the invasion of the blastocyst. The tissue proteinases, gelatinase B and urokinase-type plasminogen activator (uPA), are produced by the mouse trophoblast giant cells at the time of embryo invasion (day 7.5 of development). Proteolysis is probably curtailed by the expression of the proteolysis inhibitor TIMP-3 expressed in uterine decidual cells adjacent to the invading blastocyst (4). Other proposed roles for the decidua include a source of nutrition for the embryo, immunoprotection by serving as an immunologically privileged site, and production of hormones and cytokines required for the establishment of pregnancy.

Stromal cell proliferation and differentiation (decidualization) is initiated in response to ovarian hormones just before the expected time of implantation in humans (5) and rodents (6,7). Decidualization is accompanied by characteristic changes in stromal cell morphology, the formation of gap junctions, and the production of cellular products associated with the differentiated phenotype including alkaline phosphatase and placental lactogens (8). Within the decidua, differential gene expression occurs in the cells at the antimesometrial and mesometrial regions of the endometrium. However, when these decidual cell populations are cultured, differences between the two are lost suggesting that positional effects within the uterus are important in determining the differentiated phenotype (9).

Our research focuses on the gene regulatory mechanisms involved in the control of stromal cell proliferation and differentiation. In this chapter, these two topics have been artificially separated for the sake of brevity. However, it is our view that proliferation, differentiation, and apoptosis are intimately linked. The referenced literature in this chapter is biased toward the mouse and rat models because they are amenable to experimental manipulation. Analogous cell types, however, are present in both human and rodent decidua (10) suggesting that the molecular mechanisms that control decidualization are conserved among species.

Control of Uterine Cell Proliferation

After ovulation the uterus is reorganized to prepare for implantation of the blastocyst. The endometrium is comprised of three major resident cell types known as the luminal and glandular epithelial cells and endometrial stroma (Fig. 23.1). Stromal cells are fibroblast like cells that are scattered throughout the stromal extracellular matrix. The uterus also contains smooth muscle and endothelial cells (Fig. 23.1) (11) along with a variety of immune cells (12,13). The role of immune cells in the uterus has been reviewed recently (14) and is beyond the scope of this chapter. Endometrial cell proliferation is controlled by ovarian hormones (15). In the rodent uterus epithelial cells proliferate in response to estrogen for the first few days after ovulation. At day 3 of pregnancy in the mouse (15) and day 4 of pregnancy in the rat (16) there is a proliferative switch from the epithelia to the uterine stoma. This switch is dependent upon progesterone (16). The case for progesterone control of stro-

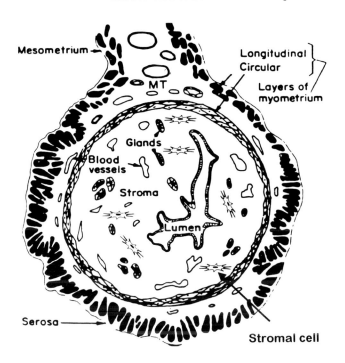

Mesometrium

Longitudinal
Circular

Layers of
myometrium

MT

Glands

Blood
vessels

Stroma

Lumen

Serosa

Stromal cell

FIGURE 23.1. Diagram representing a cross section through the uterus of the rat. The endometrium is comprised of three major resident cell types, the luminal and glandular epithelia and the stromal cells. Stromal cells are scattered throughout the extracellular matrix labeled stroma in this diagram. The myometrium contains both longitudinal and circular muscle. MT, mesometrial triangle. After Finn, Res in Reprod 1987;19:3–4.

mal cell proliferation in the human endometrium is less well characterized. However, stromal cells show a second wave of proliferation in the last days of the menstrual cycle (17). Progesterone receptors are present in stromal cells at this time (18), suggesting that progesterone action controls this late wave of stromal mitosis. The dependence of uterine stromal cell proliferation on progesterone is an unusual primary function for this steroid because progesterone is normally considered the hormone promoting cellular differentiation. This progesterone requirement for stromal cell proliferation may have evolved to ensure that decidualization occurs temporally with ovulation. Progesterone action on uterine cell proliferation is an area in reproductive biology that is not well studied from a mechanistic point of view (19).

While it is clear that some steroid responses in uterine cells result from hormonal stimulation of various growth factors and their receptors (20–22), it is now evident from breast cancer cell studies that sex steroids can directly control cell cycle regulatory proteins (23). This aspect of hormone action in uterine cells is virtually unexplored. A host of growth factors have been mapped to various cell types in the endometrium of the human, rodents, and domestic animals, and several reviews summarizing their distribution are available (20–22). Work in our laboratory (24) focuses on the fibroblast growth factor family, and specifically on basic fibroblast growth factor (bFGF) because of its importance in controlling cell proliferation and angiogenesis in a variety of cells and tissues (25). The distribution of bFGF mapped in rat uterine cells during the periimplantation period suggests that this growth factor coregulates uterine cell proliferation (24). Basic FGF localizes intracellularly in rat epithelial and stromal cells at days 2 and 3 of pregnancy and in the extracellular matrix. This finding is somewhat surprising because bFGF normally resides in the extracellular matrix and not within cells of adult tissues (26). Basic FGF distinctively localizes to the apical surface of epithelial cells in the rat and mouse (24,27). This pattern of localization suggests export of the growth factor into the uterine lumen. Although bFGF lacks a classical consensus signal peptide (28), it has been reported in the luminal flushings of pregnant pigs (29) and rats (24). Interestingly, bFGF is expressed in the epithelium of pregnant pigs but not cycling gilts (30).

Labeling of stromal cells in vivo results in the appearance of ^{3}H thymidine in decidual cells (16) conclusively demonstrating that they are the progenitors of decidual cells. Therefore, central to understanding the onset of decidualization is identifying the mechanisms by which progesterone controls stromal cell proliferation. It seems likely that progesterone could influence the production of growth factors or their receptors thereby stimulating stromal cell proliferation. Consistent with this view, changes in the cellular distribution of rat uterine bFGF coincide with the shift in endometrial proliferation from epithelium to stroma. To further clarify hormone-growth factor interactions in the uterus, pregnant rats were treated with the progesterone receptor antagonist RU-486 to block implantation (31). The number of cells in mitosis at days 3 and 4 in the different cellular compartments was counted. The immunohistochemical distribution of progesterone receptors and bFGF was determined. Because the concentration of progesterone in circulation and the quantity of progesterone receptors in the rat uterus are low during early pregnancy (32), we anticipated that expression of progesterone receptors would be restricted to specific target cells thereby enabling a low quantity of receptor to illicit a biological response. The temporal and cell-specific distribution of progesterone receptors during early pregnancy and in RU-486-treated rats revealed that some luminal epithelial cells are progesterone receptor positive at day 3 of pregnancy, while no progesterone receptors are detected in rats treated with RU-486. Moreover, the number of mitotic epithelial cells increases significantly ($p < 0.05$) in RU-486-treated rats compared to those counted in control pregnant animals (Fig. 23.2). Expression of progesterone receptors in the luminal epithelium is homogenous at day 4 of pregnancy and mitotic activity is significantly reduced. These findings are consistent with the progesterone repressor activity on epithelial mitoses that is well documented in the rodent uterus (33). In the absence of active progesterone receptor complexes epithelial cells exhibit hypertrophy at days 3, 4, and 6 of pregnancy.

Day 3

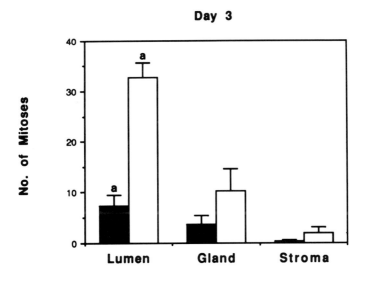

Day 4

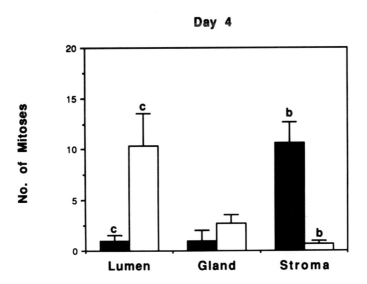

FIGURE 23.2. Changes in the pattern of cell proliferation in the pregnant rat uterus and after treatment with the progesterone receptor antagonist RU-486. Two hours before autopsy colchicine was injected s.c. Uterine horns were removed from pregnant and RU-486 injected rats at (a) day 3 and (b) day 4 post coitum. Paraffin sections were stained with haematoxylin and eosin and counts of all mitotic cells in the luminal epithelium, glandular epithelium (gland) and stroma were made on one section taken at random from one uterine horn. Solid bars represent the mean +/– SEM from pregnant rats and open bars represent the mean +/– SEM of RU-486-treated rats. Data are from three rats per group. Significant ($p < 0.05$) differences are indicated by bars with the same letter (Mann-Whitney U test). From Rider and Psychoyos (31), reproduced by permission of the Journal of Endocrinology.

The normal pattern of cell division in the rat uterus at days 3 and 4 of pregnancy is shown in Figure 23.2. This pattern is altered in rats treated with RU-486 to inhibit implantation. The progesterone-dependent switch from epithelial to stromal mitoses does not occur. Stromal cell proliferation is inhibited significantly ($p < 0.05$) at day 4 post coitum (p.c) while the epithelial cells continue to proliferate. The lack of stromal mitoses in rats and mice (34) treated with RU-486 is consistent with an absence of active progesterone receptor complexes in these cells. Comparison of bFGF expression in these same animals reveals a lack of bFGF expression in nonproliferating stromal cells. At days 3, 4, and 6 of pregnancy bFGF is present in the stromal cells of pregnant rats.

These findings correlate expression of bFGF with proliferating uterine stromal cells and further suggest that bFGF may be controlled by ovarian steroids. Uterine bFGF transcripts are present during the time of endometrial cell proliferation (days 2–4) (35). Steady-state mRNA levels are similar at each of the days examined. To investigate if steroid hormones control bFGF mRNA in the rat uterus, ovariectomized rats were treated with estrogen for 48 h followed by a single injection of estrogen, progesterone, the two hormones coinjected, or oil vehicle. Estrogen pretreatment is expected to provide adequate progesterone receptor content (36) that would otherwise be low in the ovariectomized rat uterus (37). Steroid treatments increase steady-state uterine bFGF mRNA in estrogen sensitized rats compared with vehicle control animals as measured by RNase protection. Densitometric scanning of mRNA levels reveal that estrogen increases bFGF mRNA 8.5 fold over that in the control rats, while progesterone stimulates a 27-fold increase in bFGF mRNA that is significantly greater ($p < 0.05$) than the amount measured in control animals.

Increased accumulation of bFGF mRNA levels may occur via direct binding of the progesterone receptor to the bFGF gene, because an imperfect inverted progesterone response element (38) is present in the 5'-flank of the human bFGF gene at position -878/-861(5'-TCTTATCTCCCTCAGTGT-3'). Additional studies are warranted to directly test the ability of progesterone receptors to bind potential hormone response elements and transactivate bFGF gene expression in uterine cells. Estrogen increases bFGF in human endometrial adenocarcinoma cells (39). We find that estrogen increases steady-state bFGF mRNA levels within 1 h of treatment suggesting direct regulation via the estrogen receptor response element. A search for estrogen response elements in the 5'-flank of the human bFGF gene revealed no obvious consensus sequences. However, an imperfect element at position -533/-516 contains a half-palindromic sequence (5'-GGTCAGTAAAGCAAACCT-3') which has been shown previously to promote activation of ovalbumin gene transcription in response to estrogen (40). Estrogen is required for activation, but the receptor does not bind DNA.

Biological response to FGFs occurs after interaction with high affinity FGF receptors located on target cell surfaces. Target cells also express low affinity sites for FGFs that are comprised of heparan sulfate proteoglycans (41). High affinity FGF receptors are members of the tyrosine kinase receptor supergene family (42). The proteins encoded by the four FGF receptor genes are structurally related and share similarity in their amino acid sequence. Cloning of the FGF receptor cDNAs revealed complexity of this gene family due to numerous variants that are produced by alternative splicing (42). As alternative splicing from a single gene provides a genetic mechanism to generate receptor diversity and specificity, the potential function of FGF receptor variants has been intensely investigated (43,44).

To investigate whether bFGF action in rat uterine stromal cells is mediated via FGF receptor 1 (FGFR1) and, therefore, involves a tyrosine kinase signal transduction pathway, the spatial and temporal distribution of FGFR1 during early rat pregnancy was investigated (45). Primers that anneal to FGFR1 and amplify both the full-length transcript and the alternatively spliced variant lacking the most external immunoglobulin-like domain amplified both cDNAs from the pregnant rat uterus (days 4–6). Both mRNAs are translated into protein because two isoforms of the correct molecular mass are present on Western blots reacted with an antibody that recognizes both forms of the receptor. Radiolabeled bFGF binds to uterine membranes isolated from pregnant rats. The apparent Kd (1 nM; $r = 0.92$) indicates this binding is of high affinity. Both acidic (aFGF) and bFGF displace bound bFGF when added in molar excess, whereas a 1000-fold molar excess of either EGF or transferrin does not compete. FGFR1 is present in the epithelial and stromal cells on each day of pregnancy (days 2–6). At days 4 to 6 of pregnancy the epithelial cytoplasm is uniformly reactive to FGFR1 antibody. However, FGFR1 immunoreactivity localizes in the stromal nuclei.

Binding of bFGF to its high affinity FGFR1 probably involves protein phosphorylation and specific gene transcription, but, further studies are required to identify the targets for activated receptor in the uterus. In other cell types, activation of receptor leads to a series of differential tyrosine phosphorylations that occur within minutes of ligand addition (46). Little is known about the phosphorylation substrates for FGFR1 in uterine stromal cells, but, bFGF has been shown to stimulate the proliferation of human (47) and rat (48) stromal cells in culture. In other cell types FGF receptors activate multiple signaling systems including the MAPK cascade (49). Recent evidence suggests that the effects of bFGF binding to its receptor may occur at two levels. First, activation of the receptor results in a series of differential tyrosine phosphorylation of target proteins, some of which function in the cell cycle. Secondly, FGF receptor activation may stimulate specific gene transcription directly (50) or indirectly as part of its pleiotropic actions.

Control of Stromal Cell Differentiation

Following their proliferation, stromal cells differentiate into decidual cells with characteristic changes in cell morphology (51). These changes occur spontaneously during the menstrual cycle but in rodents decidualization normally requires a signal from an implanting blastocyst. Physical stimuli such as the intraluminal installation of oil or traumatization of the endometrium are also effective decidual stimuli in rodents. During decidualization stromal cells hypertrophy and acquire the potential to function as a unit via the formation of gap junctions (52). Gap junctions serve as channels of communication between adjacent cells and provide a means for small ions to pass freely from one cell to another. Prior to decidualization, the uterine stromal cells exist as individual units lacking cell–cell contacts (see Fig. 23.1). Development of gap junctions changes the spatial relationship among these cells and is therefore likely an important aspect for decidual function. Formation of gap junctions is essential during development of both amphibian and mammalian embryos.

Decidual nuclei are polyploid because the chromosomes fail to separate at metaphase. Endomitosis, while not common in mammalian cells, takes place in trophoblast cells (reviewed in (53)) and in bone marrow megakaryocytes during their differentiation (54). In the latter case, Datta et al. (54) showed that endomitosis is a function of the uncoupling of DNA replication and mitosis since endomitotic cells fail to form active mitosis promoting factor (MPF). Although endomitosis is associated with terminally differentiated cells, it is not clear if this phenomenon is a means to ensure specific gene amplification or if it serves to reprogram DNA for terminal differentiation. Decidualization begins in the antimesometrial aspect of the endometrium but as decidualization progresses, decidual cells surround the developing blastocyst providing a barrier between the blastocyst and the remainder of the endometrium (55). In rodents, stromal edema takes place after blastocyst attachment and is shortly followed by decidualization. Stromal edema persists in mice injected with actinomycin D to inhibit transcription, but decidualization is delayed for approximately 30 h (56).

Differentiation during development is regulated by coordinated cell–cell and cell–extracellular matrix interactions (57). The extracellular matrix acts through its integrin receptors promoting changes in cytoskeletal organization and cell shape to stimulate cellular differentiation (58). Stromal cells are surrounded by the stromal extracellular matrix. During decidualization in the rat, alterations occur in extracellular matrix proteins including fibronectin (59–61). Rat fibronectin is encoded by a single gene (62). Alternative splicing of exons EIIIA (A), EIIIB (B), and the V region results in mRNAs in which exons A and B are present or absent while the V region can be present, partially present, or absent (63). Cellular fibronectins are produced by many cell types and reside in the basement membranes and the extracellular matrix. The functional significance of fibronectin isoforms is unclear; however, several lines of evidence suggest differential expression of the isoforms during development and in adult tissues (62,64). At day 6 of pregnancy in the rat uterus, fibronectin mRNAs encoding the V95 and A regions preferentially localize to the antimesometrial zone of the subepithelial stroma (61). Accumulation of these mRNA variants is dependent upon decidualization but the embryo is not required. Moreover, although there is an initial reduction in fibronectin content at the site of implantation (59,60), hyaluronidase-treated samples of day 6 pregnant uterus fixed in 2% paraformaldehyde show increased fibronectin content in the subepithelial stromal compared to the surrounding endometrium.

Cell–extracellular matrix interactions are mediated by a family of surface receptors called integrins (reviewed in (65)). The integrin receptors are transmembrane glycoproteins comprised of two subunits. There are 16 α subunits and 8 β subunits that can assemble into different receptor combinations. The α4 subunit associated with β1 or β7 subunits bind fibronectin and vascular cell adhesion molecule-1 (VCAM-1). Mouse embryos lacking the α4 subunit because of target mutagenesis implant but fail to form a chorioallantoic placenta (66). Embryos deficient for VCAM-1 show similar allantois defects suggesting an essential role for α4integrin/VCAM-1 interaction in the fusion process (67). Mouse embryos lacking the α5 subunit implant but development fails after the implantation reaction (68). As there are several receptors for each extracellular matrix protein (65), these results are equivocal regarding the role of uterine fibronectin specifically in embryo implantation. However, mouse decidual cells in culture express α5β1 integrin (69), and changes in fibronectin mRNAs specifically occurs during decidualization (61). Together these findings suggest that maternally produced fibronectin is involved in decidualization and thereby indirectly affects embryo implantation.

Alterations in stromal cell shape and motility during decidualization (51) suggest reorganization of the stromal cell cytoskeleton. Changes in cytoskeletal assembly may promote transcription of genes involved in differentiation by releasing mechanical restraints to DNA unfolding, changing transport rates of proteins from cytoplasm to nucleus, or altering the function of transcription factors that are associated with the nuclear protein matrix (70). The actin supergene family encodes a number of protein isoforms that help to control the shape and the motility of nonmuscle cells (71). Evidence implicating nonmuscle actin in cell migration comes from cell injury and repair analysis. Cells cultured on defined matrices in the presence of bFGF shift their isoactin mRNA and protein profiles (71). Isoactin mRNAs contain domains within their 3' untranslated regions which are isotype specific. This permits identification of actin-isoform specific mRNAs within complex tissues. Cytoskeletal actin genes are controlled by estrogen in the immature (70) and mature ovariectomized (Fig. 23.3) rat uterus. During the early attachment of decidual cells to culture dishes, stress fibers colocalize with fibronectin in decidual cells (69). Treatment of cultured decidual cells with cytochalasin B to disrupt actin microfilaments results in morphological changes including retraction of cytoplasm and development of numerous thin filopodia. These results suggest that the actin cytoskeleton is important in maintaining decidual cell morphology. However, because the cells were decidualized before culture, these experiments do not clarify the potential role of the cytoskeleton in the process of decidualization. Cytoskeletal changes during

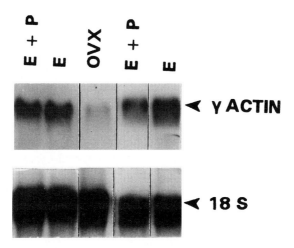

FIGURE 23.3. Estrogen increases cytoplasmic γ actin in the rat uterus. Sexually mature rats were ovariectomized and rested for 10 days. Some rats were pretreated with estrogen for 48 h (lanes 1 and 2). Animals were injected s.c. with estrogen (E, 0.6 μg) or estrogen and progesterone (E + P, estrogen, 0.6 μg, progesterone, 2 mg) coadministration. Control animals (OVX) were injected with sesame oil vehicle. The uterine horns were removed 6 h after hormone administration and total RNA was isolated. The RNA was size fractionated by agarose gel electrophoresis and transferred to a nylon membrane. Cytoplasmic γ-actin mRNA was detected using a radiolabeled cDNA constructed from the 3' untranslated region of a rat γ-actin cDNA (ATCC number 37768). This same blot was hybridized with a radioactive 18S ribosomal RNA cDNA to control for assay variation. Lanes 1–3 contained 20 μg of total uterine RNA from estrogen sensitized rats. Lanes 4 and 5 contained 10 μg of total uterine RNA from ovariectomized rats without estrogen pretreatment.

decidualization probably include alterations in the composition of intermediate filament proteins in addition to changes in cytoplasmic actin. Vimentin and desmin expression increases during rat decidualization (73,74), and such changes may strengthen decidual cells against the mechanical stresses associated with their differentiation. Since these cytoskeletal interconnections physically link the cell surface to the nuclear matrix they may facilitate signal transduction from the cell surface to the nucleus.

Future Directions

In species that require invasive implantation including the human, formation and regression of the decidua entail essential uterine changes necessary to accommodate the conceptus. These uterine directed events are required for embryo implantation, yet little is known about the molecular mechanisms involved. A major roadblock to progress on this biological problem is the lack of culture systems in which cells are suitably regulated by steroid hormones. Complex tissues like these uterine epithelial cells are often connected to each other via junctional complexes. Epithelial cells in the endometrium are polar and express different proteins at the apical and basal regions. Recapitulating these features in culture is difficult. For example, while uterine epithelial cells grown on solid substratum present an attractive surface for blastocyst attachment the process is independent of steroid hormones, unlike the process in vivo. Epithelial cells grown on filters develop polarity and blastocyst attachment does not occur in the presence of estradiol similar to the conditions of normal pregnancy (75). It is not clear, however, if this model can be hormonally manipulated to encourage attachment.

Although cultured epithelial cells lack appropriate hormonal regulation, recent analysis of uterine stromal cells in culture demonstrates progesterone-dependent control of proliferation is maintained (76,48). Stromal cells can be synchronized in serum free medium and stimulated to proliferate significantly in response to several growth factors if progesterone is included in the medium (48). Nontransformed stromal cells thus provide an important model to identify hormone-growth factor control of cell cycle regulatory proteins in the uterus. Because cellular differentiation and apoptosis are intimately connected to cell cycle events, it is crucial to study the mechanisms involved in cellular differentiation in the context of cell cycle regulation. Preliminary studies in our laboratory suggest differences in cytoskeletal proteins between proliferative and quiescent stromal cells (Jones and Rider, unpublished data). This model system holds great promise for understanding stromal cell differentiation in the context of cell cycle regulation.

A normal part of the implantation process involves programmed cell death in response to steroid hormones. Apoptosis of the luminal epithelium occurs as the embryo passes through the epithelial layer to the stroma. In addition, decidual cells undergo apoptosis to accommodate the growth of the conceptus. Bcl-2 was the first protein identified in the multi gene family of proteins that regulate apoptosis (77). Recent evidence using a hormone-dependent rat uterine epithelial cell line suggests progesterone prevents apoptosis by altering the ratio of alternatively spliced transcripts from the bcl-X gene (78). Bcl-X is a homologue of Bcl-2 and produces two mRNA variants. Progesterone shifts the ratio between the two different forms in favor of the long transcript variant (bcl-X_L) that inhibits apoptosis. It will now be important to confirm that these alternatively spliced mRNAs are produced in the epithelial cells of pregnant animals and that the alternatively spliced mRNA variants are translated into protein. These results, however, suggest a molecular mechanism whereby progesterone receptor expression at day 4 of pregnancy in the rat (31) could protect epithelial cells from apoptosis. Progesterone receptors in the uterine epithelium are not detectable by immunocytochemistry at day 6 of pregnancy (31). Epithelial cell apoptosis may be induced at this time because of the loss of progesterone receptors leading to a shift from bcl-X_L to bcl-X_S transcripts.

Perhaps the greatest challenge for understanding uterine changes during implantation and early pregnancy is to develop coculture systems in which interactions between epithelial and stromal cells can be studied. Recent results from studies using targeted mutagenesis to analyze individual gene function reiterates the importance of cell–cell interactions in the uterus (79,80). Tissue recombinants between wild type cells and cells lacking the estrogen receptor via targeted mutagenesis clearly show that uterine epithelial cell proliferation in the mouse is mediated by estrogen receptors in the uterine stroma (79). Similar studies in prostate suggest that epithelial mitogenesis in both estrogen (uterus) and androgen (prostate) target organs are stromal mediated events (79). Mice lacking the *Hoxa-11* gene by targeted mutagenesis show defects in uterine cell proliferation and decidualization. *Hoxa-11* transcription is restricted to mesenchymal cells but the induction of leukemia inhibitory factor (LIF) in the glandular epithelial cells of *Hoxa-11* mutants is absent (80). Contemporary technology including targeted mutagenesis, PCR and improved culture systems will continue to provide new and exciting information about specific gene function in implantation. The next decade is expected to provide great progress in understanding the signal transduction cascades necessary to coordinate cell–cell and cell–extracellular matrix changes in the uterus that are essential for uterine decidualization and blastocyst implantation.

Acknowledgments. The author is grateful to past and present members of the laboratory who have contributed to the work referenced in this chapter. I thank Jim Swafford (UMKC) for help with the figures and Marilyn Evans (Immunology Research Lab, St. Luke's Hospital) for reading the manuscript. Our research has been funded in part by grants from the National Institutes of Health (HD28038, HD23896) and the University of Missouri Research Board.

References

1. Chang MC. Development and fate of transferred rabbit ova or blastocyst in relation to the ovulation time of recipients. J Exp Zool 1950;114:197–225.
2. Amaroso EC. Placentation. In: Parks AS, ed. Marshall's physiology of reproduction. London: Longmans, 1952:127–311.
3. Pijnenborg R, Robertson WB, Brosens I, Dixon G. Review article: trophoblast invasion and the establishment of haemochorial placentation in man and laboratory animals. Placenta 1984;2:71–92.
4. Harvey MB, Leco KJ, Arcellana-Panlilio MY, Zhang X, Edwards DR, Schultz GA. Proteinase expression in early mouse embryos in regulated by leukaemia inhibitory factor and epidermal growth factor. Development 1995;121:1005–14.
5. Noyes RW, Hertig AT, Rock J. Dating of the endometrial biopsy. Fertil Steril 1950; 1:3–25.
6. Martin L, Finn CA. Hormonal regulation of cell division in epithelial and connective tissues of the mouse uterus. J Endocrinol 1968;41:363–71.

7. Psychoyos A. Uterine receptivity for nidation. Ann New York Acad Sci 1968;476: 36–42.

8. Rasmussen CA, Orwig KE, Vellucci S, Soares MJ. Dual expression of prolactin-related protein in decidua and trophoblast tissues during pregnancy in rats. Biol Reprod 1997;56:647–54.

9. Gu Y, Gibori G. Isolation, culture and characterization of the two cell subpopulations forming the rat decidua: differential gene expression for activin, follistatin and decidual-related prolactin protein. Endocrinology 1995;136:2451–8.

10. Bell SC. Decidualization: regionalization differentiation and associated function. Oxf Rev Reprod Biol 1983;5:220–71.

11. Goodger AM, Rogers PAW. Uterine endothelial cell proliferation before and after embryo implantation. J Reprod Fertil 1993;99:451–7.

12. Finn CA, Pope MD. Infiltration of neutrophil polymorphonuclear leucocytes into the endometrial stroma at the time of implantation of ova and the initiation of the oil decidual cell reaction in mice. J Reprod Fertil 1991;91:365–9.

13. Kachkache M, Ackner GM, Chaouat G, Noun A, Garabedian M. Hormonal and local factors control the immunohistochemical distribution of immunocytes in the rat uterus before conceptus implantation: effects of ovariectomy, fallopian tube secretion, and injection. Biol Reprod 1991;45:860–8.

14. Hunt JS. Immunologically relevant cells in the uterus. Biol Reprod 1994;50:461–6.

15. Finn CA, Martin L. Patterns of cell division in the mouse uterus during early pregnancy. J Endocrinol 1967;39:593–7.

16. Galassi L. Autoradiograph study of the decidual cell reaction in the rat. Develop Biol 1968;17:75–84.

17. Ferenczy A, Bertrand G, Gelfand MM. Proliferation kinetics of human endometrium during the normal menstrual cycle. Am J Obstet Gynecol 1979;133:859–67.

18. Lessey BA, Killam AP, Betzger DA, Haney AF, Greene GL, McCarty KS. Immunohistochemical analysis of human uterine estrogen and progesterone receptors throughout the menstrual cycle. J Clin Endocrinol Metab 1988;67:334–40.

19. Clarke CL, Sutherland RL. Progestin regulation of cellular proliferation. Endocrinol Rev 1990;11:266–301.

20. Pollard JW. Regulation of polypeptide growth factor synthesis and growth factor-related gene expression in the rat and mouse uterus before and after implantation. J Reprod Fertil 1990;88:721–31.

21. Guidice LC. Growth factors and growth modulators in human uterine endometrium: their potential relevance to reproductive medicine. Fertil Steril 1994;61:1–17.

22. Rider V, Piva M. Role of growth factors of uterine and fetal-placental origin during pregnancy. In: Bazer FW, ed. Endocrinology of pregnancy. Totowa, New Jersey: Humana Press, 1998.

23. Musgrove EA, Hamilton JA, Lee CSK, Sweeney KJE, Watts CKW, Sutherland RW. Growth factor, steroid, and steroid antagonist regulation of cyclin gene expression associated with changes in T47-D human breast cancer cell cycle progression. Mol Cell Biol 1993;13:3577–87.

24. Carlone DL, Rider V. Embryonic modulation of basic fibroblast growth factor in the rat uterus. Biol Reprod 1993;49:653–65.

25. Basilico C, Moscatelli D. The FGF family of growth factors and oncogenes. Advan Cancer Res 1992;59:115–65.

26. Cordon-Cardo C, Vlodavsky I, Haimovitz-Friedman A, Hicklin D, Fuks Z. Expression of basic fibroblast growth factor in normal human tissues. Lav Invest 1990;63:832–40.

27. Wordinger RJ, Smith KJ, Bell C, Chang I-FC. The immunolocalization of basic fibroblast growth factor in the mouse uterus during the initial stages of embryo implantation. Growth Factors 1994;11:175–86.

28. Mignatti P, Morimoto T, Rifkin DB. Basic fibroblast growth factor, a protein devoid of secretory signal sequence, is released by cells via a pathway independent of the endoplasmic reticulum-golgi complex. J Cell Physiol 1992;151:81–93.

29. Brigstock DR, Heap RB, Barker PJ, Brown KD. Purification of heparin-binding growth factors from porcine uterus. Biochem J 1990;266:273–82.

30. Gupta A, Bazer FW, Jaeger LA. Immunolocalization of acidic and basic fibroblast growth factors in porcine uterine and conceptus tissues. Biol Reprod 1997;56: 1527–36.

31. Rider V, Psychoyos A. Inhibition of progesterone receptor function results in loss of basic fibroblast growth factor expression and stromal cell proliferation during uterine remodelling in the pregnant rat. J Endocrinol 1994;140:239–49.

32. Vu Hai Mt, Lagged F, Milgrom E. Progesterone receptors in the rat uterus: variations in cytosol and nuclei during the oestrous cycle and pregnancy. J Endocrinol 1978;76:43–8.

33. Martin L, Das RM, Finn CA. The inhibition by progesterone of uterine epithelial proliferation in the mouse. J Endocrinol 1973;57:549–54.

34. Cullingford TE, Pollard JW. RU 486 completely inhibits the action of progesterone on cell proliferation in the mouse uterus. J Reprod Fertil 1988;83:909–14.

35. Rider V, Carlone DL, Foster RT. Oestrogen and progesterone control basic fibroblast growth factor mRNA in the rat uterus. J Endocrinol 1997;154:75–84.

36. Savouret J-F, Rauch M, Redeuilh G, Sar S, Chauchereau A, Woodruff K, et al. Interplay between oestrogens, progestins, retinoic acid and AP-1 on a single regulatory site in the progesterone receptor gene. J Biol Chem 1994;269:28955–62.

37. Kraus WL, Katzenellenbogen BS. Regulation of progesterone receptor gene expression and growth in the rat uterus: modulation of estrogen action by progesterone and sex steroid hormone antagonists. Endocrinology 1993;132:2371–9.

38. Bailly A, LePage C, Rauch M, Milgrom E. Sequence-specific DNA binding of the progesterone receptor to the uteroglobin gene: effects of hormone, antihormone and receptor phosphorylation. EMBO J 1988;5:3235–41.

39. Presta M. Sex hormones modulate the synthesis of basic fibroblast growth factor in human endometrial adenocarcinoma cells: implication for the neovascularization of normal and neoplastic endometrium. J Cell Phys 1988;137:593–7.

40. Gaub MP, Bellard M, Scheuer I, Chambon P, Sassone CP. Activation of the ovalbumin gene by the estrogen receptor involves the fos-jun complex. Cell 1990; 1267–76.

41. Klagsbrun M, Baird A. A dual receptor system is required for basic fibroblast growth factor activity. Cell 1991;67:229–31.

42. Johnson DE, Williams LT. Structural and functional diversity in the FGF receptor multigene family. Adv Cancer Res 1993;60:1–41.

43. Shi E, Kan M, Xu J, Wang F, Hou J, McKeehan WL. Control of fibroblast growth factor receptor kinase signal transduction by heterodimerization of combinatorial splice variants. Mol Cell Biol 1993;13:3907–18.

44. Werner S, Duan D-SR, de Vries C, Peters KG, Johnson DE, Williams LT. Differential splicing in the extracellular region of fibroblast growth factor receptor 1 generates receptor variants with different ligand-binding specificities. Mol Cell Biol 1992;12:82–8.

45. Rider V, Piva M, Cohen ME, Carlone DL. Alternative splicing and differential targeting of fibroblast growth factor receptor 1 in the pregnant rat uterus. Endocrinology 1995;136:3137–45.

46. Zhan X, Hu X, Friesel R, Maciag T. Long term growth factor exposure and differential tyrosine phosphorylation are required for DNA synthesis in BALB/c3T3 cells. J Biol Chem 1993;268:9611–20.

47. Irwin JC, Utian WH, Eckert RL. Sex steroids and growth factors differentially regulate the growth and differentiation of cultured human endometrial stromal cells. Endocrinology 1991;129:2385–92.

48. Piva M, Flieger O, Rider V. Growth factor control of cultured rat uterine stromal cell proliferation is progesterone dependent. Biol Reprod 1996;55:1333–42.

49. Friesel RE, Maciag T. Molecular mechanisms of angiogenesis: fibroblast growth factor signal transduction. FASEB J 1995;9:919–25.

50. Newberry EP, Willis D, Latifi T, Boudreaux JM, Towler DA. Fibroblast growth factor receptor signaling activates the human interstitial collagenase promoter via the bipartite Ets-AP1 element. Mol Endocrinol 1997;11:1129–44.

51. Finn CA. Biology of decidual cells. Adv Reprod Physiol 1971;5:1–26.

52. Kleinfeld RG, Morrow HA, DeFeo VJ. Intercellular junctions between decidual cells in the growing deciduoma of the pseudopregnant rat uterus. Biol Reprod 1976;15:593–603.

53. Ilgren EB. Control of trophoblastic growth. Placenta 1983;307–28.

54. Datta NS, Williams JL, Caldwell J, Curry AM, Ashcraft EK, Long MW. Novel alterations in CDK1/Cyclin B1 kinase complex formation occur during the acquisition of a polyploid DNA content. Mol Cell Biol 1996;7:209–23.

55. Rasmussen CA, Orwig KE, Vellucci S, Soares MJ. Dual expression of prolactin-related protein in decidual and trophoblast tissues during pregnancy in rats. Biol Reprod 1997;56:647–54.

56. Finn CA, Bredle, JCS. Studies on the development of the implantation reaction in the mouse uterus: influence of actinomycin D. J Reprod Fertil 1973;34:247–53.

57. Damsky C, Sutherland A, Fisher S. Extracellular matrix 5: adhesive interactions in early mammalian embryogenesis, implantation, and placentation. FASEB J 1993;7:1320–8.

58. Werb Z, Tremble P, Damsky CH. Regulation of extracellular matrix degradation by cell-extracellular matrix interactions. Cell Diff Develop 1990;32:299–306.

59. Grinnell F, Head JR, Hoffpauir J. Fibronectin and cell shape in vivo: studies on the endometrium during pregnancy. J Cell Biol, 1982;94:597–606.

60. Glasser SR, Lampelo S, Munir MI, Julian J. Expression of desmin, laminin and fibronectin during in situ differentiation (decidualization) of rat uterine stromal cells. Differentiation 1987;35:132–43.

61. Rider V, Carlone DL, Witrock D, Cai C, Oliver N. Uterine fibronectin mRNA content and localization are modulated during implantation. Devel Dyn 1992;195:1–14.

62. Hynes RO. Fibronectins. New York; Springer Verlag, 1990.

63. Schwartzbauer JE, Tamkun JW, Lemishka IR, Hynes RO. Three different fibronectin mRNAs arise by alternative splicing within the coding region. Cell 1983;35:421–31.

64. Pagani F, Zagato L, Vergani C, Casari G, Sidoli A, Baralle FE. Tissue-specific splicing pattern of fibronectin messenger RNA precursor during development and aging in rat. J Cell Biol 1991;113:1223–9.

65. Hynes RO. Integrins: versatility, modulation, and signaling in cell adhesion. Cell 1992;69:11–25.
66. Yang JT, Rayburn H, Hynes RO. Cell adhesion events mediated by ˆ4 integrins are essential in placental and cardiac development. Development 1995;121:549–60.
67. Gurtner GC, Davis V, Li H, McCoy MJ, Sharpe A, Cybulsky MI. Targeted disruption of the murine VCAM1 gene: essential role of VCAM-1 in chorioallantoic fusion and placentation. Genes Devel 1995;9:1–14.
68. Yang JT, Rayburn H, Hynes RO. Embryonic mesodermal defects in $\alpha5$ integrin-deficient mice. Development 1995;119:1093–105.
69. Babiarz B, Romagnnano L, Afonso S, Kurila G. Localization and expression of fibronectin during mouse decidualization in vitro: mechanisms of cell:matrix interactions. Devel Dyn 1996;206:330–42.
70. Ingber DE. Fibronectin controls capillary endothelial cell growth by modulating cell shape. Proc Nat Acad Sci USA 1990;87:3579–83.
71. Herman I. Actin isoforms. Curr Opin Cell Biol 1993;5:48–55.
72. Hsu C-Y, Frankel FR. Effect of estrogen on the expression of mRNAs of different actin isoforms in immature rat uterus. J Biol Chem 1987;262:9594–600.
73. Glasser SR, Julian J. Intermediate filament protein as a marker of uterine stromal cell decidualization. Biol Reprod 1986;35:463–74.
74. Mani SK, Julian J, Lampelo S, Glasser SR. Initiation and maintenance of in vitro decidualization are independent of hormonal sensitization iv vivo. Biol Reprod 199;47:785–99.
75. Julian J, Carson DD, Glasser SR. Polarized rat uterine epithelium in vitro: responses to estrogen in defined medium. Endocrinology 1992;130:68–78.
76. Cohen H, Pageaux J-F, Melinand C, Fayard, J-M, Laugier C. Normal rat uterine stromal cells in continuous culture: characterization and progestin regulation of growth. Eur J Cell Biol 1993;61:116–25.
77. Oltvai ZN, Korsmeyer SJ. Checkpoints of dueling dimers final death wishes. Cell 1994;79:189–92.
78. Pecci A, Scholz A, Pelster D, Beato M. Progestins prevent apoptosis in a rat endometrial cell line and increase the ratio of bcl-X_L to bcl-X_S. J Biol Chem 1997;272:11791–8.
79. Cooke PS, Buchanan DL, Young P, Setiawan T, Brody J, Korach KS, et al. Stromal estrogen receptor (ER) mediate mitogenic effects of estradiol on uterine epithelium. Proc Nat Acad Sci USA 1997;94:6535–40.
80. Gendron RL, Paradis H, Hsieh-Li HM, Lee DW, Potter SS, Markoff E. Abnormal uterine stromal and glandular function associated with maternal reproductive defects in Hoxa-11 null mice. Biol Reprod 1997;56:1097–105.

24

Regulation of Hormone Receptor Gene Expression in Endometrium

Nancy H. Ing and Jane A. Robertson

The hormonal responsiveness of a cell is dictated by its complement of hormone receptors. In the cyclic female mammal, the response of the uterus to oscillating concentrations of estrogen and progesterone from the ovary is dictated by the expression of the estrogen and progesterone receptor genes within the uterine cells. The main regulators of estrogen and progesterone receptor genes are the hormones, estrogen and progesterone. Both the current and the previous cycle of steroid hormone influence are important in regulating expression of the steroid hormone receptor genes. This review focuses on the molecular mechanisms of estrogen and progesterone receptor regulation in endometrium of livestock species during the estrous cycle and early pregnancy. This, along with steroid regulation of oxytocin and prolactin receptor genes, among others, synchronizes endometrial gene expression with the changing needs of developing embryo(s).

Steroid Hormones and the Estrous Cycle

With few exceptions, female mammals demonstrate repeating cycles of receptivity to mating until pregnancy is attained. These cycles coordinate mating behavior, ovulation, and the oviduct and uterine environments to facilitate conception and the needs of the early, free-floating embryo(s) prior to placentation (1). The timing and readiness of the maternal environment to nurture embryos is regulated similarly across mammalian species by the ovarian steroid hormones: estrogen from follicles and progesterone from corpus luteum. That these are sufficient has been demonstrated with the successful use of steroid-treated, ovariectomized animals as recipients in embryo transfer studies. The steroid replacement therapy must include treatment mimicking a full estrous cycle before the current estrous period to create a uterine environment conducive to pregnancy (2). This is likely to relate to the decreased fertility seen naturally during initial periods of cyclicity: at puberty, after seasonal anestrus, and after parturition. The reasons for the requirement for delayed and acute effects of ovarian steroid hormones on endometrium for successful pregnancy are unclear, but may relate to regulation of hormone receptor genes.

Embryo transfer studies also demonstrated the requirement for synchrony between embryos and the uterine environment. Whether using ovary-intact animals or ovariectomized animals treated with steroid hormones as recipients, transferred embryos do not survive in uteri that are more than one or two days out of synchrony (3). This implies that the steroid hormones modulate endometrial gene expression uniquely for each day of the estrous cycle. Because plasma levels of estrogen and progesterone are not particular to each day of the estrous cycle, differential gene expression is probably the result of regulation of the endometrial estrogen and progesterone receptors.

Regulated Expression of Hormone Receptor Genes in the Uterus

A key variable to steroid modulation of gene expression in endometrium is the regulated expression of estrogen and progesterone receptor genes. These nuclear receptors bind the membrane-permeable steroid hormones and transduce the signals by altering gene expression (4). The expression of the receptor genes in endometrium is primarily under the control of the steroid hormones, estrogen and progesterone (5). In general, during the follicular phase when estrogen influence dominates, expression of estrogen receptor and progesterone receptor genes is high. In contrast, expression of the receptor genes is low in endometrium during the luteal phase, when progesterone influence dominates. Although we do not know exactly how many receptors are required in a cell for a response to a steroid hormone, it is clear that cells with more receptors are more responsive: that is, they are able to respond to lower doses of hormone and/or are able to elicit greater or more responses to one dose of hormone (6). So, the endometrium reacts to the oscillating levels of estrogen and progesterone during the estrous cycle based on its concentrations of estrogen and progesterone receptors. This regulation of steroid hormone receptors at the tissue level may explain how the steroid hormones orchestrate the changing pattern of gene expression during the estrous cycle and/or early pregnancy.

The Preovulatory Surge of Estrogen

Our laboratory studies regulation of endometrial genes early in the estrous cycle and pregnancy. Estrogen is the greatest steroid influence during the follicular phase of the cycle. In all of the mammals examined, the preovulatory surge of estrogen up-regulates the expression of estrogen receptor and progesterone receptor genes in the uterus. Presumably, this primes the uterus for subsequent hormonal responsiveness, changes in gene expression, and growth. Therefore, our laboratory has focused on the molecular mechanisms of estradiol regulation of estrogen receptor and progesterone receptor genes in endometrium as a first step toward understanding the integral roles of steroid hormones in the process of pregnancy.

Our animal model is the ewe, ovariectomized after exhibiting several normal estrous cycles during the breeding season and rested two or four weeks. To simulate the preovulatory surge of estrogen, each ewe receives one 50 µg injection im of estradiol 17β. This dose was chosen from the work of Miller and Moore, who successfully used it as part of the steroid replacement therapy to prepare ovariectomized ewes as recipients in embryo transfer studies (2). In addition, this dose generates 60 pg/ml serum levels 6 h postinjection, consistent with concentrations found in the ovarian vein during proestrus (7). Further, the concentrations of estradiol in endometrial tissues of the treated ewes are similar to those in endometrium of ovary-intact ewes at Day 1 of the estrous cycle (8).

Estradiol Up-Regulates Estrogen Receptor and Progesterone Receptor mRNA Concentrations

To initially describe the effects of estradiol on estrogen receptor and progesterone receptor gene expression in the endometrium of ovariectomized ewes, a time course study was performed (7). Groups of six ewes were hysterectomized 6, 12, 24, or 48 h after estradiol injection. Control ewes were injected with vehicle (charcoal-stripped corn oil) 24 h prior to hysterectomy, while treated ewes were injected with 50 µg estradiol. Endometrial RNA was analyzed for estrogen receptor and progesterone receptor mRNAs on Northern blots and in ribonuclease protection assays, respectively, using cRNA probes we cloned from sheep endometrium. Estradiol increased the concentration of estrogen receptor mRNA in endometrium five-fold at 24 h postinjection. Progesterone receptor mRNA concentrations increased more modestly with estradiol treatment: by 66% at 12 h postinjection. These results are consistent with the increased endometrial concentrations of estrogen receptor and progesterone receptor mRNAs and proteins demonstrated during the preovulatory period of ovary-intact, cycling ewes (9).

Most Uterine Cells Respond to Estradiol

To determine which uterine cell types (luminal and glandular epithelium, endometrial stromal fibroblasts, and/or myometrium) up-regulated estrogen receptor and progesterone receptor mRNAs, uterine cross-sections from the ewes on the time course study were subjected to in situ hybridization (10). In the absence of estradiol treatment, most uterine cells of ovariectomized ewes had low to moderate levels of estrogen receptor and progesterone receptor mRNAs. In response to estradiol injection, most uterine cell types increased expression of the estrogen receptor and progesterone receptor genes. As above in the ribonuclease protection assay and Northern blot analyses, the progesterone receptor mRNA was up-regulated earlier than estrogen receptor mRNA (at 12 h compared to 24 h). The exceptions were that estradiol did not increase estrogen receptor mRNA concentrations in luminal epithelial or myometrial cells. These cells responded, however, in ewes primed with estrogen and 14 days of progesterone before the estradiol challenge. In the other uterine cells, this attempt to recreate the steroid influences of a previous estrous cycle augmented the increase in estrogen receptor mRNA.

Immunohistochemical analyses of uterine cross-sections from the time course ewes using the estrogen receptor antibody H222 and the progesterone receptor antibody MA411 (Affinity Bioreagents; Neshanic Station, NJ) indicated that receptor protein levels rose consistent with increased mRNA concentrations in the various uterine cell types (10). Concentrations of both progesterone receptor and estrogen receptor proteins were elevated at 24 h postestradiol. However, at 48 h after estradiol injection, only estrogen receptor protein concentrations remained elevated. These results are consistent with the up-regulation of estrogen receptor and progesterone receptor gene expression in uterine cells of cyclic ewes during the periovulatory period (11).

"All-or-None" Effects of Estradiol

To determine if up-regulation of estrogen receptor and progesterone receptor gene expression was maximal with the 50 μg dose of estradiol, we performed a dose response and a double challenge experiment with estradiol (12). In the former, 25, 50, and 100 μg doses of estradiol were administered to ovariectomized ewes 24 h prior to hysterectomy. In the latter experiment, 50μg doses of estradiol were administered at both 48 and 24 h prior to hysterectomy. Our hypotheses were that a higher dose of estradiol or a second estradiol challenge (when more estrogen receptor protein was present) would enhance the up-regulation of estrogen and progesterone receptor genes. However, both were incorrect. It appeared that estradiol, in any dose or treatment regimen, elevated the estrogen receptor and progesterone receptor mRNA concentrations similarly in the endometrium. Thus, the estradiol effects appeared to be "all-or-none" in character.

Antiestrogens Fail to Block Estradiol
Up-Regulation of Estrogen Receptor mRNA

To define the role of the estrogen receptor protein in the up-regulation of estrogen receptor and progesterone receptor mRNAs, we used estrogen receptor antagonists. The first one we tested was tamoxifen, the antiestrogen most commonly prescribed to women. Although tamoxifen is known to have mixed antagonist/agonist actions relative to estrogen, we were interested in its effects on estrogen and progesterone receptor genes in endometrium because it predisposes women to steroid-responsive, endometrial cancers. In our ovariectomized ewes, an injection of 20 mg tamoxifen up-regulated estrogen receptor mRNA concentrations in endometrium (8). When used in conjunction with estradiol, tamoxifen did not antagonize or add to estradiol's effects on the estrogen receptor gene, but it antagonized estradiol's up-regulation of the progesterone receptor gene.

Next, we obtained a "pure antagonist" of estrogen receptor, ICI 182,780, from Zeneca Pharmaceuticals (Macclesfield, Cheshire, England). Endometrium was treated locally via indwelling uterine catheters for six hours before and after estradiol injection, with 6 ml/h of 10^{-7} M ICI 182,780 in 1 mg/ml ovine serum albumin in phosphate-buffered saline. Endometrium was collected at hysterectomy 18 h after estradiol injection. Northern analyses of endometrial RNA indicated that ICI 182,780 alone up-regulated estrogen receptor mRNA concentrations and, when used with estradiol, did not antagonize or add to estrogen receptor up-regulation (unpublished data). However, ICI 182,780 treatment did not up-regulate concentrations of glyceraldehyde phosphate dehydrogenase mRNA, as estradiol does (see below). Therefore, the antiestrogen ICI 182,780 acts as a partial estrogen agonist in sheep endometrium.

The mixed agonist/antagonist actions of tamoxifen and partial agonist actions of ICI 182,780 may be explained in several ways. Since tamoxifen alone up-regulates estrogen receptor gene expression, it will appear to be an estrogen agonist. However, tamoxifen also prevents estradiol up-regulation of the progesterone receptor, therefore it will appear to be an antagonist. A second is that the complement of cellular cofactors that interact with estrogen receptor may not distinguish between estradiol-bound and tamoxifen-bound receptors and allow productive complexes to form on some estrogen-responsive genes, while the reverse may be true on another subset of genes. Lastly, radically divergent molecular mechanisms for estrogen regulation of endometrial genes (below) may allow some effects of estrogen to be mimicked by antiestrogens bound to the estrogen receptor while others are blocked.

Molecular Mechanisms of Estradiol Action

The mechanism by which estradiol up-regulates progesterone receptor gene expression is well-characterized and has served as a paradigm for steroid hormone activation of transcription. The progesterone receptor genes of the human and rat both contain two estrogen-inducible promoters (13,14). We demonstrated that the sheep progesterone receptor gene is activated by estradiol treatment in runoff experiments with endometrial nuclei from our time course ewes (7).

In sharp contrast, our nuclear runoff experiment showed that transcription of the estrogen receptor gene was *not* activated by estradiol (7). Therefore, the molecular mechanism for the increase in estrogen receptor mRNA concentration must be posttranscriptional. The most likely mechanism is by estradiol stabilizing the estrogen receptor mRNA. Regulated message stability is rapidly being recognized as a powerful mechanism involved in control of gene expression (15). The best characterized example of hormone-modulated message stability is estrogen stabilization of vitellogenin mRNA in frog liver, where a single dose of estrogen extends the message half-life from 16 to 600 h. Dr. David Shapiro's group identified an RNA sequence element within the 3′ untranslated region of the message that is responsible for stabilization by estrogen and is currently cloning the binding protein responsible for estrogen-modulated stability (16). Both human estrogen and progesterone receptor mRNAs have extensive 3′ untranslated regions that each contain 13 AUUUA sequences, identified as instability elements in short-lived oncogene mRNAs (17). Therefore, estrogen and progesterone receptor mRNAs appear to be targeted for short half-lives, which could make them very sensitive to post-transcriptional regulation. Interestingly, the human estrogen receptor mRNA carries a sequence element that is homologous to the stability elements in vitellogenin mRNA, so it may be stabilized by estrogen similarly.

To determine whether estradiol enhances the stability of estrogen receptor mRNA in endometrium, we collected endometrium at 18 h postinjection, during the time of increasing estrogen receptor mRNA concentrations (18). Endometrial explants were cultured with 75 μg/ml 5,6-dichloro-1-β-D-ribofuranosylbenzimidazole (DRB), which inhibited 90% of transcription. With the majority of transcription effectively blocked, declining concentrations of mRNAs were analyzed in endometrial explants cultured for 0, 3, 6, 9, and 12 h. Estradiol treatment extended the half-life of estrogen receptor mRNA from 7 h to more than 24 h, similar to the five-fold increase in steady state estrogen receptor mRNA concentrations in endometrium. This effect was specific for estrogen receptor mRNA, because message stabilities of progesterone receptor, glyceraldehyde phosphate dehydrogenase, and c-fos were unaffected by estradiol.

However, c-fos mRNA exhibited uncharacteristic stability in explant cultures, which was attributable to DRB artifactually ablating its major pathway of degradation (19). We were concerned that estrogen receptor and progesterone receptor mRNAs, with their 13 AUUUA instability elements, might also have demonstrated artifactual stability with DRB treatment. Therefore, endometrial RNA was labeled in vivo by injecting a pulse of thio-uridine into the uterine lumen of ovariectomized ewes via indwelling catheters 14 h after the estradiol injection. The pulse-labeled thio-RNA was purified on organomercurial columns (Affigel 501; BioRad, Hercules, CA) from endometrium collected at 18 and 24 h postestradiol and analyzed on replicate slot blots for estrogen receptor, progesterone receptor, glyceraldehyde phosphate dehydrogenase, and c-fos mRNAs, as before. The in vivo results for estradiol effects on message stability were strikingly similar to those determined in the in vitro explant cultures: estradiol stabilized only the estrogen receptor mRNA. The only differences were that progesterone receptor and c-fos mRNA half-lives were shorter in vivo, implying that both are degraded by a common pathway that is inhibited by DRB. Currently, we are analyzing the 4 kb 3′ untranslated region of the sheep estrogen receptor mRNA for sequence elements and binding proteins involved in the estrogen modulation of its stability.

Progesterone Regulation of Receptors in the Luteal Phase of the Estrous Cycle

The up-regulation of estrogen receptor gene expression by estrogen is unusual because most hormones down-regulate their receptors to limit the endocrine response. The up-regulation is possible because it is followed by progesterone in the luteal phase of the estrous cycle, which down-regulates estrogen and progesterone receptor gene expression in endometrium. In fact, when progesterone influence is dominant, during the luteal phase of the estrous cycle and pregnancy, progesterone receptors are nearly undetectable in luminal and superficial glandular epithelium by immunohistochemistry (10). In these cells, progesterone responses may be restricted by low progesterone receptor concentrations, or may occur via paracrine signals from neighboring stroma or deep glandular epithelium that retain immunoreactive progesterone receptor (10).

The molecular mechanism by which progesterone down-regulates estrogen receptor and progesterone receptor genes probably involves the progesterone receptor repressing transcription, similar to how the closely related glucocorticoid receptor represses genes involved in inflammation (20). It is notable that, of the two forms of the progesterone receptor protein in the human and the rat, the A form is more effective at repressing transcription than the B form (21). Therefore, characterization of the protein forms of progesterone receptors in reproductive tissues, as well as their hormonal regulation, will be important to determining the actions of progesterone.

Late in the estrous cycle, the progesterone repression becomes self-limiting because of declining progesterone receptor concentrations (22). This, probably assisted by low levels of estrogens from developing follicles, increases estrogen and progesterone receptor concentrations in endometrial cells. After progesterone from the corpus luteum declines, estrogen receptor and progesterone receptor concentrations are fully released from repression and can be up-regulated once again by the preovulatory surge of estrogen at the start of a subsequent estrous cycle.

Steroid Regulation of Oxytocin and Prolactin Receptors in Endometrium

Estrogen and progesterone affect the expression of numerous endometrial genes, either directly or indirectly (23). In fact, glyceraldehyde phosphate dehydrogenase, cyclophilin, and actin mRNA concentrations, considered to be constitutive in other systems, increase in the endometrium in response to estradiol treatment (12).

Two hormone receptor genes in endometrium that are critical to early pregnancy are the oxytocin and prolactin receptors (22). Oxytocin, via its receptors, triggers the production of the luteolytic pulses of prostaglandin by the endometrium. Although previous work indicated that estrogens up-regulate oxytocin receptor gene expression in endometrium (24), estradiol treatment did not increase oxytocin receptor mRNA concentrations in our ovariectomized ewes. Others found that estradiol treatment of ovariectomized ewes failed to increase oxytocin receptor protein concentrations in endometrium (25). This suggests that declining progesterone influence is more important than estrogen in up-regulating oxytocin receptor gene expression. Because of its suppression by progesterone, oxytocin receptor concentrations generally follow those of estrogen and progesterone receptors: high in follicular phase of the estrous cycle and low in the luteal phase. The depression of all three hormone receptors in the luteal phase has led to the term "progesterone block" describing the lack of endometrial responsiveness to hormones (26).

Endometrial prolactin receptors are known to be important to early pregnancy in the pig, but their transduction of prolactin and placental lactogen signals is probably important to most mammalian species (22). Because prolactin concentrations in plasma are relatively constant during early pregnancy of the pig, it appears that prolactin effects on endometrium are primarily regulated by altering prolactin receptor concentrations. Estrogens from pig embryos up-regulate expression of the prolactin receptor gene in endometrium. In rabbit endometrium, progesterone up-regulates prolactin receptor (27). Production of many endometrial secretory proteins, including uteroferrin in the pig and uteroglobin in the rabbit, require the action of prolactin along with steroid hormones (22), probably because of regulation of hormone receptors.

Receptor Regulation by Embryonic Products During Maternal Recognition of Pregnancy

In the earliest days of pregnancy, hormone receptor regulation in endometrium is the same as in the first half of the estrous cycle: up-regulation by estrogen, down-regulation by progesterone. Then, as progesterone influence wanes, the uteri of ungulates responds to oxytocin by producing pulses of prostaglandin that lyse the corpus luteum. For maternal recognition of pregnancy, the embryo must communicate its presence to the endometrium to block the prostaglandin pulses and spare the corpus luteum. To do this, embryos secrete species-specific products that regulate expression of hormone receptor genes in endometrium.

Ruminant conceptuses produce large amounts of interferon-τ during the time of maternal recognition of pregnancy (28). Interferon-τ is an antiviral molecule, which, like estrogen, modulates gene expression of tissues in two ways: transcriptionally (via the Janus kinase-signal transducers and activators of transcription pathway) and posttranscriptionally by inducing an RNase. The former mechanism is used by interferon-τ to suppress transcription of the estrogen and oxytocin receptor genes two-fold in endometrium (29). In this way, interferon-τ is proposed to suppress endometrial responsiveness to oxytocin and to prolong the progesterone block, and preclude the generation of prostaglandin pulses. This spares the corpus luteum and allows the establishment pregnancy.

In the pig, estrogen produced by the embryos is the signal for maternal recognition of pregnancy (3). In fact, estrogens are produced by most embryos before and/or during the time of maternal recognition of pregnancy. Embryonic estrogens up-regulate prolactin receptors in endometrium as a part of maternal recognition of pregnancy in pigs and may thus support the cooperative actions of prolactin and progesterone and the progesterone block (27). It is also possible that embryonic estrogens further down-regulate estrogen receptor gene expression in endometrium, as seen in animals given pharmacological doses of estradiol. This occurs by transcriptional repression via a sequence within the coding region of the estrogen receptor gene (30). The ultimate result of estrogens from the pig embryos is the rerouting of uterine prostaglandins from an endocrine direction (into the uterine vasculature to destroy the corpus luteum) to an exocrine direction (into the uterine lumen). The molecular mechanisms linking hormone receptor regulation by embryonic estrogens and rerouting of prostaglandin pulses are not clearly defined, but appear to involve prolactin-induced calcium ion cycling in the endometrium (22).

Future Possibilities for Therapeutic Interventions

To produce food for the growing numbers of consumers, livestock producers are being asked to produce more meat more efficiently with fewer resources and low environmental impact. Advances in reproductive management can rapidly enhance productivity: increasing the numbers of pregnancies per animal and/or the number of offspring per pregnancy. For example, estrus synchronization is a multimillion dollar component of the livestock industry because it reduces the time and work required to artificially inseminate a herd with semen from superior sires. However, many of such therapies employ pharmacological doses of hormones, which are likely to down-regulate the very hormone receptors required for successful pregnancy (31). Therefore, these treatments result in reduced fertility, which severely limits their desirability. Knowledge of how hormones regulate endometrial hormone receptors may allow the more judicious use of hormonal therapies for reproductive manipulations, such as estrus synchronization, superovulation, and embryo transfer.

Fertility could be improved by reducing early embryonic losses, estimated to be as high as 40% in most livestock species (32). Only about 15% of the embryos lost are genetically flawed, so the rest may be a result of asynchrony of the embryo and the uterine environment (3). Reproductive therapeutics could enhance fertility by relaxing the requirement for synchrony between the embryo(s) and the uterus. Treatments with exogenous hormones involved in maternal recognition of pregnancy (e.g., estrogen or interferon-τ) might allow less synchronous embryos to survive, resulting in more pregnancies and/or more offspring per pregnancy.

Knowledge of gene and mRNA sequences instrumental to molecular mechanisms of early pregnancy opens the door to intervention with oligonucleotide therapeutics. These include such colorfully named compounds as "triplex," "antisense," and "hammerhead ribozyme" oligonucleotides, which bind to regulatory sequences and interfere with their function (33). Although future applications might enhance fertility, the limits of our current knowledge make interrupting fertility more practical. For example, antisense oligonucleotides directed to bind the stability sequence of estrogen receptor mRNA could displace the binding protein, destabilize the message and prevent up-regulation of estrogen receptor gene expression in endometrium. Such a therapy would likely prevent pregnancy and be useful in regulating fertility in humans and animals.

Summary

The estrous cycles of female mammals is a well-choreographed dance of molecular regulation of endometrial genes, directed by estrogen and progesterone from the ovary. During the follicular phase of the estrous cycle, estrogen up-regulates hormone receptors. Then during the luteal phase, progesterone represses them. To initiate a subsequent estrous cycle, the endometrium escapes the progesterone block. However, this dance culminates with the entrance of the embryo, which steals the show by prolonging the period of progesterone dominance during implantation and subsequent development. The fact that early embryonic death is common implies that the choreography between endometrial gene expression and the needs of the embryo is not perfect and could be improved by therapies based on knowledge of the molecular mechanisms critical to the success of pregnancy.

Acknowledgments. The authors wish to thank Dr. Troy Ott for critical manuscript review.

References

1. Sorensen AM. Estrus and the estrous cycle. In: Animal reproduction: principles and practices. New York: McGraw-Hill, 1979:234–67.

2. Moore NW, Miller BG, Trappl MN. Transport and development of embryos transferred to the oviducts and uteri of entire and ovariectomized ewes. J Reprod Fertil 1983;68:129–35.

3. Pope WF. Uterine asynchrony: a cause of embryonic loss. Biol Reprod 1988;39:999–1003.

4. Ing NH, O'Malley BW. The steroid hormone receptor superfamily: molecular mechanisms of action. In: Weintraub B, ed. Molecular endocrinology: basic concepts and clinical correlations. New York: Raven Press, 1995:195–216.

5. Clark JH, Schrader WT, O'Malley BW. Mechanisms of action of steroid hormones. In: Wilson JD, Foster DW, eds. William's textbook of endocrinology. Philadelphia: Saunders, 1992:35–89.

6. Webb P, Lopez GN, Greene GL, Baxter JD, Kushner PJ. The limits of the cellular capacity to mediate an estrogen response. Mol Endocrinol 1992;68:157–67.

7. Ing NH, Spencer TE, Bazer FW. Estrogen enhances endometrial estrogen receptor gene expression by a posttranscriptional mechanism in the ovariectomized ewe. Biol Reprod 1996;54:591–9.

8. Robertson JA, Bhattacharyya S, Ing NH. Tamoxifen acts as an estrogen agonist in the endometrium of the ewe. Biol Reprod 1997.

9. Ott TL, Zhou Y, Mirando MA, Stevens C, Harney JP, Ogle TF, Bazer FW. Changes in progesterone and oestrogen receptor mRNA and protein during maternal recognition of pregnancy and luteolysis in ewes. J Mol Endocrinol 1993;10:171–83.

10. Ing NH, Tornesi MB. Estradiol up-regulates estrogen receptor and progesterone receptor gene expression in specific uterine cells. Biol Reprod 1997;56:1205–15.

11. Spencer TE, Bazer FW. Temporal and spatial alterations in uterine estrogen receptor and progesterone receptor gene expression during the estrous cycle and early pregnancy in the ewe. Biol Reprod 1995;53:1527–43.

12. Zou K, Ing NH. Oestradiol up-regulates oestrogen receptor, cyclophilin, and glyceraldehyde phosphate dehydrogenase mRNA concentrations in endometrium, but down-regulates them in liver. J Steroid Biochem Mol Biol 1998;64:231–7.

13. Kastner P, Krust A, Turcotte B, Stropp U, Tora L, Gronemeyer H, Chambon P. Two distinct estrogen-regulated promoters generate transcripts encoding the two functionally different human progesterone receptor forms A and B. EMBO J 1990;9:1603–14.

14. Kraus WL, Montano MM, Katzenellenbogen BS. Identification of multiple, widely spaced estrogen-responsive regions in the rat progesterone receptor gene. Mol Endocrinol 1994;8:952–69.

15. Ross J. Control of messenger RNA stability in higher eukaryotes. Trends Gen 1996;12:171–5.

16. Dodson RE, Shapiro DJ. An estrogen-inducible protein binds specifically to a sequence in the 3' untranslated region of estrogen-stabilized vitellogenin mRNA. Mol Cell Biol 1994;14:3130–8.

17. Wreschner DH, Rechavi G. Differential mRNA stability to reticulocyte ribonucleases correlates with 3' non-coding (U)nA sequences. Eur J Biochem 1988;172:333–40.

18. Ing NH, Ott TL. Estradiol up-regulates estrogen receptor-alpha messenger ribonucleic acid in sheep endometrium by increasing its stability. Biol Reprod 1999;60:134–9.

19. Shyu A-B, Greenberg ME, Belasco JG. The c-fos transcript is targeted for rapid decay by two distinct mRNA degradation pathways. Genes Devel 1996;3:60–72.

20. Savouret JF, Rauch M, Redeuilh G, Sar S, Chauchereau A, Woodruff K, Parker MG, Milgrom E. Interplay between estrogens, progestins, retinoic acid and AP-1 on a single regulatory site in the progesterone receptor gene. J Biol Chem 1994;269:28955–62.

21. Katzenellenbogen BS. Estrogen receptors: bioactivities and interactions with cell signalling pathways. Biol Reprod 1996;54:287–93.

22. Bazer FW, Spencer TE, Ott TL, Ing NH. Regulation of endometrial responsiveness to estrogen and progesterone by pregnancy recognition signals during the periimplantation period. In: Dey SK, editor. Molecular and cellular aspects of periimplantation processes. New York: Springer-Verlag, 1995:27–47.

23. Ing NH, Tsai SY, Tsai MJ. Progesterone and estrogen. In: Gwatkin RBL, ed. Genes in mammalian reproduction. New York: Wiley-Liss, 1993:271–91.

24. Vallet JL, Lamming GE, Batten M. Control of endometrial oxytocin receptor and uterine response to oxytocin by progesterone and oestradiol in the ewe. J Reprod Fertil 1990;90:625–34.

25. Zhang J, Weston PG, Hixon JE. Role of progesterone and oestradiol in the regulation of uterine oxytocin receptors in ewes. J Reprod Fertil 1992;94:395–404.

26. McCracken JA, Schramm W, Okulicz WC. Hormone receptor control of pulsatile secretion of PGF2a from the ovine uterus during luteolysis and its abrogation in early pregnancy. Anim Reprod Sci 1984;7:31–56.

27. Chilton BS, Mani SK, Bullock DW. Servomechanism of prolactin and progesterone in regulating uterine gene expression. Mol Endocrinol 1988;2:1169–75.

28. Bazer FW, Spencer TE, Ott TL. Interferon tau: a novel pregnancy recognition signal. Am J Reprod Immunol 1997;37:412–20.

29. Spencer TE, Bazer FW. Ovine interferon tau suppresses transcription of the estrogen receptor and oxytocin receptor genes in ovine endometrium. Endocrinology 1997;137:1144–7.

30. Kaneko KJ, Furlow JD, Gorski J. Involvement of the coding sequence for the estrogen receptor gene in autologous ligand-dependent down-regulation. Mol Endocrinol 1993;7:879–88.

31. Wright PJ, Malmo J. Pharmacologic manipulation of fertility. Vet Clinics North Am: Food Animal Prac 1992;8:57–89.

32. Zavy MT, Geisert RD, eds. Embryonic mortality in domestic species. Boca Raton, FL: CRC Press, 1994:1–224.

33. Song CS, Jung MH, Supakar PC, Chen S, Vellanoweth RL, Chatterjee B, Roy AK. Regulation of androgen action by receptor gene inhibition. Ann NY Acad Sci 1995;761:97–108.

Author Index

Subject Index

PROCEEDINGS IN THE SERONO SYMPOSIA USA SERIES

Continued from page ii

PROCEEDINGS IN THE SERONO SYMPOSIA USA SERIES

ISBN 0-387-98806-8

EAN

9 780387 988061 >